What does a person need to know to cope with cancer? The health section of bookstores and websites are filled with "how to" books for dealing with cancer—from one or another perspective. But NONE give the pragmatic, commonsense approach that Dr. Fleishman provides in his *Learn to Live Through Cancer* book. He has drawn on his remarkable experience in oncology to answer the big questions like "What can I make of my life now?" But what is uniquely great is that he can just as comfortably describe what should go into a Smoothie Shake! Doctor Common Sense Fleishman has told it all! And, provided a model for coping and recording information you need to know and think you will remember—but we won't! At last, a truly practical approach to a complex and difficult topic!

—*Jimmie C. Holland, MD, Wayne E. Chapman Chair in Psychiatric Oncology, Attending Psychiatrist, Department of Psychiatry & Behavioral Sciences, Memorial Sloan-Kettering Cancer Center, New York, New York*

Finally we have an exceptional guidebook for people who have just learned that they have cancer and want to know the ins and outs of cancer treatment while maintaining good quality of life. Dr. Fleishman, an internationally recognized expert in cancer care, has long been the "go to" doctor for other physicians who have questions about cancer treatment effects. His 40 years of practical experience have been distilled in this book infused with his kindness and gentle humor.

—*Mary Jane Massie, [...] ter; Professor of Cl[...], New York, New Yo[...]*

We in the treatmen[...] understand guide which [...] ay. Dr. Fleishman has...m[...] cer deal with it in a manner [...] upon his long experience [...] with both the day-to-day [...] ly for the patient, but for [...]

—*Kanti Rai, MD, [...] Center, New [...] School of Mea[...]*

LEARN TO LIVE THROUGH CANCER

LEARN TO LIVE THROUGH CANCER

WHAT YOU NEED TO KNOW AND DO

Stewart B. Fleishman, MD

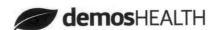

Acquisitions Editor: Noreen Henson

Production Editor: Dana Bigelow

Compositor: Apex CoVantage

Printer: Bang

Visit our website at www.demoshealth.com

Medicine is an ever-changing science. Research and clinical experience are continually expanding our knowledge, in particular our understanding of proper treatment and drug therapy. The authors, editors, and publisher have made every effort to ensure that all information in this book is in accordance with the state of knowledge at the time of production of the book. Nevertheless, the authors, editors, and publisher are not responsible for errors or omissions or for any consequences from application of the information in this book and make no warranty, express or implied, with respect to the contents of the publication. Every reader should examine carefully the package inserts accompanying each drug and should carefully check whether the dosage schedules mentioned therein or the contraindications stated by the manufacturer differ from the statements made in this book. Such examination is particularly important with drugs that are either rarely used or have been newly released on the market.

Library of Congress Cataloging-in-Publication Data

CIP data is available from the Library of Congress.

Special discounts on bulk quantities of Demos Medical Publishing books are available to corporations, professional associations, pharmaceutical companies, health care organizations, and other qualifying groups. For details, please contact:

Special Sales Department
Demos Medical Publishing
11 W. 42nd Street, 15th Floor
New York, NY 10036

Phone: 800–532–8663 or 212–683–0072
Fax: 212–941–7842
E-mail: rsantana@demosmedpub.com

Made in the United States of America

11 12 13 14 15   5 4 3 2 1

CONTENTS

Foreword

It is a great privilege, as one of Dr. Fleishman's mentors, to write the Foreword for this special book for patients with cancer. I met Dr Fleishman when he came to Memorial Sloan-Kettering Cancer Center in the 1980s to work with our small Psychiatry Service faculty to learn about the complex psychological and physical problems experienced by patients coping with cancer. He quickly became adept at understanding and treating the psychological and social problems of patients, as well as the more serious problems with psychiatric disorders. It also quickly became clear that he had a keen interest in how to help patients control the range of distressing symptoms that often accompany cancer, like fatigue, pain, insomnia, nausea, and GI dysfunction with diarrhea or constipation. Doctors often are so focused on the "big picture" that they overlook the day-to-day toll that persistent uncontrolled symptoms have on patients' ability to tolerate the needed treatment. The quality of life can be completely lost and patients become demoralized when they feel that no one is able to control a troublesome symptom.

Dr. Fleishman went on to Long Island Jewish Hospital where he became the consultant for the busy Oncology Service and he delved further into how to help patients with advanced illness and their families navigate the shoals of health care. Many of the hassles have to do with phone calls and bitter dialogue at times with health and drug insurance companies that are often unsympathetic to callers who are distressed and exhausted. Dr. Fleishman took on trying to make sense of the drug and insurance rules to help patients through these trials. He then moved to Beth Israel where he organized the range of services for patients that spanned the medical to the financial to the psychological.

It was in this last situation that he began to think through a simple model—with an acronym of LEARN—that encompassed the issues for patients in a commonsense way so they could understand and could keep the needed information in a personal health record—a totally new concept, but a critical one for informing each doctor of current medications and treatments. I am impressed with the forms and space for notes that are included in the book. The LEARN Model puts things into five areas: to Live (clearly the first goal), Education (know the basics of what is important), Activity (where exercise and level of work and play should be), Rest (important for refreshing oneself), and Nutrition (important to both illness and well-being). The suggestions in each area are so basic and so down-to-earth that they seem as if we knew them already—but we don't.

I am so proud, as an early mentor, of Dr. Fleishman's work and the fact that he has taken his experience over a career and put it into a program that any patient can follow with both pleasure and guidance. The essence of wisdom is to take the complex (and frequent jargon) of a field and turn it into "plain English" for people to use. Dr. "Common Sense" Fleishman has done just that with this book. I believe it will become a classic in how to cope with cancer, ranging from the abstract and existential to the everyday troublesome symptoms.

Jimmie C. Holland, MD
Wayne E. Chapman Chair in Psychiatric Oncology
Attending Psychiatrist
Department of Psychiatry & Behavioral Sciences
Memorial Sloan-Kettering Cancer Center
New York, New York

Acknowledgments

An endeavor such as this guide is very definitely not a one-man show. Thousands of people: colleagues, patients, families and good friends have taught me what I am passing on here. I have been blessed with mentors in my personal and professional life who have given me access to a fount of information and taught me the skills to cobble the facts together, all while inviting me to be a part of their journey. Their altruism works in that they too can "give forward" through my efforts, benefiting countless others from their experience. Mentioning names means I may omit some meaningful ones, so please excuse any omission.

First to my parents Mariane and Bill for rooting me in the technical aspects of our family pharmacy, fostering the abilities to communicate effectively and diplomatically, and prioritizing "helping others" as a core life value; my family: Bruce, Herbert, Iris, Jeffrey, Sharon, Severine, Lynne, Nan, David, Ira, Naomi, and Linda in this life-long journey in which we have found that the more you give the more you get.

Next to my medical mentors—Doctors (all): Jimmie Holland, who is the founder of the field of psycho-oncology and mentor par excellence; Mary Jane Massie who taught me how to clarify the message; Lynna Lesko, Kanti Rai, Ronald Blum, Arthur Sawitsky, Louis Harrison, Mark Persky, Moses Nussbaum, Roy Sessions, Russell Portenoy, Manjeet Chadha, Suzan Naam, Kenneth Hu, Sheldon Feldman, Jean-Marc Cohen, Warren Enker, Martin Karpeh, Roy Sessions, Wendi Lovenvirth, Andrew Evans, Ronald Ennis, Stephen Malamud, Bruce Culliney, Peter Kozuch, Seth Cohen, Sharon Rosenbaum-Smith, Susan Boolbol, Laurie Kirstein, Mark Smith, Arnold Katzoff, and Howard Berkowitz who all put theory into practice every day to save and improve so many lives, then teach us all how to do what they do; and Sarah Schwartzbord Gelberd who has helped me to clarify, question, nurture, and learn over more than thirty years of camaraderie.

To so many non-physician colleagues that have taught me so much and set the bar higher and higher: Elise Carper, Thelma Myers-Navarro, Cindy Turkeltaub, Diane Serra, Diane Blum, Carolyn Messner, Victoria Rosenwald, Bridget Bennett, Darren Arthur, Nancy Bourque, Lori Schwartz, Carolyn Cassin, Anne Moses, Marilyn Bookbinder, Jason Bishop, Susan Gold, Carol Farkas, Neva Solomon, Nayo Akowe, Enid Stecker, Rosie Hylton, Damien Francois, Sandy Lansinger, Myra Glajchen, Christine Jones, Carol Lowe, Cesar Espineda, George Handzo, Randye Retkin, Howard Gelberd, and Deborah Korzenik whose oncology social work, nursing, nutrition, legal, and leadership skills embody the finest professional principles each and every day; Victoria Schlegel, Jeff Jacomowitz, Barbara Brownell, Sue Fredericks, with extra-special gratitude to Elayne Feldstein — word-smith and thought-smith educators whose need to understand pressed me to understand more and explain better; our wonderful string of Continuum students with special mention to Dimitri Yukvid and Erica Silen for their help on the Survivorship Project and Jus Chadha on the nutritional section; Ellen Clegg and Allen Levine who put "chemo-brain" into my brain and into the daily lexicon.

And to scores of patients, some long-term cancer survivors and some not, whose trust and search for life after cancer has served as my beacon. Special mention to Jeffrey Fleishman, Barbara Brownell and Elayne Feldstein whose own survivorship underscores that cancer affects all of us without exemption and whose personal and professional advice has helped disseminate this work into the print and electronic worlds.

Special mention to the grateful patients and foundations who have helped throughout my career to promote projects and services in order to afford me the opportunity to learn from patients, families and colleagues. These include: The Millman Family, The New York Community Trust, The Pechter–Machis Family, The Michelle Klipstein-Cohen Foundation, The Schnurmacher Foundation, The Nagorski Family, The Brody Family, The Alvin Smith Family, The Sandford Simon Family, The Stein Family/Balm Foundation, The Brodoff Family, The Karpas Family, The Joel Finkelstein Family Foundation, the American Cancer Society, the Cancer and Leukemia Group B cooperative clinical trials group, the American College of Surgeons Commission on Cancer, and the Federation of Jewish Philanthropies. Cancer research cannot be pursued in current times without the support from the pharmaceutical industry, that has been able to foster some of my research without bias: Abbott-Ross, Celgene, Merck, Solvay, and Sapphire Corporations.

All of us providers are also patients during our lives. I would like to thank those who have helped my parts to work well enough to set these words to paper: Ben Zane Cohen MD, Jay Wisnicki MD, Suzanne Bellante OD, Peter Halper MD, David Gorman MD, Donald Kastenbaum MD, Nate Schulman MD, Ira Finegold MD, and Bruce Haber DDS.

With the advances in cancer medicine and biology, perhaps all oncology specialists will seize the lion's share of symptom management and support when the majority of patients will present with curable diseases.

Thank you all.

A Few Words About Language

More than just political correctness, the treatment of cancer involves many people, and their titles are continually evolving.

To be concise without sacrificing inclusiveness, certain group identifiers are shorthand for a variety of titles. Please be assured that no one is being left out of the village that it takes to care for someone with cancer.

"Provider" encompasses physician, nurse, social worker, psychologist, pharmacist, optometrist, nutritionist/dietician, technician, tumor registrar, physical, occupational, speech or stoma therapist, research assistant, information specialist, patient navigator, pastoral care chaplain, educator, or volunteer. Cancer is a condition treated by professionals coming from a multitude of disciplines working together in an interdisciplinary manner. Their services can exist because of administrators, administrative assistants, policy makers, legislators, donors, and visionaries who all make our complicated system function.

"Family" or **"caregivers"** includes our nuclear families, blood relatives, marital families, extended family, friends who are our family of choice, neighbors, acquaintances, fellow congregants, fellow travelers, and anyone who extends their hand and largesse to us when we are in need, over the span of a lifetime, occasionally or even just once.

In the spirit of gender equality, most times **he**, **she**, **he or she**, **he and she** or **(s)he** should be read as acceptable surrogates for each other, unless clearly gender-specific.

So please read "provider" and "family" and gender-related pronouns in this wider context.

The Fine Print

The information provided in this book is of general interest. Since the situations involving cancer and its treatment can vary from individual to individual, your providers can help you individualize the care, using what is pertinent for you. Be sure to check if any of the interventions discussed apply to you or not, or need to be customized in some way.

LEARN TO LIVE THROUGH CANCER

Part I

Why This Book?

1 Survivorship Begins at the Time of Diagnosis: What You Need to Know and Do Now

WHEN RECOVERY STARTS

Perhaps the hardest place to begin is at the beginning, especially if you don't know when that is. When does cancer start? At the very start, it is too small to detect and affect the rest of the body. When it grows, diverting oxygen and nutrients and leaving behind waste products, it pushes on a nerve fiber or enters a bone causing some symptom—pain or discomfort—and then prevents something from working properly. Or it puts the body into a state of overdrive that causes fatigue and weight loss. It is hard to know when to start that clock. That makes it even harder to know when recovery starts. The goal of this guide is to integrate a system of recovery from whenever the clock starts. This is a revolutionary concept. When no one survived their cancer, why would anyone put efforts into recovery? As treatments improved, survivorship lengthened and became more widespread. Most of us—patients and professionals—were grateful for such improvements and in that celebration took to rest as an interim reward, waiting to either get better or, hopefully, not get sicker. The idea of nurturing and directing a survivorship period was premature and way out of the box.

When the period of survival lengthened and more people began to live with cancer, professionals and patients intuitively looked at various existing models of recovery. We used the postoperative period after surgery or a stroke for comparison. What can you do after even successful surgery but rest, eat, control the pain, and ease back to where you were before, being a little more shopworn? With the improved success in the recovery from strokes, physical medicine and rehabilitation led the way, bolstered by the growing personal fitness movement. When the bleeding or clotting stopped, pushing to reinvigorate muscles and reconnect to the stimulation from close-by nerve fibers meant hard work. "No pain, no gain," "push-push-push," and do "a little more each time" were solidified as guiding principles. It became clear after the fact that a basic difference in the biology of cancer and stroke made this model less than effective for cancer. In cancer, the body weakens and many times uses more calories than it takes in. The stroke rehabilitation model without some adaptation uses up more calories than at rest without replacement, worsening already fatigued muscles and losing important body mass. Pushing a lot extends fatigue and can be counterproductive.

So neither the postoperative model nor the stroke model works with the biology or mind-set of people with cancer. It can be assumed, but perhaps overstated, that the improvements in survivorship with breast cancer provided the impetus to look more critically at our models in all cancers. Taking an active role extends the advocacy for

3

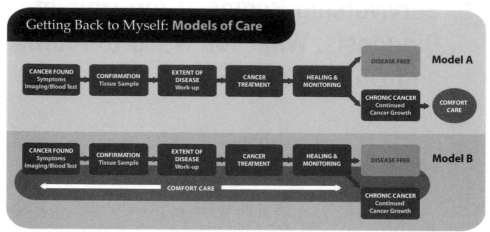

Model A: Comfort care recommended after chronic cancer is disagnosed. **Model B:** Comfort care included as part of treatment from initial diagnosis.

patients to get second opinions and organ preservation surgery, leading to a harder look at life after cancer to overcome the residual effects of illness and treatment.

From my more than 25 years of professional experience in the field specializing in supportive care of patients with cancer, numerous patients and their families have asked for access to guidance *in advance* to lead them through the beginning of treatment and then the recovery process. What you have in your hands now is a systematic version of what patients and families have taught me over the years. Even with such wide variation in how cancer is detected and the course of treatment, there are certain types of experiences that patients have in common. The tools developed grow from that cumulative experience with many patients.

Such influences on how we go about designing recovery treatments moved us all to a more sophisticated plan involving a *preemptive strike: Don't wait to get better; work to make it happen.*

This graphic contrasts two models of care: one that provides *comfort* after treatment that has not controlled the cancer (the *old Model A*) and the *new Model B* using adapted rehabilitative techniques all the way through. Of course, comfort should be maximized all along, it just needs to run in conjunction with curative care treatments. A window of extraordinary opportunity has opened for the millions of cancer survivors to ease the burdens of cancer treatment even before symptoms begin.

RECOGNITION OF EARLY SYMPTOM INTERVENTION IN THE MEDICAL LITERATURE

The idea of *early* attention to minimize the symptoms of cancer and its treatment has slowly gained recognition in the professional literature. A 2010 multicenter study showed that additional attention to cancer-related symptoms during the treatment of lung cancer both increased survival and quality of life. A similar idea has been brought forward in 2010 by Eduardo Bruera and David Hui in the *Journal of Clinical Oncology*. In a presentation at the National Cancer Institute's State of the Science Conference on Symptom Management in Cancer in 2002, I similarly advocated for the integration of supportive care all through the course of treatment. (See Resources & Worksheets section, p. 319 "Integrating Supportive and Palliative Care in the Trajectory of Cancer.")

Who Is a Cancer Survivor?

The National Coalition of Cancer Survivors has defined *survivorship* simply: "It starts on the day of diagnosis and continues for a lifetime." Yes, cancer may have started years beforehand, but one did not live with the knowledge, fear, or responsibilities.

AM I A SURVIVOR?

I am a cancer survivor if I have been found to have cancer. The period of my survivorship starts from the time of diagnosis and extends through the rest of my life. My family, friends, and caregivers who are affected by the cancer can also be considered *survivors*.

What Do We Know about Cancer Survivors as a Group?

Quite a lot. The National Cancer Institute developed its Office of Cancer Survivorship in 1996 and has helped fertilize programs throughout the country. Numerous private organizations—the American Cancer Society, Cancer*Care*, and the American Society of Clinical Oncology to name some big ones—have made massive efforts to share information. The Lance Armstrong Foundation is one of many private foundations that have directed hard-collected monies into this area.

We also know that most people, once they suspect or find out they have cancer, have a predictable emotional reaction that often stuns them. It is part of the process. Stoicism may be what appears on the outside, but on the inside, most people, when they will speak candidly, are frightened and angry. Some people, when they can put their feelings into words (which is not usually immediate), report feeling "devastated." However, they are often thinking and fearing what Dr. Jimmie Holland (*the founder of the field of psycho-oncology*) calls the "Five Ds": worries about dying, dysfunction (organs and ways of coping aren't working well), discomfort (pain), disability (not being able to do the things we enjoy or the tasks necessary for daily life), and dependence on a system that we all believe needs improvement.

Cancer becomes an experience of the tissues, the mind, the spirit, the family, and the community. Certain commonalities emerge when we look at those who fare best: they have the most fixable cancers (i.e., best response and long-term survival from treatment); they have demonstrated past and/or present individual resiliency; and they have actual social support provided by those they love or sometimes even paid care assistants.

DR. JIMMIE HOLLAND'S FIVE D'S OF CANCER

Whether they are able to put it into words or not, most people when cancer is suspected or actually confirmed think or worry about the following:

Dying

Discomfort (pain)

Dysfunction

Disability

Dependence

FLIGHT OR FIGHT?

The
LEARN
System©

p. 248
What Is
Important
to Me

One could argue that this is the ideal time to do a personal inventory. One could also think it is the worst time: "I have enough to do." Bad time. Like going on a diet—no good time but likely the best time. What have I been through in life thus far? How did I do it? Be specific...list mentally or on paper—exactly how?

Use the "What Is Important to Me" worksheet at the end of this book.

Some people learn what they can and try to weigh the options. Some people just shut down emotionally and go into automatic pilot—just getting through, without self-examination. That's OK, except for the next questions. What is important to me *now?* I will need to invest immediately in my quality of life for a potentially longer term to have a longer life. Exactly how bad may I feel now? What is the emotional cost? What is the hazard of not doing anything? What if I haven't shown resiliency in the past? Does that mean I start from scratch? Maybe—yes. Does that mean I am doomed and nothing will help me? That's a very rare situation. Most of us can find some area of success or inner strength, with a little direction.

The enduring thoughts that you have *now* most likely are the meaningful ones. You will be asked to quiet the noise outside for a few minutes. Turn off the cell phone, the television, and the Internet just briefly; close the door and focus on your own values. The worksheets will help. More to come before you are ready.

OFFICIAL RECOGNITION OF CANCER SURVIVORS' TASKS

From Cancer Patient to Cancer Survivor—Lost in Transition

The Institute of Medicine (IOM) is a quasi-private entity with strong governmental connections. It tackles hard, controversial health issues to raise the public's awareness. In its landmark 2006 report, *From Cancer Patient to Survivor—Lost in Transition,* the IOM looked critically at the steadily increasing number of cancer survivors, which is growing each year, cataloging which services will be needed, identifying the research agenda to define the needs, and showcasing the existing model programs in the United States. The goal of the IOM report is to define and improve quality of care for survivors.

The report identifies four of the essential components of survivorship care: prevention, surveillance, intervention, and coordination of care. It reports that cancer survivors are often lost to systematic follow-up within our health care system and that opportunities to effectively intervene are missed. Many people finish their primary treatment for cancer unaware of the information they—and their primary care providers—need to know: specifically, identifying the heightened health risks as a result of having cancer and treatment, and planning for future health care needs. The IOM report focuses on what is needed now and what our fragmented delivery system can actually provide. The IOM Report underscores the lack of awareness of what, if anything, can be done to nurture recovery as well as minimize the late effects of cancer and/or treatment. It further characterizes that fragmentation in information between providers stifles communication, and reduces provider awareness. However, simply discussing the phenomenon will be increasing patients' expectations.

FOUR ESSENTIAL COMPONENTS OF SURVIVORSHIP CARE

The Institute of Medicine identified the following essential components of survivorship care in its report, *From Cancer Patient to Survivor—Lost in Transition:*

Prevention

Surveillance

Intervention

Coordination

The IOM report falls short in that it carefully examines the role of clinicians, researchers, and the health care delivery system but does not suggest what specific steps patients and families can take. The carefully considered and wonderful suggestions are done for/to patients.

The next logical questions are to ask, What can patient and family do *now?* What do patients and families need to know and do (or not do) to improve their rebound from cancer and their quality of life after cancer? Should it be the providers that suggest and guide? Who should do so? What information do we have? How good is the information? What tools have been already developed? What is the hazard of developing survivorship programs that may not have been fully vetted in clinical trials thus far? How can we all, providers and patients, adapt what we know about the recovery from other illnesses? What is the role of a formal survivorship plan to encourage active collaboration?

The gaps in the recommendations in *From Cancer Patient to Survivor—Lost in Transition* have been in large part the stimulus for this book's follow-up treatment: the LEARN System.

THE LEARN SYSTEM

This system is a way of organizing the care from providers combined with the things that I must know and do to have the best quality of life and help the healing and recovery after a cancer diagnosis. There are five components:

Living

Education

Activity

Rest

Nutrition

Using the tools and suggestions in the LEARN System, right from the day of diagnosis and onward, you and your family and friends will better know what to expect and how to proceed.

COMMON SENSE OR PREVENTIVE MEDICINE?

The backbone of the LEARN System is supported by basic *healthy living* suggestions: increased activity, encouraging effective rest, good nutrition, and improved understanding can make a big difference in your quality of life during the time you are undergoing initial testing and treatment. These ideas should not be new to you. They have been the basic *prescription* from primary care providers and cardiologists for many years: eating a diet based on whole grains and vegetables more than red meats, minimizing processed foods made from enriched white flour and sugar products, increasing physical activity, having adequate and restorative sleep, and gaining solid health information and perspective on the situation. These health maintenance techniques are standard content in most health magazine articles and standard preventive medicine advice during your yearly checkup.

Application of the LEARN System during cancer treatment is innovative. Most people kick back when feeling tired and frightened, indulge in comfort foods, and wait to feel better. Just as modern cancer research has proven new drugs and devices to cure or control cancer through the standard clinical trial, portions of such a program are being tested in clinical trials with promising results. Although the clinical trial is the gold standard in deciding what care is helpful (or reimbursable by insurance companies), a complete package of these interventions has not been tested. But it makes very good sense to adopt these changes now.

Healing in medicine is said to result from both the *art* and *science* of the field. Using these common sense, safe, and heart healthy methods now has helped many patients. The alternative is to wait—wait to feel better after treatment, or wait for clinical trials testing the combination intervention to be done with 20 years' delay until any long-term consequences can be discovered. Use this opportunity now.

Most primary care providers and cardiologists will encourage these same, good habits. By choosing to invest time, energy, and maybe some expense in our recovery, we enter the realm of an area of medical care that often gets short shrift: balancing the short-term *quality of life investment* versus the potential *long-term gain*. Sounds like a lesson right out of an economics textbook? Well, yes and no. It is important because when we start to think about what we have to do to get better, it brings us to consider many things we do not necessarily do already. Some critics of this type of more active recovery plan think it is just a way to maintain the semblance of control that can fool people into thinking they can really do something about cancer. Oftentimes, the perception of feeling you can do something *is* important. It is actually the reason why placebos work to some extent. You are doing something important for yourself. And at the very least, you are opening up enhanced communication between providers, extended family and friends, and even with government regulators and insurance carriers.

Learn to Live Through Cancer: What You Need to Know and Do puts the tools and concepts of cancer medicine in your hands so that you can use them throughout your treatment. Here is one tool you can use right now, and you will find it helpful all throughout your treatment.

Asking "How Are You?" All Through Your Care
(and Wanting a Real Answer)

Many times, we ask each other, "How are you?" as a matter of course. It can be an opening line when we meet someone, and many times, it is a question that doesn't look for a genuine answer. Our usual response is, "I'm OK" or "Fine" as a social courtesy. In the world of cancer treatment, having someone ask, "How are you?" and wanting more than a cursory answer happens thousands of times each day in oncologists' offices and cancer centers around the world. Many of the *technological* advances in cancer medicine are available to help control symptoms that arise either from the cancer, the treatment, or both. Accessing them often requires a reminder tool such as the *distress thermometer* when a lot needs to be done during a short follow-up visit.

The distress thermometer (right) was developed in the late 1980s and early 1990s by a committee composed of disparate members with one goal in mind: improving the quality and effectiveness of care provided to patients with cancer. Its sponsor was the National Comprehensive Cancer Network, a not-for-profit alliance of the world's leading cancer centers. Its major focus was to produce a set of accepted clinical practice guidelines for use by patients, clinicians, and other health care decision makers. I was asked to become a member of a

The
LEARN
System©

p. 250
Distress
Thermometer

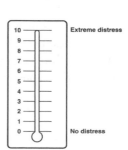

The
LEARN
System©

p. 251
Important
Blood Tests
You Need to
Know About

multidisciplinary panel examining the psychosocial issues pertinent to the spectrum of cancer illnesses. The distress thermometer and specific guidelines to help care for patients is slowly becoming adopted for use with patients treated in a variety of settings, from private practice oncology offices to clinics and cancer research centers across the United States.

Different components of comfort become more important at different points in treatment. At the time cancer is discovered, getting good information and worrying about practical matters, others in your life, and the future often need attention. At the start of treatment, it may be the prevention of nausea or control of pain. It may be help with insurance benefits. When treatment is finishing, it may be returning to work or school and wondering when your taste will return to normal.

In order to more effectively pay attention to comfort throughout the course of treatment, targeted assessment tools have been developed and tested. Your treatment center may use a form or questionnaire or ask you about these points during your visits. Knowing what is uppermost in your concerns and how important it is to you is the first step in good care. Such a tool, known as a distress thermometer, identifies the most significant elements of comfort during cancer treatment.

The acceptance of a tool like the distress thermometer further motivated producing a system to guide care from the day that someone finds out about having cancer to throughout the survivorship period.

If your oncologist's office or treatment center does not use a tool like this, you can use the list in the Resources section as a guide to know what can be brought to his or her attention or to the attention of your oncology nurse. Rating symptoms on a scale of 0 to 10 is an often-used shorthand in medicine. A rating of 0, 1, 2, or 3 means *mild.* A rating of 4, 5, or 6 is *moderate,* and a rating of 7 or above signifies *severe,* requiring immediate attention. The thermometer concept is one with which we are all comfortable. The list below the thermometer can key you and your caregivers in to the kinds of things to look for *before they happen* so you know what you *may* expect and know to alert your providers. (See the worksheets at the end of the book for this form.)

Looking at the items on the distress thermometer acquaints you with the type of experiences that commonly happen before, during, and after treatment. The list is varied. Some of the items are more important to each of us, others less so. The components that are important change over time, but a set of underlying themes, or values, belonged to you before you knew about the cancer and is enduring.

In medicine, the idea of a *baseline* is important so one can determine if a treatment or intervention of any type is effective. Although it may seem out of place, a short detour to outline your own personal values will be helpful to you, your family, and your providers throughout the course of your care. In my experience, it is helpful to think these values through before any decisions are made, if you have the opportunity to do so. Try to think about the themes we will highlight in Chapter 3, and then we will hop back on the expressway of modern cancer treatment.

2 Getting the Most Out of This Book

Although there are many cancer books out there, and lots of information dwells on the Internet, the purpose of this book is to provide some guidance for an unanticipated visit into a very closed world. It is a strange place, with its own culture, language, and procedures. Just as you may use a travel guide to learn about a new city before you leave home to visit it, so can you use this book to learn about cancer, the way it is treated, and what you can do to recover better and faster. You can read it from cover to cover or jump a little ahead and see what the next steps are. Or you can carry it with you and read it on the way to your appointments. However, it is best used in advance, when you can think things through a bit, and it is with that eye that My Recovery Plan was made. My Recovery Plan is a practical way to approach your recovery from cancer and its treatment. It features the LEARN System and a set of worksheets to use before and through treatment. My Recovery Plan asks you to ask yourself some hard questions to help you participate in care decisions more easily. Waiting until the trip to your first chemotherapy appointment is OK, but it is far more effective to do so before then. The reward is a potentially faster and better recovery, but not necessarily an easier one due to the additional work.

The LEARN System©

p. 247
My Weekly Recovery Planner

Chapters 1–3 are for *right now* with information you need to know and what you need to do at the time of your cancer diagnosis. It outlines the steps to set up your treatment and how the system works. From the very moment of diagnosis, you are focusing on your treatment and your recovery. *You will see that working on healing and recuperation begins not after you finish treatment, but as you are preparing for the consultations with the various oncology specialists and the rest of your health care team.*

Chapters 4–8 walk you through the consultation process and the beginning steps of treatment with detailed advice born out of many years of clinical and research practice. It takes you through the many details you will need to know right at the start of treatment and through the first weeks to months of treatment with an emphasis on practicalities and an understanding of our health care system with regard to cancer.

Chapters 9 and 10 help you to have important information at your fingertips *as and before* you need it. Deciding with whom to share your situation takes a bit of planning, and some rehearsal will make a difficult task at least a little easier, but likely a lot easier. With the explosion of online information, some of what you will inevitably read involves complementary and alternative therapies. *Complementary techniques* (those used alongside standard treatments) have only recently become accepted in today's health care market. Some followers of *alternative treatments* ask that they be used *in place of* proven treatments that are the backbone of mainline cancer treatment, so you need some introduction to these concepts from the start. Well-meaning advisors tend to recommend many of the complementary and alternative approaches, which we are coming to understand and use more effectively. Some could even say that the focus of this book, which incorporates healing and recuperation right from the start, is a complementary approach that enhances the best of modern, effective cancer treatment. Although it may be *complementary* to your cancer treatment in the sense of accompanying it, its principles are mainstream.

As many aspects of your life change with cancer and its treatment, the subsequent sections deal with those with which you need to be familiar as they directly impact both quality of life as well as survival. Learning about specific symptoms (many derived from the distress thermometer) and ways to control them, information about how your body's hormones may be affected by cancer and its treatment, and the day-to-day skills to help you *find your way back* comprise the following sections of the book.

The final chapters serve as a helpful guide to the next phases of recuperation with a full, partial, or minimal response to treatment. The last chapters discuss ways that you can give back to those who helped you and give forward to future generations of cancer patients.

■ *It seems that there's homework here. Did I misunderstand?*

Homework, well yes. You take a pop quiz by just going to each appointment. Finals, no. Term paper? Well, there is a journal to keep. But it won't be graded.

■ *My doctors, nurses, and other providers are not familiar with the LEARN System. How can they help?*

The foundations of the LEARN System are based on sound clinical practices, the Institute of Medicine report, and guidelines that are publicized by the most respected professional associations that benchmark care. The program draws from the best elements of cancer treatment, the introduction of *wellness* into modern medicine, and the techniques that other branches of health care currently use. *Wellness, recovery,* and *rehabilitation* have only recently been used in cancer treatment. Using My Recovery Plan and the LEARN System incorporates elements of these fields earlier in the course of treatment, adding value to the treatment you receive to control your cancer, not replacing it.

You are not expected to teach your providers, but truth be told, providers learn from patients every day. Medical school professors constantly remind us all that it is called the *practice of medicine* because we all continually learn from our encounters, and that experience makes us more curious and benefits future patient care. Refer your providers to a companion guide, *Manual of Cancer Treatment Recovery: What the Practitioner Needs to Know and Do* (forthcoming).

The following two cases certainly do not validate an intervention as well as a clinical trial, but the contrast between AA and BB was astounding. Their experience though is typical of the difference between the two approaches. It may be unimaginable to adopt a more healthy approach to eating and activity right after you find out about the cancer and the need for treatment. But the more proactive and early adoption of such healthy living habits made it easier and faster for BB to bounce back.

Using a system that plans for recovery right from the start can help in a number of ways. By keeping an eye on the recovery process from the start, you are a step ahead

CONSULTATION IN A BOX: A TALE OF TWO NEIGHBORS

Two women, AA and BB, were each diagnosed with breast cancer within a month of each other. AA had her surgery first and, being satisfied with her care, recommended that BB see the same oncology team, who luckily were also providers on BB's health insurance plan. Though friends and neighbors for eight years, they approached their treatments differently even though they were both given the same chemotherapy and radiation therapy plans. BB was fearful of gaining weight and becoming tired from inactivity throughout her chemotherapy and radiation therapy after surgery, so she made sure to be active every day that she could, walking each morning the weather allowed and using small free weights with an exercise video. She resisted the urge for starch-filled comfort foods when her appetite returned after each chemotherapy treatment, substituting more protein and whole grain snacks. She met with the physical therapist to learn how to avoid arm swelling after surgery and the nutritionist for direction. She reluctantly joined an online support and information group, becoming one of its regular contributors. AA figured that she would wait until her treatments were over, suspending her health club membership until she felt well enough to go back.

Despite their mutual support for each other during their treatment and even coming to follow-up appointments together so that family members would not miss work, BB recovered much more quickly. She gained 4 pounds over the six-month period of chemotherapy and radiation therapy but felt as well as one can after treatment. She was able to disregard the tingling in her hands and feet after chemotherapy, and she was able to get back to work within weeks of her last day of radiation. She had spoken up about her hot flashes and gotten some medication to suppress them. The information she learned in an online chat group kept her on track.

AA was suffering more, unable to walk easily due to her fatigue and 25-pound weight gain. She was tired, and tired of being tired, while the feelings of isolation grew. Six months after her last day of radiation, she saw the same physical therapist and nutritionist that BB saw, feeling it was time to get back to herself.

by the time the treatment is up. Knowing how to do just that can be accomplished by beginning to formulate My Recovery Plan and understanding how doing so early on makes it so much quicker and easier when treatment is finished.

Over the coming weeks and months, you will be using a number of worksheets, focusing on improving communication between you and your providers, and setting realistic goals. A small time investment in the basic parts of the LEARN System, knowing what you value most, and using the worksheet tools will help you through the rigors of treatment more easily.

WORKSHEETS? IS THIS FOR REAL?

The
LEARN
System©

p. 248
What Is
Important
To Me

p. 247
My Weekly
Recovery
Planner

p. 252-259
My Recovery
Plan
Communicator

p. 251
Important
Blood
Tests

p. 277
Your
Personal
Health
Record

The following worksheets, which appear at the end of the book, are designed to make your life easier and to overcome many of the obstacles outlined in the Institute of Medicine report.

1. "What Is Important to Me": Helps you really think about your own philosophy: how you think through serious decisions, how much of a short-term quality of life investment you are willing to make for long-term survival; the importance of comfort to you; and your comfort level with risk taking It is worth reviewing from time to time.

2. "My Weekly Recovery Planner Using the LEARN System": Helps you take stock of what you need to know and do, as well as what has been accomplished. Spend a few minutes a week. That's it.

3. "My Recovery Plan Communicator": It is in your best interest for each of your providers to know what the rest of your medical team is up to. Short of a unified electronic medical record, this is a good system. These sheets are composed of the bare minimum information for safety so as not to be burdensome. Make many copies of the one that applies to you.

4. "Important Blood Tests You Need to Know About": Knowing a little med-speak and what the tests are for will help you become more familiar with how your treatment is being monitored.

5. "Your Personal Health Record": Provides tools that can focus the information you will eventually need to know and bring back to your primary care providers who are unlikely to have direct access to your oncology records. The "Personal Health Record" will help you collect information you will need immediately and for a long time: the type of cancer diagnosed, treatment received, what you need to do now, and what your providers will need to know in the future. At the back of the book, you will find personal health record worksheets specific for many types of common cancers, as well as a general template form that can be used for less commonly experienced cancers.

3 Setting Your Goals

WHAT IS MOST IMPORTANT TO ME NOW?

Think Hard about Your Goals of Care

Most likely, your goals right now are to live, to live without symptoms of cancer or lingering effects of treatment, and to recover as much and quickly as possible. What may worry you in the middle of the night? It may be frightening, but let's anticipate now: What will I have to sacrifice from short-term comfort for a better chance to successfully treat the cancer? What's my personal philosophy? I never knew I had one or I never thought about it.

GOALS OF CARE

Live in comfort

Live as long as possible (*length* of life)

Live without symptoms of cancer or treatment (*quality* of life)

How much am I willing to risk now, for how much gain later? Health outcome researchers call such a question a "standard gamble." It is similar in many ways to what we need to do when we look at how to invest savings. First, do the risks exist, and what are they? Then, how much risk can I safely experience? How much is there to endure for an improved outcome? Hopefully, what you can achieve is a cure—be cancer free forever. This is called *long-term survival or disease-free survival.* Does the treatment proposed slow down the time until the cancer comes back (called *time to progression*)? That's quantitative—a quantity of time. What will my quality of life be during those periods? Will I be left with side effects of treatment that will go away or that are permanent? Will my energy be restored? How much of it? For how long?

Such are the complicated equations. What is important to one person may be less important to another. These types of value judgments are very individualized and even change over the course of a lifetime.

We generally don't stop in our everyday comings and goings to think about questions like this. When faced with a sudden cancer diagnosis, initially we are too stunned and afraid to do so. Yet from the beginning, our providers need to know what is in our personal comfort zone and which current comforts we will invest for more tomorrows, whether they are better or not.

The
LEARN
System©

p. 248
What Is
Important
to Me

The "What Is Important to Me" worksheet (at the back of the book) is what you can complete and present to your medical provider to help your team understand your personal values. It's best to complete it now so you can use it as a guidepost throughout the steps of your treatment and recovery. If you cannot complete it, at least *think about the items* so that you may complete it soon. Patients have universally said that they welcomed the opportunity to think about what is important to them right from the start. Using such a tool, and involving your family and close friends, is an effective springboard for thought and discussion. You may want to review the tool from time to time.

From Hard to Harder

No one wants to think that the treatment plan they are about to undertake will be anything less than successful. But yet, there's this pervasive feeling out there that everyone with cancer dies anyway. So how do you proceed in this world of uncertainty? You will ask yourself time and time again, and your answers may change. But you really do have to consider your future now. Do you want to think now about what would happen to you in an emergency? Are your finances in order? Who would speak for you if you are unable to speak for yourself?

The rules and laws in every state are different. Many states separate financial decisions from health-related choices due to specific federal laws. Some states honor living wills (a document that allows you to state what you don't and do want). Some states ask you to name a person to speak for you, like a power of attorney for financial transactions—a health care proxy. In some states, no one (even a spouse or parent) can speak for you unless they are deputized in writing. The discussion is important (not just the paperwork). Every state specifies something, reflecting the local interpretation of the federal Patient Self-Determination Act of 1991. You will likely be asked for the document on hospital admission and at a first office visit.

Get this done: discuss with family and friends, sign the papers and put them away, and then spend your full attention on treatment and getting better. Find out what your state needs. Then spend some time thinking it through. You can always change your mind—as long as you can, then the documents or the forethought may not be necessary. But the forethought is constructive, so you learn about your own personal philosophy. When we hear that having cancer is a growth experience, as unusual as that sounds, this is what folks are referring to.

Why Now?

Cancer treatment used to be an entirely inpatient hospital experience. Now, many patients never spend one night in the hospital; so much is done on an ambulatory basis. This has spread much of the responsibility to family and friends, most of who are untrained to handle it. The expense is also now shared with budgets for transportation, meals, and other personal care items. That hospital gown that reveals all to the world is the butt of generations of jokesters, but it was provided and washed by the hospital staff. Even the food—whether good or unappetizing—is prepared by someone else, who also cleans the dishes. Not so at home.

Families and friends generally *over*estimate the distress of a loved one. Providers, incidentally, often *under*estimate. The technological revolution has made more information available to patient communities with electronic access or advocacy groups to teach the information. The consumer movement has made medical care more of an interchange on a level playing field than in previous generations. Breast cancer patients led the way for greater input by people living with the disease. Women objected to the full mastectomy, which included removal of all of the breast tissue along the lymph nodes and muscles under the arm. Such was the standard and the only type of surgery that was done. Then the extent of the surgery got smaller, frequently now confined to removing the tumor and just a bit of surrounding tissue. Personal preference is now a factor in decision making, with information found in books, online, and in supermarket tabloids. But there is a new partnership between provider and patient born in the world of breast cancer, with increasing survivorship and improving quality of life for many. Advances have fostered improvements in quality of life after treatment, by focusing on organ preservation, chemotherapy, and radiation therapy before surgery that allows more minimal procedures than in the past. Now there is more potential to rehabilitate. What started in breast cancer now occurs in many, but not yet all, cancers, so thinking about what to do to recover from treatment becomes more of a factor.

■ *This is hard for me: Who can help?*

For thinking through a personal philosophy, start informally and locally. Though difficult, begin with a frank discussion with family members or friends who are important to you and whose opinions you trust. Many families have found that a discussion over food eases the tension. Try to set some time aside when the television and computer are off and children and dependent elders are occupied. Those who care about you may dismiss the discussion, finding it pessimistic or morbid, with a simple reassurance "not to think this way and everything will be fine." Adult children typically are reluctant in these situations.

If geography prevents a face-to-face discussion with those best able to do so, make an appointment to speak over the telephone. Many home phones can conference between a few places so that everyone is on the phone at once. Ask that full attention be focused with minimal outside distraction.

If you are unsure how to start, use your own words to say:

> - "I need your help to make some important treatment decisions now."
> - "I'd really like to discuss my treatment choices with you so that it is clear in my own mind, and I can put it down on paper."
> - "In the rush of finding out about the cancer, I haven't had a moment to stop and think about what is really important to me. I need your help to do so."
> - "Not that any of the doctors have said so, but in case there is an emergency, I want you to know what I would do." Or "I am unsure what I would decide, so I want to figure it out with you now."

These discussions are not easy. It is easier just to avoid them. If you can't bring yourself to start it off, ask someone who could to be there with you at the table (or on the telephone). In some communities, the clergy play a pivotal role in such personal and family matters. In cancer centers around the country, the clergy do not only get involved when someone is dying and needs last rites. No matter what their religious affiliation, putting major decisions in a life context involves basic clergy skills. For those who have been in some sort of counseling or therapy, someone who knows you can help jump-start thinking and short-circuit the process as well.

It should be clear to you and those who care about you that discussions about what is important in life is *not solely about end-of-life care or getting older.* If you or family, friends, or spiritual advisers are unable to start the conversation, you or they may be too frightened or superstitious to discuss such important ideas openly.

CONSULTATION IN A BOX: CAN WHAT I DO AT WORK HELP ME HERE?

An intuitive patient, himself a chief operating officer of a large corporation, was used to having discussions about new products or developing ideas with trusted staff and stockholders. He believed that a leader must prepare to guide the discussion with a lot of advance thinking, which may often be internal and solitary, so that a formulated idea can be presented for input and advice. Looking at decision making from a setting different from personal health care, he drew the parallel and welcomed the chance to think about what was important to him—like he did with his company before developing a new product just as investing lots of time and stockholder funds.

One of the ways he knew that his company's decisions remained faithful to its goals and values was to periodically review the original thoughts to make sure the company stayed on track. He welcomed the chance to do the same with his health care in a personal inventory and penciled in his responses before the family discussion.

It's best to go through these ideas now, saving them for the future when you will appreciate seeing how far you have come.

$\underline{4}$ Understanding Cancer

The word *cancer* is used in everyday language as a metaphor for so many things. Let's start with the official definition from the National Cancer Institute:

cancer (KAN-ser)

A term for diseases in which abnormal cells divide without control and can invade nearby tissues. Cancer cells can also spread to other parts of the body through the blood and lymph systems. There are several main types of cancer. Carcinoma is a cancer that begins in the skin or in tissues that line or cover internal organs. Sarcoma is a cancer that begins in bone, cartilage, fat, muscle, blood vessels, or other connective or supportive tissue. Leukemia is a cancer that starts in blood-forming tissue such as the bone marrow, and causes large numbers of abnormal blood cells to be produced and enter the blood. Lymphoma and multiple myeloma are cancers that begin in the cells of the immune system. Central nervous system cancers are cancers that begin in the tissues of the brain and spinal cord. Also called malignancy.

Cancer affects the whole body, the individual, the family, the workplace, the schoolroom, the congregation, the village, the town, the city, the state, the region, the country, the continent, and the ecosystem.

WHEN HEALING BEGINS: PREVENTION IS THE BEST TREATMENT

It is very much out of place to say it after cancer is diagnosed, but the best prevention against cancer is not to get cancer at all. Some cancers are preventable by avoiding exposures to radiation, alcohol, and tobacco products and through regular exercise and proper nutrition. Some can be discovered through screening tests, and some are found by chance.

FINDING CANCER

Getting an X-ray or scan for an unrelated reason sometimes finds small cancers, those too small to be giving symptoms yet small enough to be cured. Ovarian cancer is sometimes found when a woman is not getting pregnant on demand. Lung cancer can be discovered in someone without symptoms who is getting a routine chest X-ray for a new job. A screening test may be done on purpose (taking a stool sample and checking it for hidden blood on routine physical exam). There may be a nonspecific symptom, be it pain, fatigue, or unexplained weight loss. That symptom may even be attributable to something else. Indigestion happening regularly may be simply indigestion, or it could be a symptom of pancreatic cancer.

HOW CANCER IS DISCOVERED

Suspicious symptom such as pain, change in growth, change in bowel patterns, or finding a lump or growth

General symptoms: weight loss, tiredness

Blood tests

Imaging

Screening tests (mammograms, breast self-exams, breast exams done by a skilled provider, digital rectal exams with prostate-specific antigen blood tests, for example) grow in and out of favor as more is learned about their accuracy in finding small cancers.

Current Screening Guidelines

The American Cancer Society recommends screening tests specific to gender and age. These guidelines change every few years as new information is learned about the patterns of cancer in a population.

For people *aged 20 or older* having periodic health exams, a cancer-related checkup should include health counseling and, depending on the person's age and gender, might include exams for cancers of the thyroid, oral cavity, skin, lymph nodes, testes, and ovaries.

Ages 20-29

MEN

Colon Cancer Testing: for those with a family history of colon cancer or polyps

WOMEN

Breast Exam: every three years. As part of the exam, talk to your health care professional about your risk for breast cancer.

Pap Test (Cervical Cancer Testing): every one to two years, depending on the type of test

Colon Cancer Testing: for those with a family history of colon cancer or polyps

Ages 30–39

MEN

Colon Cancer Testing: for those with a family history of colon cancer or polyps

WOMEN

Colon Cancer Testing: for those with a family history of colon cancer or polyps

Breast Exam: every three years

Mammogram: because of family history, genetic tendency, or

   A lump or thickening of tissue anywhere in the breast

   Skin dimpling or puckering of the breast

   A nipple that is pushed in (inverted) and hasn't always been that way

   Discharge from the nipples that comes out by itself and is not clear in color, staining your clothing or sheets

   Any change in the shape, texture (raised, thickened skin, for example), or color of the skin (should be screened with MRI in addition to mammograms)

Pap Test (Cervical Cancer Testing): every one to three years, depending on the type of test

Ages 40–49

MEN

Colon Cancer Testing: for those with a family history of colon cancer or polyps

Prostate Cancer Testing: African American men and men with close family members with prostate cancer should talk with their doctor about the benefits and limitations of testing beginning at age 45 so they can decide if they want to be tested.

WOMEN

Colon Cancer Testing: for those with a family history of colon cancer or polyps

Breast Exam: every three years

Mammogram: every year. An MRI may be added if there is a lump or thickening of tissue anywhere in the breast.

   Skin dimpling or puckering of the breast

   A nipple that is pushed in (inverted) and hasn't always been that way

   Discharge from the nipples that comes out by itself and is not clear in color, staining your clothing or sheets

   Any change in the shape, texture (raised, thickened skin, for example), or color of the skin

Pap Test (Cervical Cancer Testing): every one to three years, depending on the type of test you get and past results

Ages 50–64

MEN

Colon Cancer Testing: Start testing at age 50. Talk with a health care professional about which tests are best for you and how frequently tests should be done.

Prostate Cancer Testing: Men should talk with their doctor about the benefits and limitations of yearly testing beginning at age 50 so they can decide if they want to be tested.

WOMEN

Colon Cancer Testing: Start testing at age 50. Talk with a health care professional about which tests are best for you and how frequently tests should be done.

Breast Exam (performed by a doctor or nurse): every year

Mammogram: every year. Report any breast changes to your doctor or nurse without delay. An MRI may be added with a lump or thickening of tissue anywhere in the breast.

   Skin dimpling or puckering of the breast

   A nipple that is pushed in (inverted) and hasn't always been that way

   Discharge from the nipples that comes out by itself and is not clear in color, staining your clothing or sheets

   Any change in the shape, texture (raised, thickened skin, for example), or color of the skin

Pap Test (Cervical Cancer Testing): every one to three years, depending on the type of test you get and past results. Pap testing after a total hysterectomy is not necessary unless the surgery was done for cervical cancer.

Ages 64 and older

MEN

Colon Cancer Testing: testing recommended. Talk with a health care professional about which tests are best for you and how frequently tests should be done. *Covered under Medicare.*

Prostate Cancer Testing: Men should talk with their doctor about the benefits and limitations of yearly testing so they can decide if they want to be tested. *Covered under Medicare.*

WOMEN

Colon Cancer Testing: testing recommended. Talk with a health care professional about which tests are best for you and how frequently tests should be done. *Covered under Medicare.*

Breast Exam (performed by a doctor or nurse): every year

Mammogram: every year. Report any breast changes to your doctor or nurse without delay. *Covered under Medicare.*

Pap Test (Cervical Cancer Testing): every one to three years, depending on the type of test you get and past results. *Covered under Medicare.* If you are 70 and over, you may stop testing if you have had three normal Pap tests in a row and no abnormal Pap tests in the past 10 years. Pap testing after a total hysterectomy is not necessary unless the surgery was done for cervical cancer.

Examples of situations leading to diagnosis are heard all of the time in the primary provider's office, on the commuter bus, or in the supermarket line: "I was trying to get pregnant and couldn't. Something showed up on my ovary." "I had a cough that didn't go away, so after a set or two of antibiotics, the doctor sent me for an X-ray or CT scan, and a (spot, lump, lesion) was seen." "On my routine checkup, when I had my rectal exam the stool sample showed hidden blood when it was tested." "During my period, I always check my breasts in the shower and felt something. It didn't go away after a few days, so I went to my gynecologist (or family doctor)." "I was applying for a new job, and the employee health service insisted I get a chest X-ray since I had been vaccinated against tuberculosis after I was born and my skin test is always positive." "The dentist saw something on my tongue when I was having a cleaning, and he sent me to an oral surgeon for a biopsy."

Knowing about Screening Can Help Your Friends and Family

In addition to guidance from a primary care provider, living through cancer with someone you love is strong motivation to detect cancer early through screening based on age and gender. You can help family and friends by making sure they are screened and do what they can to prevent cancer or detect it early.

Conventional Wisdom Is Not Always Up-to-Date

What is important to state over and over again is that cancer is not an automatic death sentence. To this day, there remains a belief that once someone gets cancer, death will be caused by the cancer before it would occur from natural causes or another illness and it is inevitable. *It is just not so.* Treatments are not helpful to everyone all of the time, but many cancers have very effective treatment. Commonly, people still lower their voice when saying the word *cancer,* as if it was a superstitious rite and showing such respect provides us each with a little immunity.

Why Not Just Recommend Whole Body Screenings for Everyone?

Wouldn't it make more sense to spend our health care dollars to find cancers that are small and most fixable? Yes—maybe. Scanning tools are getting better, so good that it is hard to tell if what is seen is a beginning cancer or an innocent spot, something benign or even nothing, an *artifact* but not in the sense of archeology. An artifact in medicine is something that is suspicious for cancer but turns out to be an errant drop of contrast pumping through a small blood vessel just as the image is captured. Or perhaps a benign cyst has been in your liver for whole life, but no one ever scanned you to find it before. Or it may be scarring in the lining of the lungs from the bronchitis that bordered on pneumonia when you were an infant.

By using scans as screening tools to detect cancers early, we oftentimes find things that we mistake for cancer but that turn out to be harmless. The resulting uncertainty could often be followed by taking a sample biopsy under more scanning and leaving a scar, having additional procedures with some risks attached and then finding out only afterward it was insignificant. On the other hand, the scans themselves may be carcinogenic or otherwise harmful. Weighing the true public benefit versus cost is a challenge. Other obstacles exist for screening: some insurance companies include screenings as part of their benefits, while others don't. Some of the preparations are exhausting, such as for a colonoscopy, which involves completely cleaning out your bowels and needs someone available to pick you up when you are done since you will have received light anesthesia. Worrying between the time the test is done and the time the results are in is always nerve-racking. The concern about the unknown effects of additional exposure to the radiation used in some scanning makes a recommendation for uniform total body scanning controversial. Newer technology such as sound waves in sonograms or magnetic imaging can eliminate radiation exposure while offering a glimpse into inaccessible body parts or surfaces.

HOW AM I SURE IT IS CANCER?

Biopsy (examination of a tissue sample under a microscope and other laboratory testing) is the only definitive proof of cancer.

Weighing the Gold Standard: Is the Biopsy Necessary?

Yes, virtually 100 percent of the time. As the saying goes, "If it looks like a duck, walks like a duck, sounds like a duck…" The same applies here. Despite the improvements in imaging that can look even clearer than the view during surgery, biopsy confirmation is crucial for everyone. No one wants to be treated for the wrong illness. No provider or institution wants to offer it. The field has advanced with the help of technology and human know-how. Smaller samples can be obtained under sonogram or imaging-guided approaches. Old-fashioned glass slides, like from your high school biology class, are still made. However, they are subjected to rigorous inspection with the advantages of modern optics and electron microscopy. Tissue samples can be tested for certain antibodies and genetic patterns, many of which are as specific as a fingerprint.

Unless there is a very specific situation, if you are offered treatment without a biopsy, a second opinion is ever more critical.

Not All Cancers Are the Same: How Does That Affect What Treatment Will Be Recommended?

With modern advances in electron microscopy, testing specific DNA chains of genetic patterns, and the discovery of receptor cells on the surfaces of cancer cells, it is most correct to view cancer not as one disease but as a spectrum of cell growth abnormalities. The names become very confusing, as some identifiers are traditional throwbacks to the days when technology was limited to old-fashioned light microscopes.

What Actually Causes Cancer?

With the genetic information for cancer in the cell's nucleus (DNA and RNA; remember the first day of 10th-grade biology all of a sudden?), future generations of cells receive the cancer DNA, not the healthy cell DNA. Sometimes slowly and sometimes more quickly, the cells that make up body tissues and organs do not work properly and after a while can cause symptoms. "I have a headache that hasn't gone away in two weeks." "I can't breathe." "I have cramping and pain with each bowel movement." "I can't urinate properly." These are some common symptoms that bring cancer to medical attention. Sometimes, a suspicious sign (a *sign* is objective, something that can be felt, heard, seen, or measured; a *symptom* is something you sense such as pain) causes a series of tests (a work-up) that discovers something wrong in its earliest form. Sometimes that occurs by chance.

Due to a combination of hereditary predisposition and environmental damage, the faulty DNA is formed and continues to be passed on to future cell generations. Those abnormal cells collect in a *tumor*, which takes up space. The tissues cannot do the necessary jobs that they were supposed to do. If the tumor is detected when small through screening or by chance, fewer of the body's functions are interrupted, making it easier to remove or inactivate the tumor with chemotherapy, radiation therapy, surgery, or other treatment.

If Cancer Is Found to Start in One Place and Travel to the Bone, Is It Bone Cancer?

The place the cancer starts determines not only the name but how it grows and what type of treatment it responds to, so it keeps its name of origin. For example, if cancer starts in the lungs and spreads to the bone, it would be lung cancer that has spread or *metastasized* to bone, not bone cancer. The cells that grow in the bone are lung cancer cells and are unwelcome guests. Most types of cancers prefer certain microclimates in different parts of the body. Searching for cancer in those places is somewhat predictable. Lung cancer often metastasizes to bone, liver, and brain, but rarely to the prostate or ovaries, for instance. An *extent of disease work-up* refers to the search for cancers, focusing on the predictable places once the initial spot is discovered to judge the proper course of treatment.

Since people differ, the effect of even one type of cancer is different on different people. Many factors, including age at diagnosis, general health circumstances, and the functions of specific organ systems all determine how cancer can affect any one of us. Due to these person-to-person differences, few people go through treatment in exactly the same way. But general trends are mostly shared, making the experience of others valuable to each of us.

■ *I have heard about personalized cancer treatment: What is it?*

The newest forms of technology have *almost* gotten us to the point where cancer treatment becomes a personalized one. *Personalized* here refers to treatment for a specific genetic makeup that defines an individual's tumor rather than treating a class of cancer. The term *personalized medicine* is sometimes confused with receiving care in a way that takes the personal factors such as emotional, spiritual, and practical aspects of life into account. Personalized medicine will more correctly be able to predict whose tumors are more likely to respond to certain treatments instead of recommending what is thought to be best for a certain type of cancer.

CANCER AS A CHRONIC ILLNESS

A recently established general optimism about survivorship has allowed us all to speak about cancer as a chronic illness rather than a fatal one. The *chronic illness* concept involves needing one treatment followed by another or even maintenance treatment over many years to avoid a recurrence or relapse. Societal attitudes change slowly.

5 Preparing for the Initial Consultations and Treatment

MY INSURANCE

Money is not the politically correct place to start, but it is practical and unavoidable. Although each of us may have certain personal opinions about health care as a right and mandatory medical insurance coverage, at least for the present, it drives our care. Thankfully, the landscape is changing. You need to understand more about your insurance, more than you ever did. Sit down with some uninterrupted time and read the policy highlights from the insurance carrier or employer. Some basics are important: Do you need to see specialists only in the network, or are you free to go anywhere? Can you only see a specialist if you are referred by your primary care provider? Is there a case management service, sometimes called *disease management* or *coordination,* at your insurance company? Often these folks can be very helpful in making sure the right services can be accessed; sometimes less so. What are deductibles? Deductibles are what you have to pay before your insurance will consider any charges, often at the beginning of the calendar year. Co-pays are the payments made at each visit, generally 10–40 percent of the allowed charge. Can tests can be ordered by each specialist or only advised by them and ordered by the primary care provider? Are there yearly limits? Lifetime limits? If you are lucky enough to have double insurance through a family member, does that mean you can collect on each claim twice because you pay double premiums? *No.* There is *coordination of benefits* so that the policies work together.

Do you have a prescription plan? Does it cover generic drugs only, or is there a preferred list of medications (the *formulary*)? Is chemotherapy covered? Is radiation therapy covered? Do you have a hospice benefit if needed? Find your insurance cards; get duplicates if misplaced.

■ *I have no insurance: What are the options in my hometown?*

There are some accredited cancer centers out there (see http://www.facs.org/cancerprogram) that take sliding scale payment or offer free care. Investigate accredited cancer programs at teaching hospitals associated with medical schools in your community or close by—they may have sliding scale clinics. If a teaching program is not close by, each county in the United States has at least one hospital that accepts you for care irrespective of ability to pay. Some of these programs are located at larger centers, and others in a separate building. If you cannot locate the county or state-funded program in your area, contact the mayor's office or the state health department for direction. No health care institution can deny emergency services under federal laws. Although cancer is a life-threatening illness, most patients are not in diagnosed at the point of emergency.

■ *Second steps: I bet a lot happens behind the scenes. I don't want to be clueless. What is the process?*

Our ideal model often stems from what we have seen on television shows: a primary care provider who knows you does all of the testing, brings you into the office, and has unlimited time to sensitively explain if it's cancer or not and the next steps to take. He or she then calls you at home that night to see how you have understood the information and offers personal support, sends you to a trusted colleague, close by at an accredited cancer center that takes your insurance, has an immediate appointment, and is a specialist with that particular kind of cancer. That's not usually what happens in real life.

Such seamless care does happen, although we don't know how often. We do know that for some the transition is rockier with multiple chances for deviation from such an ideal model. Parts of the ideal model *do happen.*

The entry point into cancer treatment can be through a variety of doors. Important to the concept of multimodal treatment, with medical oncology, radiation oncology, or surgical oncology defined as the core cancer specialties. No matter whom you meet first, unless it is truly an emergency, an *interdisciplinary team* of specialists should meet to collectively come up with an opinion and a *treatment plan,* which is sometimes unanimous and sometimes divergent.

Such cross-talk takes place at a meeting with an old-fashioned name, the "Tumor Board." Each of the core specialists is there along with a radiologist to help interpret the imaging, such as scans, X-rays for the group, and a pathologist to clarify the slides that are projected onto a large screen for all to see. Depending upon the facility, a host of others may attend to have input, including nurses and research assistants to see if there are available clinical trials, which may help point the discussion to the most up-to-date treatment. Often a symptom management expert to anticipate special needs in treatment of pain, fatigue, or nutritional care is in attendance.

Each patient's pathology biopsy slides, imaging, and story are combined in a shorthand uniform classification system, known as the process of *staging.* Much is misunderstood about the numbers with older systems still in use beside the newer, more complex system. The *stage* is an indication of where the cancer has spread, but **does not** tell how well the cancer will respond to treatment. The current gold standard is the seventh edition of the American Joint Committee on Cancer (AJCC). The present system is more detailed than the traditional stage 1, 2, 3, or 4 cancers. *It is extremely important to realize that the stage does not take into account how sensitive a type of cancer is to treatment, or whether a treatment will work. It is not synonymous with survival.* That can't be said enough times. *It is extremely important to realize that stage does not take into account how sensitive a type of cancer is to treatment or whether a treatment will work.* Staging cancer is a complex process, different for each type of cancer.

Frequently, the emotional reaction to hearing, "Stage IV" drowns out the facts, catapulting someone already frightened to believe they are in a hopeless situation. Make sure to clarify the exact meaning of the stage assigned with your oncologist. Resist jumping to the wrong conclusion. It will cause unnecessary grief.

STAGE ≠ SURVIVAL

A cancer stage indicates where the cancer cells are found.

It does NOT indicate if the cancer will respond to treatment.

It does NOT indicate rates or length of survival.

With this information, and the eyes and experience of the attendees, choices about a treatment plan are debated. The choice of modality—surgery, chemotherapy, radiation therapy, hormonal therapies—and the order to be recommended is vital, since discussion before treatment starts makes use of one of the most effective innovations in cancer treatment. Organ preservation may put chemotherapy and/or radiation therapy *first* to shrink the tumor to allow a smaller surgery. More chemotherapy, radiation therapy, or both often follow surgery. Sometimes very small dose of chemotherapy is used *during* radiation therapy to amplify the radiation, reducing the amount of radiation used with equal or better effect, which is less damaging to healthy tissues.

This type of discussion becomes even more essential than it seems at first glance. It virtually forces the treatment team to anticipate recovery needs right from the start. Do you need to see the dentist or meet the physical therapist and nutritionist *before* or just *when starting* treatment? Equally important is that it removes the bias of the provider, so no matter which provider is seen first, be it the surgical, medical, or radiation oncologist, that provider's specialty does not automatically dictate what treatment is offered or in what order treatment is given to increase the chance of an organ-sparing plan. This type of innovation, namely, communication and respect among subspecialty colleagues, is one of the most powerful tools to fight cancer. Yet it does not make the front page of a newspaper above the fold with top importance, and it will not sell commercial time on the network news.

Such cross-talk is an important advantage of treatment at an *approved* or *accredited* cancer center or program. Three well-respected professional organizations have detailed accreditation processes. The most common is the American College of Surgeons Commission on Cancer (ACoS CoC) with more than 1,400 accredited programs across the country. These programs account for 71 percent of patients treated for cancer in 2007. To achieve accreditation, at least 10 percent of cases need to be reviewed in advance, which is the bare minimum. Larger centers review almost all of the patients unless the beginning of treatment is an emergency. The National Cancer Institute also accredits stand-alone cancer research hospitals that are not always embedded in a general hospital, known as a comprehensive cancer center. A major difference between those two types of cancer centers is that a comprehensive cancer center does laboratory research in addition to the patient-centered clinical trials. The American College of Radiology visits radiation therapy centers in addition to the other two groups to examine safety and treatment practices. Some may be familiar with the Joint Commission of Accredited Hospital Organizations (JCAHO), which surprisingly is a spin-off of ACoS CoC.

TEAM MEMBERS YOU MAY NEVER MEET

There are many people you will never meet. Some may even bill for their services, an unusual feature that can and does occur in the business of medicine. A pathologist will review each of the biopsy slides, conducted at the place where the biopsy was actually done or for a second opinion if it was read somewhere else. This is almost an absolute rule; no one is treated without verifying cancer through a biopsy report. Seeing something that "appears to be cancer" or "looks like cancer" is not sufficient. The radiologist plays a vital role in defining how big the initial tumor is, if it has spread in the local area or is visible in other areas of the body, but such *indirect* information does not have the confidence of a biopsy report. Modern imaging has so exceeded the limitations of our vision using the naked eye, making it invaluable in treatment. A larger surgery may be proposed if the cancer is not visible in any other part of the body. It is the job of the radiologist to harness the technology, advising the team in the right direction. The radiologist can even suggest which tests should be done, avoiding those that may not show enough or that duplicate what's already known. Sometimes even meeting the radiologist is by chance, only to be told that the doctor who ordered the test will get the report. As frustrating as that may seem, a report out of context may not be helpful in any way except to reduce the waiting time to find out the results.

If you are to have radiation therapy, a lot of *treatment planning* goes on behind the scenes by highly trained people who map the direction and the length of the actual radiation treatment, to get it where it's needed and avoid the healthy tissues. Doctoral-, master's-, and bachelor-degreed physicists are there to work out the minutest detail. Any time you receive chemotherapy, whether in the hospital or in an ambulatory center, a pharmacist is involved. He or she will check each written order at least once, or even more, and make sure your height and weight dictate the amount of chemotherapy. The pharmacist will mix the chemotherapy to prevent it from spillage and spoilage. He or she will also double-check that all of the medications are compatible with what is prescribed by other providers and even advise about supplements that should or should not be used during cancer treatment.

It is your responsibility to coordinate all of your appointments and get them approved by your insurance company, verifying deductibles and co-pays, and identifying which provider is in-network or out-network. This may seem unfair, but at the present time, this is the way it is. Pre-certification coordinators, assistants, billers, secretaries, and office managers have different titles in different settings, but all help to orchestrate a complex world of appointments and bureaucracy.

TEAM MEMBERS YOU WILL LIKELY MEET SOON

If you need to tap the experience of someone who has been through cancer treatment, oncology-specialized social workers can put you in touch with veteran patients, point you in the right direction, lend a hand with practical and personal matters unlike a than a family member can, unless there just happens to be one in the family. Some social workers help coordinate care at hospital discharge; others in the office arrange home care, supplies, or in some areas even transportation. Cancer is in many ways a family issue, and social workers can lend a trained ear and experience. Meeting a veteran patient who can answer questions more personally is a good practical approach.

Weight loss or weight gain at the wrong times can be fatal, and that's not an exaggeration. Many cancer centers have on-site (or can refer you to) oncology nutritionists or dieticians who can help monitor weight and recommend nutritional changes. Recovery after cancer is an underutilized area of a nutritionist's skills, but ever-so important. Dieticians or nutritionists who know cancer work in collaboration with the other treatment team members to aid the survivor. Knowing what to read and what not to read is a responsibility shared by all with some centers having information specialists that advise the best (and worst) sources of information. Different facilities

---

TEAM MEMBERS YOU MAY MEET

Oncologist (physician specialists in cancer)
Core subspecialists: Medical Oncologist
                     Radiation Oncologist
                     Surgical Oncologist
                     Palliative Care/Symptom Management Specialist
                     Nurse/Oncology Nurse
Oncology Nurse or Advanced Practice Nurse (Nurse Practitioner)
Nursing Assistant/Technician
Physician's Assistant
Social Worker/Oncology Social Worker
Psychologist
Nutritionist/Dietician
Physical Therapist
Office Receptionist
Office Manager/Billing Coordinator
Insurance Precertification Assistants

TEAM MEMBERS YOU MAY NEVER MEET

Pathologist
Radiologist
Pharmacist
Physicist
Technicians/Assistants who work in each of theses areas

have a variety of peer counselors and sometimes veteran patients themselves who have been there and can share what they have learned. Some counselors have a pastoral care background; some are trained chaplains. This can also be a misunderstood and under-utilized group in the world of cancer centers, misunderstood in that many of us have a minister, priest, rabbi, or imam in the community or think that hospital chaplains are there to give last rites or other reconciliation rituals. Cancer affects our way of looking at our place in the world and at times our faith—or lack of it. Exploring the way we experience our world is sometimes faith-based and sometimes a universal experience. Pastoral care chaplains transcend their own faith training in a nonreligious way, mod-eled after the role of a chaplain in the military or larger police and fire departments.

INFORMATION YOU KNOW THAT THEY'LL NEED

The
LEARN
System©

p. 260
Important
Revelations to
My Treatment
Team

In the hustle of getting all of the appointments, organizing paperwork, and feeling frightened, there are certain things about each of us that would be very helpful for the treatment team to know but that may not get asked. Be prepared to supply this information even if not asked. It will be helpful. A two-part form ("Important Rev-elations to My Treatment Team") to help you organize this information is included in the worksheets.

Early and quick understanding of who you are, relevant experiences before your cancer, your coping style, and how you deal with uncertainty are a great help to the treatment team and link to center-based and community-based resources Some of these points may seem trivial, but they do count toward quality of life during treat-ment. Discomfort in closed spaces may make it hard to get imaging or radiation therapy; motion sickness or pregnancy-related nausea usually means that nausea from treatment may likely be more severe and will require stronger preventive measures; prior use of opioid (narcotic) analgesics may signal the need for higher doses to get pain relief; personal or family history of episodes of serious depressions or substance abuse may indicate the need to monitor pain medications closely as well as mood for early intervention to forestall depression (counseling and/or medications); a close blood relative having had a difficult menopause may make a patient more symptom-atic when treated with hormone blockers for prostate or breast cancer. Screening for these situations up front minimizes discomfort during treatment, making recovery easier.

6 Initial Consultation

Be prepared for delays. Saying, "I have cancer; I need to see Dr. Jones right away" won't work. All of Dr. Jones' patients do, and that is why it is so hard to get an immediate appointment. Find out exactly what to bring and what needs to be sent in advance. Some offices prefer advance delivery so the oncologist can read the materials beforehand. Others want to see the documents, imaging, and slides with the patient at the same time.

■ *Who/what do I need to bring to consultations?*

Someone from the oncologist's staff will ask for a number of reports and/or original biopsy slides, X-rays, CT scans, or PET/CT scans. The original biopsy glass microscope slides live in the pathologist's office who interpreted them, not the surgeon or interventionalist who performed the test. Due to federal privacy laws (the Health Insurance Portability and Accountability Act was bundled with a large number of privacy protections which hold for electronic transmission, paper charts, and even talking with each other), the doctor's office doesn't have authorization to get them for you, so they may be have to be requested in person or by phone/fax/e-mail with a signature or electronic permission.

Insurance Authorizations

Do you need one at all? Call your insurance company and find out. Is it on paper or electronic? Call your oncologist's office to make sure it has been received before the visit to save time and angst.

Bring a Trusted Friend or Relative

Most people retain not more than 40 percent of the information heard at an initial consult. It may be complicated, and not all of the details may be known at that time. The wisest thing to do is to bring a *scribe,* a trusted family member or friend with a few sheets of paper and new pens or pencils. He or she needs to take notes so that the details of the consultation can be reviewed later on, after the fright of the moment. The scribe may be able to ask questions for clarification that you cannot. This may sound excessive, but it works. Comparing the situation to other big decisions—buying a car, looking at an apartment or house—we usually have someone come with us as extra eyes and ears. A complex medical visit such as the initial oncology consultation is no less important. Follow the same principle!

THE CONSULTATION VISIT: WHO AND WHAT I NEED TO BRING WITH ME

Insurance authorizations if needed

A trusted family member or friend who takes good notes and ask questions on your behalf

Records whose results may be unavailable electronically

Referral note from your primary care provider

Blood test results

Imaging results (with X-ray films or images on CD)

Original pathology biopsy slides (actual glass slides)

List of all prescription medicines, over-the-counter vitamins, nutritional products, supplements

List of significant medical conditions, past surgeries with their dates

Allergies (foods, medications)

Personal information: use the forms listed below, which are provided in the worksheet section at the back of the book, and *complete them in advance of the appointment.*

"Important Revelations to My Treatment Team"

"What Is Important to Me"

"Family History Form"

The
LEARN
System©

p. 260
Important
Revelations to
My Treatment
Team

p. 248
What Is
Important
To Me

p. 262
Family
History
Form

Why They Do What They Do

Today's cancer treatment is rarely done by one doctor in one place. It is truly a group effort that needs coordination. At times, being a stranger to the world of cancer treatment, the reasons for things getting so complicated are not evident. At the risk of oversimplification from the start, it is important to understand the roles of the treatment team members and why they do what they do.

■ *What will happen at the initial consultation?*

Each office or practice has its own routines. Although not standardized, many elements are customary. After filling out much paperwork and signing forms to share information for insurance billing, you may be asked to provide much of the information you have already prepared prior to this day: medical, personal, and family histories. You will meet one of the oncologists, review some of this information, and get a full physical exam. Additional blood tests or imaging studies may be requested, depending on what you have brought with you or what was sent by the referring office. An initial plan will be discussed. This plan may involve consultations with other specialists. Having also brought the information in the "What Is Important to Me" and "Important Revelations for My Treatment Team" worksheets will help fine-tune the scope of your care right from the start of the planning process. You should be given a chance to ask additional questions. The trusted family member or friend who accompanied you is key here in jotting down what has been discussed and helping you ask questions about information that is still unclear.

TYPES OF CANCER TREATMENT

Surgery

Chemotherapy

- Intravenous

- Oral

- Local (to liver, pelvic area)

Radiation Therapy

Hormonal Therapy

Biological Modifiers

Each generalist or specialist has a trusted set of consultants whose opinions he or she respects, or who may be providers participating in the same insurance program. Hopefully, both conditions are met. The referring doctor should send information electronically on secured e-mail, by phone call, or via a note to bring on the first visit, explaining what was found, and if cancer is suspected, why. It is the job of the initial consultant to verify if there is cancer and advise the proper testing to see if the cancer has spread and where. Each suspicious cancer has its own list of tests. Few are done all in one place. If they are, then it is likely a well-oiled system in an established cancer center. The imaging and actual slides are most important as each oncologist has radiologists and pathologists they trust and work with all of the time. They want to verify that the original interpretation matches their trusted colleagues' opinions. At times, such reinterpretation is misunderstood as drumming up business for colleagues and inflating costs. Although that may be the case in a small minority of situations, it is a good idea, and in some states, mandatory, for the slides to be seen by a pathologist in the place where treatment is to be done to avoid errors.

This all takes at least days if not weeks. Once you think that something is growing where it shouldn't be or you are in pain, a universal set of reactions—fear and worry—can drive you to move ahead as quickly as possible. There are times when *time is truly of the essence:* "I can't breathe." "I haven't urinated in 24 hours." "I can't swallow." "I haven't had a bowel movement in six days." "The pain is so bad I couldn't take it anymore, and I had to go to the emergency department." If the situation is worrisome and frightening, but not an emergency, take the time to find the best place to go to begin your treatment. The public health message that has been somewhat effective—"Hit it hard. Hit it early."—is a general guideline and holds in some, but not all, situations. Take the time to get a second opinion if medically and practically possible.

Outside of the primary care provider referral, there are other ways to find the best oncologist or center for care. Television advertisements help familiarize us with what is in our own area but may not be the best for a certain kind of cancer, if it is cancer. In large metropolitan areas blessed with multiple well-known centers, each one may or may not be a *center of excellence* for each type of cancer. Often one needs to check around or have someone do so. The Internet can be helpful. There are a number of places to turn for suggestions for the primary care provider or to confirm the direction the primary care provider is recommending.

CANCER CENTER ACCREDITATION FOR ADDITIONAL HELP WITH REFERRALS

The American Cancer Society is closely affiliated with the group that accredits cancer centers (American College of Surgeons Commission on Cancer; http://www.facs.org/cancerprogram or 312-202-5085). Referrals can be made through direction on their website or by telephone.

Similarly, the National Cancer Institute's Cancer Information Service (1-800-4CANCER) can help with a selection of referrals and information in a number of languages.

WHO ACCREDITS MY CANCER CENTER?

Joint Commission of Accredited Hospitals (JCAHO)

National Cancer Institute (NCI) Comprehensive Cancer Centers

American College of Surgeons Commission on Cancer (ACoS CoC; for cancer centers and programs in a variety of settings including individual centers, networked centers, VA hospitals, teaching programs, and others)

American College of Radiology (ACR; for radiation oncology centers)

Accreditation assures you that an independent body has reviewed the qualifications of the staff and visited their facility. The reviewers meet the staff; tour key areas, such as inpatient units at hospitals, infusion suites, and pharmacies; and attend patient management planning conferences. A review of the facility's ability to make accurate diagnoses and offer multispecialty treatment has also been done. Reviewers also look at randomly selected patient charts to verify that information has been accurately reported to national databases.

■ *I am already in the hospital: What is different for me?*

The processes are the same, but the steps are even more hidden. The specialists come to your room and speak with each other even before they see you, and afterward. Coordinating care may not even be your yet-to-be medical or surgical oncologist, but a *hospitalist,* a specialist in treating general needs in the hospital and moving everything along as efficiently and smoothly as possible. It may also be a general practice physician, or a specialist in general internal medicine or family practice. Some women's care is coordinated by a primary care obstetrician/gynecologist. Under the current system, everyone admitted to the hospital has one main physician, one you may have known for years or one that was assigned to care for you in the emergency department or by your insurance carrier, who is responsible for your care while you are there. Start with him or her collecting information and learning about the treatment available in your area. With the current overhaul of our reimbursement system, it is possible that a group of providers will be your first stop, a concept now known as the *medical home.*

Being admitted to the hospital has many disadvantages as well as advantages when you are sick. Trips back and forth from home to the radiation oncologist's office are not necessary. An orderly takes you in a wheelchair or on a stretcher. In some respects, this is easier than being at home. A nurse is there if you are in pain or more nauseous to dispense extra medication. Lots of rules, and certainly not as comfortable as home, but in some ways simpler. Getting a genuine second opinion may be harder, since you are not free to travel somewhere else. Some hospitals may have Internet access in patient rooms so you can start to do some reading; some may not. Smaller hospitals often have cooperative agreements with larger academic centers in close-by cities, and with the improvements in telecommunication, consultations are even done by video-conferencing calls, which are able to transmit actual X-ray and scan images and pathology reports to a specialist anywhere.

■ *I was shocked when my oncologist asked me if I had thought about my fertility options. Why did this come up?*

This is a time-sensitive discussion. No matter how upset you are, or how difficult it is to absorb information, there is a small window of opportunity for you to weigh the options. You may be thinking to yourself, "Will I even be alive to raise a child?" Of course, that is an important question, which you can ask—and answer at a later time. The issue for *now* is doing what you can or need to do so that your options will be open later.

Please see the chapter on fertility (Chapter 23) to learn more if you are of an age where you would consider having a child when you are in good health. Your insurance carrier will help direct you as your policy details. If such a concept seems totally foreign to you right at this moment, *before* any treatment (surgery, chemotherapy, or radiation therapy), ask your family, friends, *doula,* buddy—no matter the job description—to collect information on your behalf.

■ *During the initial consultation, clinical trials and research were brought up right from the start. Does that mean it is a hopeless situation?*

Do *not* assume that if a clinical trial is mentioned right at the initial consultation it means that the oncologist is not sure what to do. Some clinical trials require that extra steps are taken right from the start, such as extra processing of a biopsy sample or timing of tests. Participation in a trial does not mean that you are being asked to accept unproven treatment without a chance at a standard regimen. It may be a way to get access to a drug or device that is close to FDA approval and would not be reimbursed by an insurance carrier. It also could reflect the newest and most effective way to treat your cancer. Ask why a trial would make sense for you instead of what is considered standard practice at the moment.

Involvement in clinical trials is another greatly misunderstood area in cancer treatment. Whether it is fear or unfamiliarity, many of us still have a media-influenced view of research, however mainstreamed it has become. Depending on our age, it may be one of the Frankenstein stories. A bright, quirky, and distrustful lone scientist believes he or she (although most often males are portrayed) can do what no one else can, such as bring a monster alive or travel through space or time. These are the stories we grow up with. They are sometimes what makes science attractive and fun when we are very young. But imagine how quickly those well-etched memories and associations are called up when we are frightened by cancer and are worried about dying. Balance those images of Dr. Frankenstein with recent history, and a reasonable person would be open at the start to see if a clinical trial could be of benefit.

TYPES OF RESEARCH STUDIES: PHASES OF CLINICAL TRIALS

Phase I Is the agent or device *safe*?

Phase II Is the agent or device *effective*?

Phase III *Compared* against the "standard" treatment, is it *more effective*?

Phase IV Measure long-term effectiveness and safety

There are many types of clinical trials. Some clearly test a new drug or procedure that has passed testing on animals but has not been tried on humans The most important feature to be tested at first is safety. Is it safe to even try experimentally? A Phase I trial looks just at that. Is it safe enough to test widely? That does not answer if it is effective. When asked to be in a Phase I trial, most often it is after all very effective and even some less effective treatments are tried. It is rare for someone to go right into a Phase I trial as their first treatment option. Phase I trials often involve small groups. Many trial drugs do not have a name but a number. But the nature of Phase I trials colors what we think of all clinical trials, which leads people to erroneously believe that all trials are testing for safety. Phase II trials are conducted after safety is verified to fine-tune the treatment for such parameters as doses or schedule. A newer variation of one drug may be substituted for the older one. Doses may start out low and automatically be increased if the lower dose is tolerated. To give access to the many people who would consider a clinical trial, sometimes one regimen is used for a few weeks on half of the participants and then switched to the second group so that no one is denied a helpful drug. When *randomization* occurs, half (or a third) of the participants get "option A" and half get "option B." It is not up to the individual investigator, nor known to him/her to which group any one patient belongs if it is a *double-blind* trial.

The placebo-controlled double-blind trial is the gold standard in clinical research. Neither the investigator, staff, nor patient knows to which arm a patient is assigned. Such secrecy is a deterrent to some investigators, especially to the folks who value being in charge. When designed, either the arms of the study are truly equivalent or it cannot move forward, and heated debates about the *equipoise* or equivalence of the choices goes on daily behind closed doors. If there is no equipoise, then having each group get the experimental drug for half of the trial is often the solution. These Phase II studies are a moderate size. Once completed, the data is entered into a computer database and is analyzed by a bevy of experts. The most promising drug or schedule then enters Phase III in which it is given to half of the participants in comparison to standard care. These trials are often large, involving thousands of participants, where individual differences are diluted by the large size of the group.

There is quite a bit of oversight of such research trials. Before anything can be offered to patients, it is reviewed by many people including a special institutional review board (the IRB) at each hospital or cancer center. Some smaller operations use a centralized IRB. IRB members include investigators, administrators, and a variety of members that must represent the community and part of the lay public. Once it is approved, significant changes in the plan need to be reapproved by the IRB. Even a flyer publicizing the study needs to be IRB approved. The IRB monitors the study's progress along the way. Any "serious adverse reaction" even thought not to be connected to the treatment being tested must be reported to the IRB. If a significant deviation from the exact plan outlined in the study occurs, it must be reported as well. This creates a huge amount of oversight and even greater amount of electronic data and paperwork that must be written and checked, then submitted and stored securely.

Perhaps at first this sounds like wearing a belt and suspenders at the same time to hold up one's pants—even the monitors have monitors. A data safety and monitoring board (DSMB) must look at results in the middle of a clinical trial. They know who is on which arm of the study and are sworn to secrecy. If a treatment is considered unsafe, or too helpful to wait for the completion of the trial, the DSMB has the authority to suspend the trial and make the results known to the general public. The existence of these two groups of experts in red tape, the IRB and the DSMB, makes the United States have the most restrictive rules for medical research. That translates into the most rules and the maximal protection for vulnerable patients. Due to the United States' history of doing research before the days of informed consent as we now know it, some claim these advantages to be grave disadvantages, particularly in the treatment of life-threatening illness. Such restrictions may keep us safe but prevent us from doing truly innovative things with a higher associated risk.

For many of us, enrolling in a clinical trial means that the treatment received whether chemotherapy, radiation therapy, surgery, or a combination is among the most up-to-date, with not only the newest drugs but also innovative approaches.

CONSULTATION IN A BOX: IS A CLINICAL TRIAL FOR ME?

A 56-year-old woman who stopped smoking 19 years ago developed a cough in the middle of a cold Northeast winter. When it didn't go away, she went to her primary care provider who sent her for a chest X-ray, which revealed a suspicious spot about the size of a quarter. Apart from the cough, she actually felt fine, although she thought she may have gotten more winded than usual at the gym. A *spiral* ultrafast CT (computerized tomography scan) can find small lesions since it takes less than a minute. This scan requires that you hold your breath for a minute, which is possible for virtually everyone. Without having to breathe in and out, the lung tissue isn't moving and smaller spots can be seen. Her scan showed the single lesion, about a centimeter (less than half an inch) in size. She was referred to a thoracic surgeon at her closest certified cancer center who explained the options. She would need a biopsy to confirm whether it was benign or cancer. If positive, she could choose between two types of surgery. The first option would be a thoracotomy in which the entry would be a large cut from the back to the front with the lesion fully visible. The lesion would be removed, and a variety of lymph nodes would be sampled. The recovery would be a few weeks, and to remove the inflammatory fluid, a tube would be inserted to be attached to a vacuum to remove as much of the fluid as possible to heal. Alternatively, the spot was small enough and in a location accessible enough to be taken out using a throacoscope (flexible tube) monitored by video camera through which the lesion itself could be removed as well as close-in lymph nodes. Just three holes in the chest wall and recovery in days instead of weeks. The disadvantage would be that the surgeon couldn't look around the rest of the lung. Such a look may actually be less necessary than in the past since the spiral CT can see such small spots. Insurance would pay for either one.

A third choice would be a clinical trial in which a newer brand of thoracoscope is being tested and the traditional road map that the surgeon uses to sample the lymph nodes in a standardized way is being altered. It is thought that these improvements would be helpful to patients and make the procedure safer, but it needs to be tested against the best standard care. That is why it is a research trial and far from the guinea pig concept.

continued

> ## CONSULTATION IN A BOX: IS A CLINICAL TRIAL FOR ME?
>
> *continued*
>
> The lesion was indeed cancerous, and the minimally invasive surgery a success. Although the size was small, one lymph node was positive, so additional treatment has been recommended, both chemotherapy and radiation therapy. Precedence exists for chemotherapy first followed by radiation therapy or having both together, with follow-up using a different type of chemotherapy. The oncologist believed that the drug regimen was optimal but was not sure, even after consulting colleagues at the Tumor Board and checking out recently published articles about the order in which the chemotherapies should be used. A clinical trial that would pay for one of the newer drugs, including an expensive one, was offered. This was certainly a way to get the most up-to-date approach with minimal cost. Besides a slew of additional paperwork to sign, a research assistant and extra nurse would be assigned to monitor the treatment, a true perk with additional explanations, phone calls to see how the patient is doing, and some reimbursement for taxis or gasoline since three extra visits would be necessary for the trial. True, there was a certain limited, but greater uncertainty with the combined and more innovative regimen. The oncologist's estimate was that the patient would easily tolerate it and might have a quicker recovery.

This patient had two chances for clinical trials and opted to do so. She mentioned her experience to other patients in the waiting room, and then on the CancerCare teleconference she joined a trial. When her treatment was done, her nurse gave her an "Ask Me about Clinical Trials" button to wear. Then someone in the supermarket asked her about the button, officially starting her stint as an ambassador for clinical trials.

■ *I want a second opinion. How can I arrange it?*

In the world of cancer treatment, second opinions are vital and routine. No matter how specific the situation and the credentials of the oncologist, there is virtually always someone else in the United States or abroad with at least similar expertise. Be wary of any cancer specialist who discourages second opinions. If the cancer is diagnosed in an emergency, such as being admitted to the hospital not being able to breathe or pass stool or urine, from a practical perspective there may not be an opportunity to have a time-out without being well enough to travel somewhere else, either close-by or faraway. Sometimes even such an emergency comes with a small window of opportunity after the initial problem is addressed and treatment is to begin. It is important to remember that until recently, surgery always came first. Now that is sometimes so, but sometimes chemotherapy and radiation therapy are advised right away to allow for a smaller surgery. That is an important information point in any first consultation. If possible, the second opinion consultant should not work in the same cancer center as the original oncologist. People who work together tend to think through problems in the same way after a while. Remember, some cancer centers are networked despite being in different buildings or hospitals. Seek the second opinion outside of such a network. If the insurance carrier delays or tries to avoid reimbursement for a second opinion, a supervisor may be helpful. Some states have laws providing automatic second opinion reimbursement for some cancers.

AT THE END OF THE CONSULTATION

At the end of your first consultation, many of your questions should be answered, and you may leave tired, perhaps frightened, and loaded with information you have not fully digested. You and your trusted representative should know what the next steps are. There may be some more definitive testing or perhaps enough information has been reviewed that a treatment plan was proposed. Depending on how urgent it is to start right away, this is the opportunity for a second opinion. The second opinion will review the diagnostic information as well as the proposed treatment plan. You or your representative may likely have more questions. This is not the last opportunity to have them answered, so make sure to have them written down. Ask that a copy of the *consultation note,* the summary of your visit that will be written, is sent to your primary care provider or the referring doctor, or both.

7 Beginning Treatment

Here is one of those situations where making complex theories understandable can be a little misleading. And lots of information published online is written to discourage the use of radiation therapy or chemotherapy by folks who may have an antitreatment agenda. Perhaps someone they themselves—or someone they love—did not have a good response to chemotherapy or radiation therapy, or it wasn't explained in a way that could be understood by a nonscientist. Or someone they loved died, with the treatment taking the blame. There is a lot of information that is both good and bad.

So let's go back to high school biology class. The body is made up of multiple *organ systems.* The integument is the skin and muscle, gastrointestinal—mouth, stomach, intestines, and so on. Organ systems are made up of organs (stomach, intestines, lungs, etc.), and organs are made up of various *tissues* such as heart muscle or lung, which are in turn composed of individual *cells.* Each cell has a *nucleus,* which contains the genetic information. This information is composed of DNA, or deoxyribonucleic acid, and RNA, or ribonucleic acid, which work in harmony to help coordinate the cell's functions. DNA and RNA are small strands of proteins that hold *genes,* which pass the directions to future generations of cells. For some cancers, such as breast, ovarian, colon, and perhaps others, there is a genetic predisposition to develop one of these cancers as the DNA is passed down through conception when a baby is formed. A similar intergenerational "gift" happens millions of times in each one of us as the cells renew so the tissues can keep doing their jobs for years. A change in these proteins or a genetic mutation can cause the message to future generation of cells to be faulty. If that tissue with a faulty genetic message is to grow wildly or to perform a different job than it was originally programmed to do, that may be understood as an *oncogene* that turns normal cells into cancer cells. For this reason, it is believed that chronic inflammation can be intimately involved with *oncogenesis*—the production of cancer genes. It may be that exposure to chemicals owed to pollution or pesticides may indeed affect the future generation of cells that start tumors (collection of cells) growing.

SURGERY

Cancer treatment in totality is designed to interrupt the transmission of the faulty cell direction to future generations of cells. Surgery was initially the only way to rid the body of cancerous tissue, to be removed from the body as fully as possible. A surgeon's keen eyesight was the only way to "get it all" by cutting a small distance into the surrounding healthy tissue, so that no cancer was visible on that cut line or *clear margins.* The best naked eye cannot see on the cellular level, and with a microscope and specialized training, a pathologist could look at the sample removed during surgery, slice it thinly, and put it on a glass slide verifying clear margins. Way back when, it was presumed that "cutting cancer spread it around," which for the most part today is *not* thought to be correct. By the time cancer has established itself well enough to cause a symptom (pain, discomfort), it has likely made a home in the immediate neighborhood (local extension), or possibly entered surrounding lymph nodes (the body's drainage system), or been caught in the high-pressure blood supply looking for oxygen and food, taking up residence in faraway tissues or organs (known as *metastasis*). Many of the existing types of treatment are designed to overcome these types of spread.

Surgery remains a mainstay of treatment. By taking out as much of the tumor as possible, the body is relieved of the extra calories the cancer uses up, freeing the energy for the rest of the body. Some the the biggest improvements in surgery use technology to help make smaller incisions (shorter healing time), or use robotics, cold temperature or intra-operative radiation therapy.

RADIATION THERAPY

Radiation was discovered and medically harnessed by Henri Becquerel and Marie Curie in the 1800s. It works today as then, with much better direction by fancy computer programming, sparing healthy tissues and pointing the radiation beam more to where it is needed, supercharged at times by new and ever-evolving technology. Radiation works by heating the tissues to *ionize* them and prevent cancer growth. It helps in the area where it is pointed but offers no protection to the rest of the body. It is very effective in many cancers and can be used under a variety of circumstances, with and without chemotherapy. Modern advances in the computer that points the radiation and spares healthy tissue, radiation seed implants, and superconcentrated doses are big advantages over the radiation of yesteryear. Seed implants when they can be done focus the radiation where it is needed without penetrating the skin and muscle outside, causing less of a skin reaction and better healing. The newest technologies offer the highest dose of radiation in the most concentrated of areas to the brain—*stereotactic radiosurgery*—and more recently to other body systems. The good effects of radiation as well as the side effects linger weeks after the treatment is finished, which is counterintuitive. Radiation therapy is given over many treatments to spare the skin and muscle, and there is something about the experience that causes fatigue or intensifies the fatigue associated with cancer. Some progressive thinkers believe that the radiation even to a limited area of the body, such as a breast lump after removal, actually stimulates proteins that spread around the body in the bloodstream known as *cytokines*. Cytokines may account for many of the side effects of cancer or its treatment on the rest of the body: pain, weight loss, fatigue, or even mood changes. For now, such speculation fits what is seen everyday: cancer and treatment make one very tired.

The process of planning and delivering radiation is highly technical with many people behind the scenes. It can take up to a few weeks for complicated treatment plans. After the plan is mapped out, now universally on computers, and bolsters are custom-made to help you maintain the correct position, there is a long simulation visit where no active radiation is used. Positioning on the table and all of the directions of the beam are checked, sort of like a dress rehearsal. Subsequent treatments are only a few minutes. Once a week, the responsible radiation oncologist will be checking in and often times ordering blood work. Patients and those accompanying them should plan to spend more "dwell time" on that day.

Some people find the experience really high-tech and are fascinated by the machinery and the precision. Others find it demoralizing and impersonal, especially those who hate small and closed spaces. Despite being in the room alone during the few minutes of treatment, there are video cameras with someone watching and listening at all times. The treatment rooms are often good-sized, offsetting the feeling of being closed-in.

Radiated tissues often become less flexible as the years go by afterward. It is common for the initial gratitude that the radiation can help save one's life to wear off when muscles get stiff and move less than expected. Use the creams recommended to keep the tissues as flexible as possible.

CHEMOTHERAPY

Chemotherapy attempts to keep cells in the initial tumor, or individual cells or cell clusters that have broken off from the original tumor, from growing. The best chemotherapy does so in a number of ways, and it is common, but not always necessary, to take chemotherapy in combinations that work together to prevent the cells that contain cancer genetic information in their nuclei to replicate as more cancer. Some chemotherapies work at different phases of the cell nucleus's duplication when it separates into two cells. Others work on destroying the cell wall, so the cancer DNA has no place to nest. Other chemotherapy enters the cell via receptors on the cell surface to discourage it from copying itself for future generations. Some block the hormone receptors on the cell membrane similarly. Even newer types of receptor blockers reduce the blood supply to the cancer cells, rendering them less able or unable to grow into future generations.

Chemotherapy has a mixed reputation. On one hand, it can be lifesaving. On the flip side, chemotherapy makes just about everyone sick to some degree, which can be blunted with a variety of medications and techniques. The average person on the street would say, "Some chemotherapy makes you throw up and lose your hair." Cancer causes tiredness. Chemotherapy causes tiredness on top of that. Tiredness or fatigue is universal in cancer. Chemotherapy travels to the faraway spots in the body, as do the cytokines, so it has become such a useful tool.

■ *My chemotherapy is a combination of drugs. Why?*

Since chemotherapy tries to stop the growth and replication of cancer cells, so far there are a few strategies that have worked the best. Some of the agents actually stop the DNA from being passed to future generations of cells. Others work by attacking the cell wall, so the genetic information loses its home, and with no place to live, dies off. Newer *targeted therapies* bind to receptors on the cell to stop it from growing. The best outcomes have so far been to combine chemotherapy drugs that work in these different ways to do the most destruction of cancer cells, relying on the combination of different chemotherapy drugs.

Fatigue and extreme tiredness were brought to medical and societal attention in the early 1990s when medications were developed and approved by the FDA that treat anemia by increasing one's hemoglobin levels by stimulating the cells in the bone marrow to make more of it. Due to the fears about contaminated blood products for transfusion, despite the safeguards that protect our blood supply, having a nontransfusion treatment for anemia became attractive and popular. Since fatigue as well as breathlessness is the prominent sign of anemia brought on by a low level of hemoglobin, it became both a sales and an educational message, forcing providers to look at fatigue more critically. Fatigue has various causes, and correcting anemia is a start, but not the sole intervention to help feel better during and after treatment.

Since chemotherapy has the biggest effect on quickly dividing cells, the roots of hair, nail beds, and the lining of the stomach are prime targets for chemotherapy to act, explaining hair loss and some of the nausea. Much of the nausea is because at least in some small amount, chemotherapy enters the brain and irritates the *chemoreceptor trigger zone,* which causes nausea or vomiting, or even both. Many of the effective antinausea drugs (*anti-emetics*) do their magic by calming down the chemoreceptor trigger zone as well as the lining of the stomach.

MINIMIZING NAUSEA AT THE FIRST TREATMENT: KNOW BEFORE YOU GO

Wear clothes that are not your favorite and may be given away after treatment is over.

Avoid eating favorite foods before treatment.

Avoid perfume or strong smells when possible.

Take diversionary activities (music, audiobook, word/number puzzles, small neat crafts).

Understand what medications should be taken the night before or morning of treatment.

Try C-bands bracelet that pushes a pressure point on your wrist.

To someone new to cancer treatment, the use of so many medications is counterintuitive. "I have so many medicines, and then medicines to take away the side effects of the treatment, and then medications to take away the side effects of the medicines to take away the original side effects." True. But many of our advances are in anti-emetics that make chemotherapy—even at higher doses and stronger combinations—more effective.

HOW ARE YOU?

Keeping track of how you are doing and feeling is a joint effort between you and your providers. Different treatment settings are set up to do so in different ways. Many offices or treatment centers will use a tool; some will not. It is important that by the time you leave from your first treatment the elements in the tool are addressed by at least one member of the treatment staff. If there is a factor that needs more attention, you and the trusted family member or friend who accompanies you should bring it up. Knowing how treatment settings differ, the best person to involve is the oncology nurse. She or he may actually use a similar checklist even informally. Use it as a guide. Oncology nurses are often the best resource when there is no social worker on staff. Many resources are in the community even in major cancer centers. Knowing who they are and how to access them is important.

PLANNING FOR THE FIRST FEW DAYS AFTER YOUR FIRST CHEMOTHERAPY

All chemotherapy drugs are not created equally. Some are hardly likely to cause nausea (such as 5 Fluorouracil, 5FU), others cause a moderate amount (such as cyclophoph-amide, or Cytoxan®, and others), and some are expected to make just about anyone nauseous (such as cis-platin [CDDP], or Platinol®, and others). Instead of waiting for the nausea to happen, a variety of medications are given to prevent as much or all of the nausea or vomiting as possible. Make sure to alert the nurse or doctor if you have motion sickness or had moderate to severe nausea during the early part of pregnancy as that knowledge may alter their advice and prescribing.

For now, make sure that you leave the chemotherapy session with a clear set of instructions about how to proceed in the next few days. This is most often done by the nurse who actually administers the chemotherapy, and sometimes by the oncologist him or herself, or both. Knowing what to do the first time is essential to make it as easy as possible for you, and this sets you up to have the least amount of nausea for the next rounds. You should leave the chemotherapy suite, if it was not done beforehand, with a set of prescriptions and instructions about what to eat and drink during the first few days after treatment. You should have some idea about how much salt you can tolerate based on your blood pressure history, if you are taking antihypertensive blood pressure drugs, and your kidney function. Ask specifically about some guidelines.

When you get home, try to doze a bit (many of the medications you got will cause drowsiness that can linger for a few hours) or do some diversionary activity to focus your attention *away from* the treatment you just had. That is different for different people. Some can immerse themselves in a movie or television program or some serious music of their liking. Reading may be difficult since some of the antinausea drugs can blur your vision (books on CD or MP3 player work well now). Just try to pass the time.

If you have gotten a corticosteroid, dexamethasone (Decadron® and others) or prednisone (Deltasone® and others), you may unexpectedly feel energetic and ready to start a project (cleaning your desk, income tax preparation). That is *not* a good idea right now. You may feel energetic, but your thinking processes may have also been blunted by the medications you just received, so do something more mindless.

Knowing how important your nutrition is, especially if you've had a corticosteroid, you may even be hungry. Eat what you can easily take in, but do not use this opportunity to bulk up. When the immediate effect of the nausea medicines wear off, that complex spicy food or large amount may then make you nauseous, so go easy. Plainer foods often are the easiest to digest during those first few days. See how you do.

If there is some residual nausea, it is easy in almost any climate to *dehydrate,* or lose a lot of fluid through the urine, stool, skin, and breath that actually makes you feel sicker. Put your efforts into replacing the fluid lost with water, flavored or plain. The amount of salt you replace (sodium in regular salt; potassium in *light salt* or electrolyte drinks like Gatorade® and others) may need to be determined by your oncologist based on your blood pressure and kidney function. If you have taken cis-platin or cyclophosphamide, you should be given a minimum amount of fluid to drink each day. During these first few days *only,* whatever food you can tolerate should be OK. Whole grain, good carbohydrates may not be what you most crave or think about as *comfort foods,* so use good judgment and indulge if you must. Weight maintenance, so crucial to the healing process, is less of an objective in these first few days.

If you are not nauseous, starting to replace good foods based upon the guidelines in the nutrition section of the LEAR*N* System (*N* is for nutrition) would be great. But if not, a few days of whatever you can tolerate is acceptable. Not dehydrating is the main goal; minimizing nausea or vomiting is the second.

As the corticosteroids wear off, your tiredness will likely increase. Keep reading. The information about what you can do is essential now.

The
LEARN
System©

p. 266
What I Am
Supposed to
Be Eating

THE BEST ANTIDOTE IS PREVENTION:
THE RECOVERY PLAN STARTS NOW

Logical thinking still confirms that the best approach against cancer is to prevent it. Taking such thought a step further, once it has been accepted that cancer and or its treatment causes a set of predictable even if somewhat varied side effects, why just wait for them to happen? Why not try a proactive, preventive approach? Prevention here will not be complete, but more on the order of damage control in the public works. If we can't stop the hurricane, cover the windows with plywood so they won't blow out. If instead we are looking at a leaking oil well, let's absorb or disperse the oil before it hits the shoreline. Such a premise gets to the heart of the My Recovery Plan using the LEARN System. A logical and helpful approach can minimize the side effects of having cancer and having it treated in the most modern ways, incorporating elements at the same time that chemotherapy or radiation therapy is starting or right after surgery.

■ *I'm starting with radiation, not chemotherapy. How will the experience be different for me?*

The routine is vastly different from the infusion suite for chemotherapy, and its own world. The goals of safety, effectiveness, and comfort are the same. Radiation

HOW DOES CANCER AFFECT THE BODY, MIND, AND SPIRIT?

Grows near original cells started (*local extension*)

Enters lymph nodes

Enters bloodstream where it gets oxygen and nutrients and gives off wastes to travel through the body

Manufactures cell proteins (cytokines) that affect many bodily functions

Weight

Energy

Appetite

Mood

Pain syndromes

USUAL, EXPECTABLE REACTION (BOTH DUE TO SITUATION AND CYTOKINES)

Why me?

It must be a mistake.

Belief it is punishment.

Anger.

therapy suites were almost always dark areas on the first floor or in the basement. The equipment is very heavy. Upscale centers try to make the areas light and attractive. You've been there already; perhaps you met the radiation oncologist in a neighboring office, but you have come once or twice to the treatment area, once for a treatment planning CT scan and another time for a *simulation* visit, or a dress rehearsal using regular light, no radiation treatment

If you are starting with radiation therapy, you have been given a series of appointments, generally Monday through Friday each week. Plan travel time and time for delays each day. Especially after the first few appointments, it is possible that it will be best if someone accompanies you. Once weekly, expect to spend extra time for a checkup visit with the radiation oncologist and oncology nurse.

THE EXPERIENCE OF MODERN CANCER TREATMENT: WHAT TO EXPECT AFTER CANCER TREATMENT

Interest in patients' experience has blossomed in recent times, owing to a number of factors: the rise in the *consumerism* movement in health care, the increased availability of information to the public on the Internet, and distrust of institutions and bureaucracies. If the start of the diagnostic process is characterized by the "Five Ds" (fears of death, dysfunction, disability, discomfort, and dependence), the end of treatment and the start of recovery is also anticlimactic, and frightening. One cannot begin to describe how physically tired and emotionally spent one becomes at the end of treatment. You will be hopeful and frightened at the same time. Treatment is over, but there is the risk of a recurrence or relapse. Waiting for a time to feel better may intuitively delay recovery and, from a quality of life point of view, may make the waiting too dependent on time and luck. As cancer may not be the only illness people have, care for the other conditions cannot be neglected and is likely to be affected by its interplay with cancer.

Diabetes is one example of such a situation. Many of the activities of daily life affect someone with diabetes who undergoes cancer treatment. Even with good control of the blood sugars, some coordination needs attention. Regular activity helps maintain good blood sugars; fatigue discourages that, so blood sugars can rise. Eating *comfort foods* may be introducing more starches into the body that cause blood sugars to rise or even fluctuate widely. Lots of salty foods may make the kidneys work extra hard. Kidneys process much of the chemotherapy in concert with the liver. Many diabetics have lessened sensation in nerve endings; many chemotherapy agents cause the same, compounding the problem and often making it more severe. People with diabetes often get gum disease or even fungal infections in closed moist areas like the toes, arm pits, groin, or mouth, which can be made worse from the reduced resistance in the body during chemotherapy or radiation therapy—and from the cancer itself. Patients with or without diabetes need to report a white "cottage cheese" type discharge from the mouth which is from *candida* and commonly called *thrush*. It can almost always be easily treated.

Why wait for these things to happen? They are not destiny but predictable. Let's work with them, plan for them, and use what is available, medically and nonmedically, to minimize their effects on daily life and keep recovery less bad, if not speed it up.

■ *What about my hair? It's really bothering me!*

One of the most disturbing adjustments you need to make quickly is to plan for potential hair loss. It is not trivial as your hair loss announces your treatment to the world before you are ready. Although it is discussed on other sections, you may want to consult a hair stylist with experience in cancer-related hair loss, so that your hair can be seen or even photographed in its usual state if your are to consider a hair replacement later on. You may not know now, nor have to decide right now if you will get a wig or use one of the other options.

Hair loss from chemotherapy is rarely permanent, but people report changes in the texture or color. Many patients choose to cut as closely as possible to the scalp without shaving (a buzz cut), but women are less comfortable and often wear hats or wigs. Men sometimes like the tough look from the buzz cut, which goes in and out of style, and some prefer to get their hair cut sooner rather than later. The scalp needs to be clean and moist, as does the rest of the body.

8 Understanding What Is Happening to You

THE FIRST DAY OF CHEMOTHERAPY

You probably didn't sleep well the night before. You are frightened. It is expected. Arm yourself with a few tools to make it through the day. Something to do that will keep your attention diverted as much as possible. That may be a book to read or a small DVD player or an iPod or similar MP3 player. Do not wear any of your favorite clothes (or else risk thinking of today whenever you put them on again). Some people will wear something they never intend to wear again and have a party to dispose of it when they are done.

You are likely to be told to eat lightly and given more specific ideas of what that should be. It may be helpful to have someone come with you for at least the first treatment, as you don't know if you will feel drowsy when it is time to leave and may need someone to guide you home, just for the moral support, or to learn the routine as well as take down information you are given verbally or in writing. Arrive early, with the idea that you may be kept waiting. You will be asked to verify certain historical facts, some of which you have already repeated to a number of providers. Yes, the system can be disjointed, and partly because of the lack of a uniform medical record, there is a lot of duplication. So either bring a sheet of paper with the information you have given to any of the oncology subspecialists at your first appointments with them, or recite the information again. Some of the duplication is also a safety check. You will be escorted into an open area with an easy chair or a bed, either in a communal area or in smaller cubicles. Some have a personal television to use. You will see a tall metal pole to hang an intravenous bag and usually a small device or two clipped onto the pole with a electronic dispenser that keeps the flow rate even. Believe it or not, you will be asked your name and date of birth and perhaps your doctor's name to avoid getting chemotherapy that belongs to someone else with a look-alike or sound-alike name.

If you have a venous access device in place (a *port,* or long intravenous access below the skin or a tube coming out through the chest wall), some clear fluid in a large bag (perhaps a quart or so, but it's likely a liter in metric terms, 10 percent bigger) will be attached through your port. After you are settled, one of the providers should verify that you are ready to start, and that includes reviewing the orders and your most recent blood work. Once that occurs (may be remote and behind the scenes), your chemotherapy nurse will carry in some syringes and smaller bags on a tray and explain what each one is. Some are anti-nausea medications given in advance (also some may be in pill form). (S)he will explain what each one is. Some are hung to drip right into the tubing, some are pushed into the tubing as a prescribed rate, and some are routed through the microcomputer that controls the flow rate (a pump).

DON'T BE SURPRISED IF YOU START
TO FEEL DROWSY RIGHT AWAY

Some of the commonly used nausea medicines at the start of chemotherapy are sedating (especially lorazepam, or Ativan®, and diphenhydramine, or Benadryl®). The nurse(s) will check in on you to see if you are having an allergic reaction to any of the medicines, few of which you are likely to have taken in the past. If you get suddenly red, hot, and itchy all over, let your nurse know right away. If not, your task from that point on is to keep occupied and divert your attention with the things you prepared and have with you. If the infusion area has Internet access or your phone works with e-mail and instant messaging, this is not the time to do banking or make any serious decisions that you would normally not make when you were sleepy or otherwise impaired. Within a short period of time with all of that fluid going in, you will likely have to go to urinate, so make sure you and your companion know how you get to the closest bathroom, probably pushing an IV pole.

After the infusions are done, you will be given some instructions about things you need to do that day and until your next appointment with the medical oncologist. Some of those instructions may involve drinking what seems to be endless amounts of water or other fluids, especially if you have gotten cyclophosphamide (Cytoxan®), ifosfamide (Ifex®), or cis-platinum (Platinol®). Take this advice very, very seriously, and be sure to do so to keep your kidney function good. If you find that later that day or the next day, you don't remember a lot of what happened, it is very improbable that you were so scared that you didn't absorb the information. The lorazepam causes some amnesia for events right after it is administered. Having your companion with you is helpful to fill in the missing pieces.

Subsequent visits will be easier. You will have learned the routines. But because of the safety rules imposed by accrediting agencies, you should always be asked two identifying facts, such as name and birth date, even though the staff may know you. Just like the television commercial for a credit card; the setting is a record store checkout register. The twenty-something associate speaking with singer Tony Bennett: "Oh, Mr. Bennett. I love your albums. I listen to you all of the time... Can I see your ID?"

I AM GETTING RADIATION TREATMENTS. WHAT CAN I EXPECT?

Radiation therapy equipment has to be very exacting, and when the technicians arrive each day, the machines are checked before they are used, and if they are even a smidgen off, maintenance performed on the scene or remotely may put the schedule behind. These delays are inevitable. Some centers will have you call in before you leave home and speak with the receptionist to see if they are running on time or late.

You will arrive and put away your coat and safely stow your belongings in a locker. Then you will be asked to get into a hospital gown over your pants or skirt. Sometimes these flimsy gowns get put on *backward*, exposing your rear. Some centers have more substantial gowns. You will probably be in a gender-specific waiting room and escorted into a treatment room, a large room with cabinets around the sides, lots of storage, and a large, somewhat imposing piece of machinery in the middle with a metal table attached to it. It looks scary. Many of the newer facilities have distracting murals on the walls or ceiling, in case you are lying down on your back and staring up. You will probably have a sheet or cushion on the metal table, and depending on the part of your body getting treatment, you will have bolsters to support you. You may even be asked that a dotted tattoo be placed on your skin to keep the aim correct. Many patients find having such a tattoo distasteful, and for some it even conjures up prisoner of war or Holocaust markings. No disrespect is intended. The idea is to keep you in the *exact* same position and place every day over the course of your treatment.

If you are getting radiation to the head and neck area, a mesh mask specially conforming to your face will be attached to the table so that you are very, very precisely in the right spot. It can seem a bit scary, like old grade-B science-fiction movies. Many facilities will have music in the room or ask you to bring an MP3 player, iPod, or CDs to play your favorites. The simulation visit is the longest visit to check your position and the settings many times over. It makes one think that all of the visits will be that long, but they are not. Treatment visits tend to be just a very few minutes. Be sure you know what you need to do that night, especially which moisturizers to apply where and how often. This is not anti-wrinkle cream. This is serious. Even if you have oily skin and never use skin cream, follow the directions you are given.

Once a week, you will be asked to stay for some extra time for a check-in visit with your radiation oncologist and nurse, sometimes called a *status check* to see how you are and if any adjustments have to be made. Other technical checks are done without you, and there are strict guidelines for them to happen often behind the scenes without your involvement.

■ *The schedule I got when I first started treatment is not worth the paper it was written on. How do I plan my life?*

Accurate planning for the future is not a skill that humans have perfected, whether it is for celebrations or natural disasters. It would seem easier to plan for a single event than an act of nature or a natural disaster. But in reality, this is not always so. Accepting that cancer treatment is done by the proverbial "it takes a village" group, coordination reduces the odds that for weeks or months, everything will be on schedule. That is burdensome to virtually everyone facing cancer treatment. Putting the facets of one's daily personal, work/school, and family life on sudden hold is hard. Interweaving a mix of human and technological delays brings planning into the realm of fiction. There are expectable patterns. On top of the expectable patterns, the only certainty is uncertainty. That is problematic for our families, our employers, and all of the people in the "village" who depend upon us. So right from the start, the road map may be there, but the speed limit is not known. It is possible that everything moves exactly as scheduled, just not probable.

You may have heard that the nausea from chemotherapy can be so bad you'll want to throw up. Is there any way to prevent this from happening? Yes. Some of the most significant technical and pharmaceutical advances in oncology have come in the prevention and treatment of nausea and vomiting. It used to be one of the two biggest obstacles in receiving full doses of chemotherapy on the most effective schedules. Why do you get nauseous from chemotherapy? There are a few reasons:

1. You hear that it happens, and you are *primed* to expect it.

2. Chemotherapy is irritating to the lining of the stomach and an area of the brain that controls nausea and vomiting, aptly called the *chemoreceptor-trigger zone* (CTZ).

Most of the effect is actually through the brain and not the stomach, so the most effective treatments affect brain chemistry. Not surprisingly, they are interconnected, which is important in this situation. The medications work by blocking the neurotransmitters that work on the CTZ: dopamine, serotonin, acetylcholine, histamine, and substance P (with its NK-1 receptor).

You read in the press often about physicians overprescribing medication and about patients, especially elderly patients, being placed on different medicines by different providers, one not knowing what the other has prescribed. Such cross-prescribing can and does cause duplicate prescriptions and unpredictable drug-drug or drug-food interactions. The message has been clearly received by many of us to take less medicine, not more. Taking less medicine also makes one feel less ill, an attractive state. Optimal prevention and treatment of nausea and vomiting requires exactly the opposite. The proper mixture of anti-nausea medicines from a variety of different drug families gives the best control but goes against what we have absorbed before.

The best prevention and control of nausea and vomiting is to take medications that block each of these chemical transmitters. The number of medicines used is based on *how* much nausea and vomiting is expectable for the combinations of chemotherapy drugs administered together. Drug regimens are categorized into *low, medium,* and *high emetogenic potential,* or the expected risk of a combination causing nausea and

---

MED SCHOOL IN A BOX:
ANTI-EMETIC (ANTINAUSEA) MEDICATIONS

These medications come in "families," and it is best for the prescribers to choose one from each category to minimize side effects and get the most desired effects.

Prochlorperazine (Compazine®), metoclopramide (Reglan®), and haloperidol (Haldol®) all work on blocking dopamine and acetylcholine, which transmit the nausea signals, as well as many others.

Ondansetron (Zofran®), granisetron (Kytril®), dolasetron (Anzemet®), and palonosetron (Aloxi®) work to block serotonin, particularly $5HT_3$. This subtype of serotonin is present in both the stomach tissues as well as chemoreceptor-trigger zone (CTZ). Granisiteron comes in both a pill and transdermal (skin) patch.

Diphenhydramine (Benadryl®) and scopolamine (TranScop® patches) are antihistamines (work on a different subtype of histamines than produced in allergic reactions). These medications also reduce the jumpiness from the dopamine blockers and should almost always be used in combination

continued

MED SCHOOL IN A BOX:
ANTI-EMETIC (ANTINAUSEA) MEDICATIONS

continued

(one from this group with any one from the dopamine group). The scopolamine patches are very helpful in managing nausea between chemotherapy cycles. Aprepitant (Emend®) blocks the NK-1 receptors of substance P to prevent being nauseous or vomiting in the first three days of the chemotherapy cycle.

Lorazepam (Ativan®) is a benzodiazepine sedative that has many other medical uses, as an antianxiety medicine. It is helpful as one of its side effects is an *anterograde* amnesia which helps not to form memories of the nausea that can come back at different times in the future unexpectedly. It also helps tremendously with *anticipatory nausea* on the morning of the chemotherapy and the night before. Picturing yourself in the chemotherapy chair and feeling queasy can make the experience even more intense. Doses of lorazepam beforehand can keep it from happening. The lorazepam can also help reduce the jumpiness from the dopamine blocker medications.

Dexamethasone (Decadron®) can help with the highly emetogenic chemotherapies to reduce the symptoms of nausea and vomiting (presumably acts like an anti-inflammatory on the CTZ, but that mechanism is not fully proven). It is often used with taxanes to reduce some of the swelling in the hands and feet that the taxanes can cause (so there are two benefits from one drug).

Dronabinol (Marinol®) and nabilone (Cesamet®) are a subtype of cannabis, the active ingredient in marijuana, and are quite helpful in managing nausea and vomiting that do not respond to the other medications for use between chemotherapy cycles.

vomiting. There are written models for different levels of emetogenesis, publicized through the American Society of Clinical Oncology (http://www.asco.org) or the National Comprehensive Cancer Network (http://www.nccn.org).

Ask for very clear instructions before your first chemotherapy so that you take the right combination. It is very important to have as much nausea- and vomiting-free time as possible during your first chemotherapy administration, so you don't get nauseous in advance for the following ones. Likewise, to avoid any learned associations with the chemotherapy, do not wear any favorite item of clothing (you may begin to strongly not like it) or eat any favorite food beforehand (same reason).

Make sure you know what to take before you leave, and that you have all of the prescriptions in writing when you leave your treatment. Also ensure that you have prior approval from your prescription insurance company for any of the prescriptions that require it (serotonin blockers, substance P blocker, cannaboids).

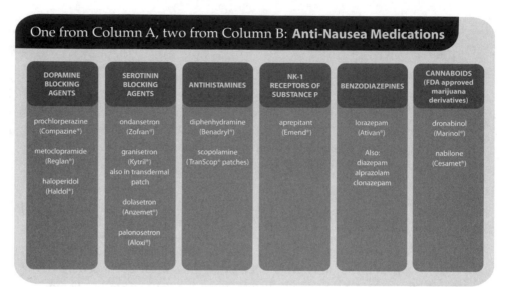

Nausea experienced before, during, or after chemotherapy is often managed using one, or a combination, of any of the medications listed above.

If in the past you have had motion sickness (car, plane, train, or bus) or significant nausea during the beginning weeks of pregnancy (dads don't count for this factor here), please let your providers know. Those conditions make you prone to stronger nausea and vomiting, so you would like them to consider that when you are getting your post-chemotherapy instructions, with the idea that they should give the higher doses for the first round to ease the ones that follow.

Non-pharmacological tools are very helpful along with the anti-emetics. They are often not powerful enough to replace them entirely (sorry). Ginger has potent anti-nausea properties in much higher concentrations than in ginger snaps or ginger ale and is available as a supplement. There are active pressure points in the wrists. Commercially sold "C bands" (also called "sea-bands" for seasickness) are made of an elastic band with two hard disks in just the right spots so the band will provide acupressure. Acupuncture has an excellent track record in preventing and treating nausea and vomiting from chemotherapy or radiation therapy.

■ *What about nausea from radiation therapy?*

Yes, radiation therapy can make one nauseous. The exact reason is not known but speculated. Radiation to the mouth, throat, or esophagus can certainly cause lots of mucus production, a funny taste, or even candida (thrush) fungal infections, all of which can bring on nausea. It may be the change in the amount of *cytokines* produced by the cancer as it is being treated. The same techniques used to treat radiation-associated nausea are the ones used during chemotherapy. There is not a treatment that is strictly FDA approved for radiation-associated nausea. Since many of the newer (translation: expensive) serotonin-blocking antinausea drugs were not tested for radiation-associated nausea, you may find that your drug plan will not authorize them without a special authorization after discussion with the provider.

Often, the nausea is a lower-level queasiness that can happen and is often best treated with the scopolamine patch or cannaboids rather than the serotonin blockers. Work with your treatment team to figure out what is best for you.

■ *Why do I feel OK on some days and really horribly on others?*

Well, none of us feels the same every day, without cancer what's more with. During treatment, it is a complicated question to answer in a general way. Not every cancer affects the body in the same way. Some types of cancer preferentially use more of the energy that sustains our body functions *(resting energy)* leaving less in reserve or for pleasurable activities. Sort of like spending more than you can earn and save. You're behind no matter what. Many of the medications used during treatment affect mood and energy. Some do rather profoundly.

Steroids—more correctly *corticosteroids*—are commonly part of the anti-nausea medications recommended before cis-platin, carboplatinum, or taxane (paaclitaxel, docetaxel) and give a boost of energy on the days taken and for a day or two afterward. As a general rule, the better you feel (energy, hungrier) on those first few days, the worse you feel afterward. Neither the immediate effect or the delayed effect is permanent.

Many other factors contribute to our energy level and general feeling of well-being during treatment: anemia (shortage of red blood cells or the hemoglobin that carries the oxygen); many hormones (thyroid hormone, estrogen, progesterone, testosterone); poor nutrition (even a single essential amino acid—the building blocks of proteins—like carnitine); too much or too little of a variety of substances that need to be in just the right balance (sodium, potassium, magnesium, calcium), an infection that is just starting; liver or kidneys overworking to digest all of the additional substances beyond our regular digestion; and medications whose action is *in* the brain (nausea medicine, pain medicines) or that incidentally affect the brain (antibiotics).

■ *Do the effects of chemotherapy and radiation therapy accumulate?*

Yes, and no, depending the level of detail with which that question is answered. There is a loophole in the understanding of this concept that sometimes gets lost in a rushed office visit or phone call. It is a controversial point. Each chemotherapy drug in its original form lasts a short period of time in the body, often a few days, and varies from drug to drug. The length of time it takes the body to absorb and digest out of its original form is known for individual drugs. But since most of the time chemotherapy is given in combination, it is not so clear-cut. In the body, most digestion of any food or drug occurs in stages with intermediate digestive products, known as metabolites (the results of metabolism—digestion). Progressive thinkers believe that those intermediate metabolites once they are chemically bound to proteins and then freed of them last for a while, even days to weeks. For many chemotherapy drugs, that is when they are most effective. Eventually they are processed so many times by the kidney and liver that they are no longer recognizable and leave the body in stool, urine, sweat, and exhaled breath. Each of the intermediate metabolites has an expectable time in the system, and pharmacologists describe this property as *half-life,* or the time it takes half of the original substance to be deactivated. Chemotherapy is given in cycles with a period of days in between each dose. That is not a random choice, nor dictated by reimbursement, but is calculated based on half-life.

Most patients say, "Just when I am almost recovered from the first cycle, it is time for my second. How discouraging." But that may not be just coincidence. If half of the first cycle is present, and you get the second cycle, the intermediate metabolites are in higher concentration. So when the third cycle is administered, it's a quarter of the first, half of the second, and so on. No wonder it seems harder to recover from subsequent cycles. It used to be thought that it was a matter of just being weary and fed up, but in conjunction with the lingering intermediate metabolites, it makes for an increasingly difficult recovery.

It has been said that the fatigue is a weird kind of confirmation that the chemotherapy is being absorbed, so it is an odd kind of affirmation. But tired is tired, and fatigue is tiredness on top of tiredness.

■ *How long does the chemotherapy last in my body after I am done?*

Another reasonable question with a complicated answer. It does not disappear from all parts of the body all at once. A sign that it is mostly being fully digested out is the reduction in fatigue, the ability to retain calories as lean body mass (muscle), and the return of growth of hair and nails. The range is variable, with a few weeks to four months as the usual time frame.

Such responses are disheartening while proceeding through treatment. No one wants to let precious time go, so there's a rush to return to normal, or feeling like one's self. But it is a process.

■ *How does radiation either before, with, or after the chemotherapy or on its own affect my recovery?*

Also a controversial concept. The immediate effect is short-lived with the adjustment of the cells to its presence taking weeks. That second part cannot be measured with a Geiger counter, but with experience. The pressure to make the time feeling sick pass as quickly as possible is the same. Some very modern approaches use combinations of smaller doses of chemotherapy with the radiation therapy, to fool the body into thinking it is getting more radiation than it is, like a transformer does to an electrical line or a megaphone to the spoken voice. That may make recovery seem even longer. Recovery from radiation therapy can often be judged by the skin on the outside of the body part radiated becoming less red and returning to its usual color. The healing inside often takes longer. A crude analogy may be cooking food in a microwave oven. The outside of the food gets hotter than the inside at first and cools faster. Same idea.

Despite the scientific description and loopholes in the theories, it generally takes about one to three weeks for the radiation to show its peak or maximum effectiveness after the last treatment and an additional three to nine weeks to return to feeling more like usual.

■ *I've read about* chemobrain. *What is it? It sounds frightening.*

Cognitive impairment from chemotherapy or even radiation therapy is a new frontier. Irreverently known as *chemobrain,* it entails being unable to record newly learned information, which results in the sense of being forgetful. Patients also say that it is harder to keep track of and do multiple things at once. It is common during treatment, owing to a variety of factors that include the direct effect of the anti-nausea medications or pain medications on alertness and learning, hormonal changes, the direct effect of the small amount of chemotherapy that seeps into the brain, and being distracted by the whole cancer and treatment process. Old information that was saved before the cancer and chemotherapy seems to remain. As we age, it becomes harder to learn new things and multitask, so part of the situation is that it makes us track what we try to disregard. This is a fascinating topic unless chemobrain is affecting you or someone you love, and something we need to learn more about. Everyone's concern is escalating and sometimes even comes up during the initial consultation. It is important to consider that this is a temporary occurrence in the majority of those that experience it. The rare individual refuses chemotherapy out of fear of developing *chemobrain.* The benefits of chemotherapy almost always far outweigh the small but real risks.

Borrowing from the advances in the treatment of traumatic brain injury, there are simple compensatory techniques that can help minimize the impact, and even medications that can help the brain compensate for cognitive limitation, but not reverse it. Believed by most (but not all) investigators that challenging the brain, especially through learning new material, is protective or even a treatment. Color-coding items, using sticky notes, putting things back where they belong (didn't Grandma supposedly say, "A place for everything and everything in its place?") either helps reenergize the brain or reduce frantic searches. Put your bag, keys, wallet, and cell phone in a defined place when you get home. If you leave your car in a parking lot, write down the number of the area or look for a landmark. When traveling to an unfamiliar place, whether in public transportation or by car, map out the route in advance. Leave extra time to avoid rushing. The use of GPS devices when driving, walking, or even on the train or bus reinforces that you are headed in the right direction. Share your struggle and the attempt to overcome it with trusted colleagues, friends, and family so they are aware. They can help!

■ *How do I know that one doctor knows what the others are doing?*

If you are receiving your care in a multispecialty cancer center (especially one that is certified by the American College of Surgeons Commission on Cancer or the National Cancer Institute), there should be a coordinated way that your information is shared between the providers. Ideally, there is an *electronic medical record* that everyone shares, so that each provider has access to initial consultation notes, office visit notes, blood work results, scan results, and biopsy results. Many cancer centers have been slow to adopt these systems, due to their compatibility (or incompatibility) with existing data collection and storage systems in the hospital networks or its state cancer registries. Without such a link or if you are being treated by providers with offices throughout

The
LEARN
System©

p. 252-259
My
Recovery
Plan
Communicator

p. 251
Important
Blood Tests

your community, it is likely they have developed a way to communicate with each other. That may entail sending printed notes in the mail, faxing documents, or using a protected e-mail system.

Since any system short of a unified electronic medical record has built-in delays, it may be unfair to ask you to help, but it is in your best interest to do so. A simple yet effective method is for you, or a loved one, is to use the "My Recovery Plan Communicator" form in the worksheets at the back of the book. There is one specific to the major types of cancer. Make some copies of it and fill in as much of it as you can. You can find out the results of the blood tests at each visit and put this on the form for the next provider. The oncology nurse or physician's assistant in each office should be eager to help you fill it out as you have made them more efficient by bringing needed information to them.

Each provider's office handles things a little differently, but the principles are the same all over. When you arrive, someone will greet you and record that you have indeed gotten to your appointment on that day. Either a file-folder chart or electronic chart will be used to record how you are doing, documenting the treatment you have gotten and what is due for the next time, as well as any prescriptions you are given or changes to what you already have. Hand your worksheet to the nurse, physician's assistant, or oncologist you are seeing.

Many practices have their own machine to measure your blood count (usually referred to as a *complete blood count* or *CBC*). If so, ask for a copy of the report it prints out or for them to note the important results (white blood count, hemoglobin level, and platelet count) for you before you leave. Most other blood work, even at large cancer centers, such as blood chemistries (a *metabolic profile, complete* or *basic* have some common elements—sodium, potassium, BUN = blood urea nitrogen and creatinine that assess kidney function, blood glucose) or tests on the comprehensive only (liver function tests, general guide of nutrition, signs of inflammation; see worksheets for a list).

■ *How does each provider know what the others have (or have not) done?*

Each office has its own way of communicating based upon the technology used, its location, and staff habits. You will become more familiar with the office routines as the weeks go by. Whether it's a short conversation in the hallway, a phone call back and forth, an e-mail written in a secure system, a fax sent to each other, or a unified electronic record, optimal care revolves around effective communication as much as professional know-how.

At your first treatment, ask how the providers in your center communicate with each other. Who should you ask? Perhaps your oncology nurse or the oncologist. Maybe it's the office manager who really knows. That will vary from place to place. Pick the Planner that applies to your type of cancer. Ask a staff member to make a copy (or you can do so in advance) and complete the few items that pertain to you. It is a simple method for back-and-forth communication between your providers that you can actually encourage and monitor. (See "My Recovery Plan Communicator" worksheet.) Fill in the parts that you can: name, date, and which of the symptoms or side effects that are occurring that day or in the previous three days. Show them the "My Recovery Plan Communicator" worksheet. This is an extremely useful and practical system. It helps you to remember what you need to share at each visit as well as prompts the questions you may have. Ask them for the information you do *not* have, and fill it in to carry to the next provider.

ADJUSTING TO MY NEW SELF

A smart man in his 30s described his adjustment after cancer as learning about "the 'new normal.'" Saying such things as "my life has changed forever" or "I'll never be the same again" means different things to different people. For some people, it may mean anything from, "I'll never take my health for granted" to "I've learned to appreciate every day and treasure it" to "I'll never be as strong, smart, or naïve in the future." Others use that term as code for accepting whatever has changed is the way it is going to be and that they have to get used to it. There are certain universal trends: Everyone worries about a *recurrence* (term used if it is a solid tumor) or *relapse* (term used for leukemia, lymphoma, or multiple myeloma). That fear is expectable. Kindly friends and family say things to deny the risk—"Stop worrying; they said everything is fine" and "Time to move on"—which seem reasonable and comforting to them but not

CONSULTATION IN A BOX: PULLED MUSCLE OR THE CANCER IS BACK

A 38-year-old woman who is a fifth-grade teacher and an aerobics instructor after school developed pain in her back three years after finishing chemotherapy for breast cancer. She felt well until the pain in her lower back got so intense she canceled her class at the gym and stayed home from school. When describing the pain in a panic, she knew that breast cancer can hide in the bones, including the spine, and she was so sure it was a recurrence in the bone and that she would be paralyzed and wheelchair bound. She pictured going to her daughter's wedding in a wheelchair being "rolled down the aisle." As an aside, she mentioned that when she was in high school, she was on the gymnastics team, and after a competition developed back pain: "...now that I am thinking about it, it felt exactly like this does. But that was years ago. They said it was a pulled muscle." Her bone scan and MRI showed no recurrence, and by the time the tests were approved by her insurance company and the results were in: she was 90 percent better. Looking back, she says, "...it must have been when I picked up a bag of groceries and the yogurt was about to splatter over the floor, so I twisted quickly holding the heavy bag to keep it from falling." Graduation scare and a rite of passage.

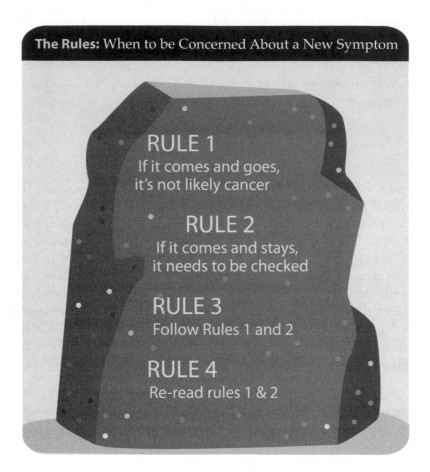

The Rules: When to be Concerned About a New Symptom

RULE 1
If it comes and goes,
it's not likely cancer

RULE 2
If it comes and stays,
it needs to be checked

RULE 3
Follow Rules 1 and 2

RULE 4
Re-read rules 1 & 2

to the individual undergoing treatment. Just as there are rituals for many life events (graduations, marriages, and hazing to join college fraternities or sororities), there is a common *graduation scare* after treatment that is likely to happen. Be prepared to identify it and muddle through. It is unpleasant and downright scary, but it is truly a rite of passage. Something happens. Perhaps it is a cough or cold that does not go away. Or it could be a muscle sprain from twisting an ankle while walking, back pain, or stomach cramps—something that could possibly be the first sign of recurrence or relapse. Naturally, many of us think the worst and get frightened and angry quickly. Revealing the feeling makes it more official, so it is often kept to oneself for a while. Especially if family and friends seem to have been losing patience with you. It is easy to picture being back in the hospital, back in chemotherapy, or getting more radiation therapy at that moment. The feeling is bad and can happen at any time. An innovative upscale supermarket in the Northeast has rules on a boulder at the store's entrance, called "Stew's Rules": Rule 1—The customer is always right. Rule 2—Follow Rule 1. Adapted for the treatment graduation rite of passage—Rule 1: If it comes and goes, it's not likely cancer. Rule 2: If it comes and stays, it needs to be checked. It may—or may not—be cancer related. As simple-minded as these rules seem, they work!

WHAT I'M THINKING ABOUT THAT I CAN'T PUT INTO WORDS EASILY

Suddenly I am expected to be a talker. I am a quiet person, and of course, I worry to myself (and it usually involves Dr. Holland's "Five Ds"—death, dependency, disability, discomfort, and dysfunction—as well as recurrence or relapse). It can sometimes precede the so-called quick feel, a small self-examination for new growth or enlarged lymph nodes. It can happen out in public, fully dressed, while driving or at work. It may not even be noticeable after perfected. Often reassuring, it can get out of hand (like being on a diet and weighing yourself a few times in a day). Sometimes I think I am not myself and am just pretending to be a healthy person Sooner or later, someone will expose me as a fraud. It's just a matter of time until that happens.

■ *I hear I will lose my hair during treatment. Can I do anything about it?*

Hair loss is one of the most obvious and public signs of cancer treatment, forcing you to advertise your situation to colleagues, acquaintances, or strangers before you are ready. There are a few things to consider.

Hair and Scalp Care Now

If your hair is starting to thin out, use a very mild shampoo like those for daily use or baby shampoo. If your hair is falling out more quickly than you can adjust to seeing it that way, a buzz cut or shaving the scalp may be the answer. If you do, keep in mind that the scalp is not used to so much exposure to light and dirt, so you need to keep it clean and use moisturizers with sunscreen (SPF 30 or higher) to keep the scalp from burning, even in the middle of the winter if you are to be outside.

If you do decide to shave your head, consider having help the first time from your barber or hair stylist. There are specially made razor handles (using standard cartridges) to make it as simple and cut proof as possible. In your community, certain hairstylists may have extra experience or sensitivity to hair loss from cancer treatment. To accommodate your special needs, they even may be able to have a wig ready overnight and know how to complete the receipt so your insurance carrier can process it for reimbursement. Do not be surprised if your scalp even hurts, as some patients have described.

The anticipation of hair loss is at times down-played, but is frought with emotion. Acknowledge it and own it, whether you cover it up with a wig or shave completely. Depending on the season and where you live, hats, caps or head coverings may be a more comfortable alternative. Having at least one ready for the day your hair starts to thin is good preparation for you and those who you meet.

Skin and Nails: The Rules Are the Same

Virtually every chemotherapy and just about all of the medications you are taking can make the skin more sensitive to the sun, so a little sun can make you very red. You will want to avoid any blistering, which can easily get infected. Clean, moisturize and use

---

CARE FOR HAIR, SKIN, AND NAILS DURING CANCER TREATMENT

Skin:

Keep clean and moisturized.

Many good products; everyone has favorites; match to climate (hot climates need *thinner* products).

Products should include sunscreen for UV (ultraviolet light rays A and B).

Try to minimize scented products.

Hair:

Keep clean and moisturized; decision when to cut hair is hard. Once cut, keep scalp clean and moisturized.

Shaved scalps need special attention; sunscreen for ultraviolet A and B is vital.

Nails:

Use gentle nail brush to clean (important as bacteria and yeast infections can hide here).

Keep nails short.

Avoid store manicures and pedicures.

Cuticles should be pushed back with soft wood (often orange wood) blunt tool, *not cut.*

---

sunscreen on exposed skin. If you are prone to acne, it can happen on your newly hairless skin, and surprisingly re-appear if you are treated with hormone blockers. Don't be surprised if body hair and even eyebrows and eyelashes thin out. Nails may get very dry and crusty from chemotherapy as well. Adriamycin can actually leave a tell-tale ring from each cycle (like a tree trunk ages). Nails can easily pick up fungal infections, so cleanliness is the rule, with short nails. Avoid any nail work done in a commercial salon to avoid infection or unnecessary cuts and bleeding.

■ *What are the* mouth sores *they mentioned to me?*

Mouth sores are small bumps throughout the mouth that occur with chemotherapy or radiation therapy to the mouth. The inside lining of the mouth is one of those tissues that reproduces itself quickly, and like hair and nails, it is affected by chemotherapy. Small bumps (stomatitis; *stoma* = Greek word for "opening"), those that produce mucous (mucositis) or candida yeast (thrush), can be controlled a good deal of the time. Every oncologist's office has its own version of *magic mouthwash.* The origin of this exotic name is unknown. An antihistamine (diphenhydramine or Benadryl®) and a topical (surface) anesthetic (lidocaine) are dissolved in a variety of different liquids (thin saline—saltwater, Kaopectate® [medical grade clay used to combat diarrhea], liquid Maalox [for indigestion], sucralfate [Carafate®]). Some formulations offer even more "magic" with some erythromycin (antibiotic) or cortisone blended in. The magic mouthwash can be used preventively or as a treatment for the mouth sores. Sometimes you'll be asked to swish it through the mouth, gargle, and spit or swish, gargle, and swallow. It should be soothing.

The ingredients can also be used separately. Lidocaine comes in a more concentrated gel to place right on top of a mouth sore that is painful in a very small spot. Sucralfate is an ulcer medicine that coats over an ulcer in the stomach to allow food to pass over it and not inflame the tissues. Sometimes referred to as *human Teflon,* referring to its nonstick properties, it does not have many interactions with other medicines or foods. Sometimes it is recommended as a preventive as well. Biotin, a natural supplement, may be helpful as a toothpaste or mouthwash.

For the white spots, or if there are pieces of white in the mucus that look like cottage cheese curds, nystatin (Mycostatin®) in liquid or in lozenges (Mycelex®) can be used. Oral antifungal medications (fluconazole, or Diflucan®) can be used preventively as before a course of antibiotics or daily, depending on your situation. Fluconazole has many interactions with other medications and some foods, so its use needs to be tracked, and liver functions should be monitored if used over a long period of time. Intravenous forms are often used in bone marrow transplantation. As nasty as this all sounds, mucositis, stomatitis, or thrush are not permanent.

9 Disclosure

■ *Who do I tell and when?*

This varies by circumstances, age, support network, and myriad other variables. It also may be different at home or work and at your place of worship. Disclosing information about having cancer is one of those double-edge swords. It may be helpful, or it may change the way others see you forever. On one hand, you do not want to be treated like you need extra help. Some people do not want to be the person who gets a seat on the bus when a twentysomething with too many earrings recognizes that you are ill and gives up his/her seat. Some people do not want to be visibly sick. On the other hand, some people are tired beyond description and would want the twentysomething to stand for a while so they can slump into the seat. Once there are visible signs of treatment—hair loss, looking pale, weight loss, and so forth—it's less of a choice. Someone will figure it out and then may ask the twentysomething to stand.

CONSULTATION IN A BOX: CANCER CENTRAL

A smart patient once said during a long day of chemotherapy that he felt like printing up calling cards with his new title, Cancer Central. "Suddenly everyone is telling me about their cancer, their daughter's camp counselor's leukemia, anyone's cancer. Like I am a magnet. It took me a long time to figure it out. At first, I thought they were trying to be supportive and share war stories. Or just let me know that they have been there themselves or for someone they loved. But it grew and grew. It is obviously something more. It almost seems magical. Tell me about your cancer, ask me how I am but don't really listen to the answer, and you get extra credit. Build up enough extra credits, and you don't get cancer; you get an exemption. Or it doesn't come back."

■ *Kid talk: How do I explain my cancer to my kids?*

"I know my kids better than anyone else, yet I can't help but cry even thinking about telling them. But I know they will figure it out." Kids sense things like that. There is some help out there. A classic booklet from the National Cancer Institute, *How to Talk to Your Kids about Cancer,* suggests words to use and what to say. Match their age, abilities, and temperament to the message. Young children think that they're personally responsible. Older kids are so self-involved with growing up that the cancer may be incidental—not to be taken personally (though hard to do). Notify the school in case there is a change in your child's habits, such as skipping school or stopping homework. The teacher and guidance counselor can step in. There may be other parents with cancer. Or staff. When specialized help is necessary, the Cancer-*Care* for Kids Program is an extremely useful resource (1-800-813-HOPE or 1-800-813-4673).

SANDWICH GENERATION: PARENTS NEED TO KNOW

Often, those in the sandwich generation are caring for parents and children simultaneously.

When diagnosed with cancer, these adult caregiver children (long distance or local) are fearful of *burdening* older parents, who themselves may be sick. They may be afraid that their parents will have a sudden heart attack and die on hearing the news or will be too upset to continue in their daily lives. Many older seniors struggle each day with reminders of mortality—they are already thinking about their own mortality but are loathe to admit it. Adult parents can benefit from the "heads up" so they can prepare themselves, or may even be of help to you on the home front or remotely. Their friends can only be their support network if they are informed.

CONSULTATION IN A BOX: MUTUAL SILENCE THAT'S DEAFENING

A woman in her 40s who is a rather successful lawyer developed early stage breast cancer that is expected more often than not to respond to treatment. She feared telling her mother, a woman in her 70s living in a well-known retirement community in Florida: "She'll just die if she hears the news." In reality, Mom had to break her tennis date and weekly dance class to pick this daughter up at the airport who "just had to visit" this weekend. She was flying from New York on a full-price ticket, so something "must have gone wrong." "I told Mom," the attorney sheepishly admitted, "who confided that she also had a small breast cancer. She had a lumpectomy and had six weeks of radiation. I thought she was going daily to the Film Festival." They laughed and then cried together, and during the night, the ambulances screeched through the Florida community, four or five times. In this senior community, everybody talks about their doctors' appointments and who has the best preparation for their colonoscopy. People are sensitized to being sick and needing care. They deal with the fright by bonding and sarcasm.

CANCER AND THE WORKPLACE

At work, the situation is somewhat different. Despite federal laws regarding nondiscrimination against people with illness or disabilities, and large corporations with similar policies, maintaining a job during a period of illness is a challenge for everyone. Patients repeatedly describe allegations of cancer-related discrimination. Sometimes referred to as the "cancer ceiling." It may be subtle, such as getting passed over for a promotion, being underemployed based upon skills and experience, or having co-workers tell you how much of your work they are taking on as you are being excluded from the daily work processes. Or maybe worse, no one expects you to do anything. The attitude is, "Just show up and don't get sick here." Your colleagues are afraid you will contaminate everyone. Some patients even find that their job has been eliminated. From the employer's side, it is difficult to keep a position open when it is unlikely the person will return to work, yet it is the law to have a similar position available at that time. And it is especially hard in small businesses on a tight budget. The Family Medical Leave Act not only covers time off to care for a family member but also time for a worker's own care. The Americans with Disabilities Act has provisions for "reasonable accommodation" while at work. For more information, refer to http://www.ada.gov.

A PLACE TO EXERCISE YOUR INFLUENCE

So much of cancer treatment is out of your control. This is one place where you can make personal choices and exert some control. The question *to tell* or *not to tell* also becomes *when to tell*. Not everyone needs to find out in one day. Ask for some friendly discretion so that you are the one to tell, if you choose, and not have a thrid party trump the discussion.

With blood relatives involved, keep in mind that many cancers have a heritable pattern. Passing the information on to them may mean earlier screening and detection, or a vigilance program to keep them cancer-free. It's your choice and a place to think more globally.

10 Why Is My Team So *Un*complimentary about Complementary Care?

■ *Just misunderstood: What is complementary care?*

In the medical subspecialties, oncology is the most advanced in providing evidence-based treatments. Not because oncologists are smarter or more inquisitive. Chemotherapy was just growing into its toddler stages after World War II, and initial treatments were toxic without the benefits of modern anti-emetics or pain medications, acceptance of using therapies that make someone so sick to get better needed proof. Thus the need grew for what we now call "the multicenter clinical trial." The multicenter clinical trial was born. Such a system sets a high standard of proof for effectiveness of any treatment. The public is right to have high expectations of treatments for life-threatening conditions such as cancer.

But the public, as well as the professional community, is frustrated by the modest gains in the treatment of some cancers and the lack of speed with which those gains were made. With the rising consumerism in American society and the availability of over-the-counter supplements that don't need any level of evidence of effectiveness aside from personal claim, a perfect storm for misunderstanding arose. Combine that with a medium like the Internet where claims are uncensored, and we have a setup for an adversarial clash. Many supplements are empowering. However, many are advertised with fake claims to cure such chronic conditions as arthritis, heart disease, and osteoporosis. Some infomercials extol the virtues of cleansing enemas and oral preparations. They sound great. Most of the infomercials have a hint of the underdog. Often these ads also inform people that *they,* meaning the medical community, won't want you to know about it. You can endorse it too and join the regular folks by buying this product. No physician visit. No prescription. No insurance forms to complete—no insurance will cover it at all. That sounds harsh but is an unfortunate reality. There is a growing field of legitimate complementary medicine practitioners and science. So far, there is solid but limited use in cancer. More needs to be done and is being done. With public advocacy, the Office of Complementary and Alternative Medicine has been embedded in the National Cancer Institute. Clinical trials are underway.

Deciding how effective complementary therapies are depends upon how they are defined. In cancer, if traditional care includes the three usual modalities (surgery, chemotherapy, and radiation therapy), what else comprises *complementary*? What about support groups, prayer, exercise, yoga, acupuncture, tai chi, Reiki? Everyone draws the line differently. So if people with cancer pray, are they utilizing complementary therapies? Or do they just go to religious services because they do anyway?

In the mid-1980s, health food stores stocked displays piled with bottles of shark's cartilage. The advertising was persuasive: "Sharks don't get cancer." Rather convincing.

No prescription necessary. No regulation. Where did the lab making the product get so much shark cartilage so quickly? What happened to the rest of the shark when the cartilage was harvested? Many unanswered questions. It was implied that shark cartilage contained something that curtailed the blood supply to the tumor. Such a theory was held by a minority of progressive investigators who did not get recognition. One modern chemotherapy, Avastin® (or bevacizumab), works in the same way. The idea was 20 years ahead of its time and legitimized by Judah Folkman.

■ *So what about faith healing? Prayer circles? Aren't they complementary too?*

Chaplain or pastoral care counselors' services are quite different from anything like faith healing. It is good to believe, and one can make a case for wanting to believe so devoutly that anything is possible. William Nolen, a prominent cancer surgeon in the 1970s visited many faith healers and chronicled his findings in a book, *Healing: A Doctor in Search of a Miracle.* He concluded that many were sham artists palming some chicken fat before "laying hands" to remove a tumor and other diversionary practices that were unethical. However, the support of a community, especially your community, is a key factor in a better quality of recovery. Knowing that everyone is thinking about your situation, praying for a good outcome, and bolstering your piece of mind is productive. Is that social networking or a prayer circle? Or is a prayer circle the oldest form of social networking?

■ *Aren't vitamins complementary treatments?*

Should the advice be different during radiation therapy or chemotherapy than afterward? Perhaps. It is believed that the same properties of super-high doses of antioxidant vitamins that may be protective against developing cancer in the first place and could help heal or minimize side effects also block the effectiveness of chemotherapy or radiation therapy. So much is not yet known about this phenomenon. The additional factor of timing becomes ever so more important. We are all so eager to finish the process and get better. Timing is important.

■ *The term* "natural" *also creates doubt in many minds. Does* natural *mean* "safe"?

Does *natural* imply "effective" or "gentle"? Heavy metals such as platinum and arsenic are poisonous yet are used in purified forms as approved chemotherapies. They are *natural.*

One common supplement with weak antidepressant properties, St. John's Wort, has a known and detrimental interaction with the taxanes, such as docetaxel (Taxotere®) or paclitaxel (Taxol®). Obviously, this supplement is to be avoided if you are receiving such treatments. This underscores the need to tell your providers about everything you are taking.

■ *Why is alternative medicine out of the mainstream?*

Alternative therapies are usually recommended *in place* of traditional therapies, not alongside them. That's *instead of.* Where most people would be uncomfortable without a prayer or two at some point in their treatment, if asked to give up treatment and pray, prayer takes on a new dimension. Other alternative treatments include enemas or detoxification regimens with the idea that cancer is due to an overabundance of toxic substances in the environment that get into us. Often the attraction is self-determination, self-empowerment, eschewing dependence on a a licensed provider. Some alternative treatments are generally outside of anyone's comfort zone, so far outside that it makes people uncomfortable. At times, something that is available in other countries has more merit than what is available in the United States. This may be a drug not yet brought to U.S. clinical trials or deemed too risky. It could mean that just the order or the way a treatment is given is changed or augmented by another modality of care, such as cooling or heating the body, or using microwave treatment. Sometimes these treatments even sound exotic. Be wary of those who believe they have the answer, particularly if no one else understands them or acknowledges them.

CONSULTATION IN A BOX: THE FIRST TRIALS OF ALTERNATIVE AGENTS

The National Cancer Institute (NCI) conducted two trials before its Office of Complementary and Alternative Medicine brought testing mainstream. One was laetrile, tested in 1982. Laetrile was made of an extract of apricot pits, and that idea sounded elegant. That a simple substance that has been discarded all along could cure a life-threatening illness is what legend is made from. However, it was found ineffective in a trial including patients with breast, colon, and lung cancer.

A second substance, hydrazine sulfate, was brought to NCI trial in the late 1980s. Hydrazine also had a simple and attractive source as a by-product of rocket fuel for a generation that was raised on Sputnik and the NASA Space Program, and oil shortages. Hydrazine was thought to be a chemotherapy substance to discourage cancer cell growth and was purported to promote weight gain with cancer-induced weight loss. Hydrazine was tested in three trials in lung and colon cancer and found ineffective to increase survival time. It was actually associated with a worsened quality of life as it had caused *peripheral neuropathy* adding to that caused by the standard chemotherapy drugs. It did not help stabilize weight when tested in a placebo-controlled double-blind trial. Each participant got the "study drug." No one knew which they had until after the study. The assignments were random. Even investigators who enrolled their own patients did not know what those patients got. One challenge to the study was that it was flawed by interactions between hydrazine and anti-nausea medicines, which was later found not to have affected the results. There was a great deal of post-study media attention, including by a tabloid magazine whose publisher's wife claimed it saved her life after being diagnosed by lymphoma and boldly refusing chemotherapy. However, she died "from an unrelated cause" months later.

Some treatments straddle between complementary and alternative: snake venom serum injections or vaccines made personally for one's own cancer. There are many.

There is political misunderstanding on all fronts. Everyone has the same goal—to cure or best treat cancer. The desire to improve the human condition is universal. The areas where groups begin to disagree are over some less fundamental points. They involve who will profit from the treatment and who bestows credibility on whom. A second element of power—the power to harness one of the major human illnesses—is attractive to those who value influence and being in the public eye. These secondary issues bring a humanistic mission to the point of being divisive and mistrusting.

The same consumerism that is part of the fabric of modern Western medicine needs to be used in the world of alternative therapies. Questioning the merits in a systematic way is key for any medical therapy.

One way to tighten the decision making is to use a strategy that is used every day in traditional medicine to see if even effective treatments should be used for a certain person in specific circumstances. Affectionately called a *BECA decision* (mnemonics got so many through college and medical school), it should be used in discussion with family and friends and then your providers. Here's what needs to be asked. Writing out the information on a pad can help the process.

B, Benefit: What is the potential benefit from either taking the treatment (or not taking it)?

E, Effectiveness: Is the proposed treatment effective? How effective? Who tested it? Is the way sensible?

C, Consent: Is it fully and really OK with the individual receiving the treatment? Is the person agreeing really and truly informed about the advantages and disadvantages of taking or not taking the treatment?

A, Appropriateness: Overall, does it seem the right thing to do? Take a step back and look at the whole situation from a few steps away. Would the average person approached in the street and given the details in a fair and balanced way say, "Sure" or "No way"?

CONSULTATION IN A BOX: HELP FROM *BECA*

Aunt Betsy is 64 years old and continues to work as an assistant in a busy law office. Six months ago, she found out that she had breast cancer, and it needed treatment. After her initial shock, and going through all of the testing, it was found to be small and in one place on the breast only. She was offered an up-to-date treatment of a lumpectomy followed by radiation therapy and hormone blockers since she had no lymph nodes involved and the hormone receptors (on the cell) were *estrogen receptor positive* and *progesterone receptor positive* (estrogen and progesterone, the most important female hormones; estrogen may encourage cancer to grow). She weathered the surgery as well as one could, with some pain at the scar site that went

continued

CONSULTATION IN A BOX: HELP FROM *BECA*

continued

away, and was frightened. After a few weeks, she began her radiation treatments, going to the center each day, being absolutely careful to apply the necessary ointments to keep the area moisturized and clean as it was getting inflamed, the expected *skin reaction* with this type of radiation. She made friends with the other patients who all came at the same time every day and was able to get her appointment in the middle of the day when someone else finished their treatments, so she could come on her lunch hour. She wore a soft sports bra for the first time in her life, and as her fears subsided and confidence that she would survive grew, she started to go for a quick lunch with two other women who had appointment times close to hers. They even called themselves, from the Broadway musical song, "The Ladies Who Lunch—Quickly" so they could get back to an afternoon's work. Even a brief lunch allowed them to share their stories. Two of the three joked about "cancer being the fountain of youth," and that really insulted the third woman. "I can't believe it, but I am going through the 'changes' again like I did when I was 48," Aunt Betsy said. Two of them got hot then cold, started to sweat, and asked to have the air-conditioning up and down in sequence within minutes. The waitress and the owner of the coffee shop joked with them, and they made the best of it.

At their weekly appointment with the radiation oncologist and advance practice nurse, the two described what was happening to them. It was common, but not universal, for women to get all of the signs and symptoms of natural menopause again, for unknown reasons, during breast cancer treatment. It is believed that both the radiation treatment, and then the hormone blockers somehow suppress the amounts of estrogen and progesterone already reduced by age, and the symptoms appear. Some patients have none; others mild or even severe effects with so many hot flashes each day they are too numerous to count. The advance practice nurse and radiation oncologist offered a variety of interventions. First, they confirmed that this was a common thing, as it would have been natural to incorrectly assume that it was somehow a sign that the cancer was growing back. Since it was happening during treatment, the women feared it was growing back quickly and fiercely. Not so. Not only have other women experienced the same thing, there are even proven treatments that do not involve estrogen or hormone supplements. Although there was not one single medication for this purpose, some medications were found to be effective, by chance, and were tested in clinical trials with good safety and good results. A majority, but not everyone, benefited with little to no side effects. When Aunt Betsy heard that the two categories of medications were used to treat depression or seizures and used for an off-label reason (not on the

continued

CONSULTATION IN A BOX: HELP FROM *BECA*

continued

official use list from the FDA published online or in the package insert), she recoiled, fearing that her pharmacist, whose daughter dates her grandson, would think that the family lines are "cursed" not only with cancer but depression and seizures. Hearing that reaction, the radiation oncologist and nurse suggested acupuncture. Aunt Betsy became dismissive again and then had a big hot flash sitting in the office. She relented. "Do you have some information that I can read about it? I remember that publisher [James Reston of the *New York Times*] had his appendix removed with acupuncture and no anesthesia," she said. And Cousin John had a bad back and got acupuncture for his back. She took the material, wiped her brow, took off her thick sweater, and went back to work.

At home, she searched online and found that acupuncture as a *complementary* treatment is widely accepted by even the American Cancer Society (ACS) and supported by a number of well-done studies. She learned that acupuncture was not approved *in place of* chemotherapy, radiation therapy, or surgery as an *alternative,* and thought it through over the next few days. Intuitively and through much discussion, she made a *BECA decision.* Aunt Betsy walked through her BECA Decision:

Benefit: About six visits; could be done after her radiation at the cancer center. Miss lunch; a maybe half-hour more of work on those days. "Some one will stick me with needles when I am awake! Will they be clean? Will I get an infection (bacteria, hepatitis, HIV)? Will the hole bleed when the needle is removed?" Burden of not doing acupuncture may be continued hot flashes or worsening ones with hormonal treatments. Cost: offered at no charge by the cancer center for just this purpose. Fear manageable; suspicion high.

Effectiveness: Supported by many clinical trials and even the conservative-thinking ACS. More than half of the people who used it get some relief.

Consent: Much reading and discussion. Informed and careful.

Appropriateness: Yes, by consensus from family, providers, and "Ladies Who Lunch—Quickly." They helped Aunt Betsy fine tune what she knew already. She's not a risk taker, and this was a low-risk procedure with a good chance of helping and virtually nonexistent long-term side effects.

BECA decision made. Aunt Betsy had a series of six acupuncture treatments, reducing her hot flashes to about once a week without taking notice. The importance of having information, knowing yourself, and thinking it through often needs someone to trade ideas and listen to your reasoning. Balancing out your fears can help you arrive at a conclusion. Part of the

continued

CONSULTATION IN A BOX: HELP FROM *BECA*

continued

advantage of approved, mainstream treatments rather than some complementary and alternative treatments is that someone—or many people—has walked through the process already, with the only part missing being the personal values. Take-charge folks who want to be in control find it irritating when bureaucracy is in charge instead of being able to make these decisions for themselves. For those who value being in charge, since the decisions about standard treatment are not in their jurisdiction, the complementary and alternative routes become more attractive even with questionable proof of effectiveness.

11 Just Finishing Treatment (and Feeling Lousy)

MY SLOWED DOWN CLOCK: DELAYED GOOD EFFECTS AND SIDE EFFECTS

How long will I feel the effects of chemotherapy? Generally, the effects of chemotherapy last from a few weeks to a few months. That's a large variation in time, and it is affected by many factors, including whether each chemotherapy drug is given by itself or in combination with others, slowing down its digestion by the liver and kidneys. It circulates many times all throughout the body to the original tumor or where cancer may be hiding. Most of the original compounds and intermediate digestive products leave the body through the stool and urine, with perhaps a bit leaving through the skin and through exhaled air. Some patients have noticed odd smells within the first few days after chemotherapy. It is possible that either a by-product is leaving through the skin or lungs, or the smell sensors in the nose and back of the throat are affected, transforming a normal smell into an odd one.

Most of the time, the period when treatment is finishing is a mixed bag. On one hand, there's the relief of the burdens of following a pretreatment anti-nausea regimen, traveling to the cancer center or oncologist's office, sitting during the infusion, and traveling home. Due to the effects of the anti-nausea medicines wearing off, some of that day and the following day can be a blur. Most people report fatigue, except if they've taken corticosteroids (dexamethasone or prednisone). Surprisingly, after the steroids, the first day or two can actually be a time of feeling energetic without nausea. That state is almost always temporary, and within a few days, the fatigue sets in again.

Virtually everyone tries to eat, following the recommendations for maintaining weight, and well-meaning family members and friends generally begin a campaign to feed. This is a great idea, but the timing may be off. Few people want to eat significant amounts of food during this time.

A puzzling period generally begins at this time. On one hand, you're relieved that this phase of treatment is over. On the other hand, there was a certain security in knowing that you were doing something very active against the cancer. Although the effects of treatment linger long after this period, it seems now as if it's "just me against the cancer," which is a lonely time, no matter who is around and what they do. The comfort of contact with the oncology team, particularly the nurses, social workers, and pastoral care staff, provides a path for questions to be answered and reassurance to be received. Otherwise, that direct access seems gone. Even the most independent individuals feel vulnerable during this period, and it is hard to avoid.

Once the anti-nausea medicine haze wears off, the predictable wondering sets in. Did it work? Are you done? Will you have to do this again? It's a common impulse to try to rush into imaging, CT scans, PET/CT scans, or anything to show that the cancer is gone. Here is one of those moments where what we see in fictional stories on television or in the movies may lead to a fictional conclusion. We've all seen these dramas and movies. In some very intense moments, the doctor throws up some X-ray films onto an old-style wall-mounted viewer box and says in amazement, "Well...it's gone. It's like the cancer was never there. You're cured!" Great drama, but not realistic.

It is disheartening to find out that scans are often scheduled a few weeks after treatment. Another one of those situations where explanation is an oversimplification. If the scans are taken too soon, is it that the cancer really responded and has stopped growing, or is the growth only temporarily suppressed, so the lesions are smaller? The gap between ending treatment and getting scanned is generally a few weeks so that what is seen is the most realistic representation of the amount of cancer left.

In real life, no growth is great, and smaller is superb. This is an easily misunderstood point. Active cancer grows. What is left may be scarring of the tissues, not new growth. Depending on the part of the body involved, that scarring may be just trivial or something that needs later attention. Scarred tissues can't function properly, but some neighboring tissues can compensate for those functions in many circumstances. The code words for no growth are *stable disease.* That is good news.

In leukemia, the parallel situation uses different words. After a strong chemotherapy regimen or a bone marrow transplant, the new cells in the bone marrow take a few weeks to grow back. An *empty* or *no cells* report of a bone marrow aspiration and biopsy signifies that new cells have not yet grown back. It is good in that all of the leukemia cells need to be killed off, but that does not tell you what happens next. Once the cells come back, testing the marrow samples by the pathologist and by looking at the DNA patterns can more definitively tell what is growing back, be it new healthy cells or resistant leukemia cells of the same family or a new cell line.

CONSULTATION IN A BOX: AN UNEXPECTED HEADACHE

MJ, a 22-year-old woman, had been living her dream in the "big city," having just graduated from a top university with a degree in business. She had worked hard in school to earn an A average and won acceptance to her first-choice school, leaving the Midwest. Her goal was to work in the nonprofit world for foundations that help underserved Americans in the South and Appalachia. Two weeks before graduation, she developed pain in her throat that did not go away. The university health service referred her to their medical school's department of otolaryngology, where an enlarged tonsil was found at the site of the pain. Scared and angry, she quickly progressed through a fine needle aspiration biopsy, many sets of CT scans and a PET scan. Her health, apart from a back injury from gymnastics at 14 years old, was fine. She did not smoke at all and drank alcohol rarely, perhaps once a month, despite the heavy drinking among her classmates. She was dating and sexually active with a guy who was heading to his MBA, and the world was as perfect as it could be until the throat pain.

continued

CONSULTATION IN A BOX: AN UNEXPECTED HEADACHE

continued

The biopsy did show cancer in the tonsil, and she spent the following six months in radiation therapy, chemotherapy, and surgery. Although she had significant pain in her throat throughout the treatment for about six weeks, she was in good physical condition, and when given information about My Recovery Plan using the LEARN System, she adopted the idea, as it was not much of a departure from how she had been living. She identified goals each week, and tracked her activity, rest, and weight, accepting interventions for each. As she approached months seven and eight, she started to feel less tired. Her weight had stabilized with a feeding tube and under the guidance of the nutritionist at her cancer center, she reintroduced foods, one by one, to strengthen her swallowing and get most of the calories through eating instead of the tube. Her parents were commuting from their home to each be with her a few weeks at a time.

A dull headache right at her hairline on the left side above her eyebrow grew more constant and then intense, and a scan showed a single spot that had not been there on the previous set of scans. She met a neurosurgeon and was extremely frightened of brain surgery, not knowing how much of her dreams would be sidelined by the cancer and its treatment. Since all of the rest of the imaging studies showed a complete response to treatment, the neurosurgeon and radiation oncologist together thought that an alternative to the surgery could be knifeless surgery, properly known as *stereotactic radiosurgery.* This is not traditional scalpel surgery at all, but a computer-guided pinpoint high-intensity radiation treatment that causes less damage than regular surgery and is done in a long one-day office visit. Her parents and boyfriend insisted she get an additional opinion, and they all traveled to another large city to meet with brain tumor experts who indeed confirmed that the stereotactic radiosurgery was one of the best options for her. The 12-hour treatment day was long, with hours of preparation by the technical staff. The procedure went well, and the steroids made her feel a bit hyper, hungry, and sleepless. What concerned her most was the difficulty she had doing two or three things at once, again sending a wave of fright through her family. As the weeks went by, she continued to heal and with quick referral to the occupational therapist was able to become more mindful of the steps for each task. She began to rebuild her skills to layer one task on another—listening to television, then adding in reading the newspaper and making her favorite iced green tea all at the same time. Indeed, with healing and some specialized intervention, her brain's neighboring tissues readopted the functions of the scarred tissue in her left fontal lobe.

One year later, her feeding tube is out, her weight is stable, and her fears have diminished with each passing scan and exam. When looking back on

continued

CONSULTATION IN A BOX: AN UNEXPECTED HEADACHE

continued

the whole situation, she admitted that as scared as she was not to eat or swallow or even talk well, the brain lesion was the most frightening. "My thoughts are my essence," she said on a follow-up visit, "and I prayed not to lose it. The occupational therapist was clear with me, explaining that I did not learn how to do anything overnight, and I needed to work, slowly and methodically in steps to regain those skills. I started to read online about people with brain injures after car accidents and how they would learn to do what they used to do beforehand. I went through the same process, and I am grateful."

Different types of cancers come with different challenges in the process of healing and recovery. The day-to-day details vary, but the principles remain the same: learn what you can about your cancer and how other people have moved through it in the past, keep up with nutrition and energy maintenance through activity and rest, and access services as early as possible to reactivate functions interrupted by treatment.

CONSULTATION IN A BOX: CANCER-FREE?

RP is a 62-year-old physician with a specialty in pathology for more than 40 years. He developed back pain that he thought was attributable to years of sitting and reading slides in a microscope and then on a large computer monitor. "My zest for exercise dwindled as I got older, and I should have paid more attention to my posture and gotten a better desk chair, but I didn't. I ignored the back pain until my annual visit to the primary care doctor, who became concerned when I explained that the pain did not go away on the weekend or on vacation, away from sitting so much. She ordered an MRI of the spine, and to our surprise, there were arthritic changes. But the blood and urine tests she did showed high protein levels, and with more testing, it was discovered that I had early (with the overly descriptive name *smoldering*) multiple myeloma." Multiple myeloma is a cancer of the white blood cells, but is not leukemia, and affects the bones and kidneys. After a second consultation at a cancer center with so much experience treating myeloma it was considered a myeloma *center of excellence,* he began chemotherapy at the cancer center at the hospital where he worked. He both liked and hated the staff recognition, sometimes welcoming the knowing smile from faces he had seen in the parking lot for years, and at other times wishing he could be invisible in the waiting room so he did not have to be social with other patients. His chemotherapy

continued

CONSULTATION IN A BOX: CANCER-FREE?

continued

was intense, and he developed yeast infections that soured his mouth and deterred him from eating. But he plowed through, sometimes with less enthusiasm than others. He felt lucky enough to have enough sick leave and some short-term disability that paid most of the family's bills, except for the promised contribution to his granddaughter's college tuition. He was eager to know how the chemotherapy was working and even looked forward to the next bone marrow biopsy, however painful it would be, to verify if the treatment was indeed effective.

The marrow test was done and read by a colleague who flashed it up on the big screen so he could see it. The marrow was read as *empty.* He thought to himself that such a finding was neither good nor bad. The myeloma white cells had disappeared as a result of the chemotherapy, but the next generation had not yet appeared. Without his specialist-level familiarity as a pathologist, he may have gotten part of the message, that the myeloma plasma cells were gone, giving a false sense of security. His providers were clear in their reporting of the results, and clarified that "empty is good" and is the first step in the body replacing the white blood plasma cells with new, normal ones.

The rest of the blood and urine tests improved. He became less anemic, and there was a reduced level of protein in the urine as the weeks went by. He started to feel better and personally learned what he had known since medical school about interpreting interim results and applying them to the long term. On the subsequent bone marrow biopsy, his results were good, and through the usual steps in the LEARN System, he returned to work nine weeks later. His concern over relapse continues while he is on maintenance oral chemotherapy.

These first few weeks are obviously a hard time in the process of healing after cancer. The fatigue and fear remain, sometimes at the same level or even more so than in the midst of treatment. The fear that the cancer can return is strong, but feeling ill prevents anyone from balancing the facts with the fears. Having "My Recovery Plan" to fall back on really counts now. Due to the degree of fatigue, level of fear, and feeling battle worn, this is *not the best time* to adopt the principles of the LEARN System without having participated all along. Earlier involvement in better rest, more activity and improved nutrition could have minimized how poorly Dr. P felt at this point. Can it be done? Yes, of course. Absolutely. Is it optimal? No.

■ *Common states of being: Why do I feel so lousy?*

You feel so lousy because cancer is a *hypermetabolic state;* it puts the body into overdrive. That uses up lots of energy and food to sustain the cancer, which leads to a downward spiral that makes you more tired and in pain, so you eat less, making you more tired, so you eat less. One goal of "My Recovery Plan" is to reverse this cycle as much as possible. Because the factors are so intertwined, interrupting the downward spiral takes a multilevel approach with the LEARN System.

■ *I worry that my memory is going: Is that chemobrain?*

The issue of *chemobrain* is a complicated and interesting one. In 1997, breast cancer patients, the best-organized self-advocates at the time, started reporting that they were having memory trouble, half-joking at first, but a serious concern. Some patients related it to the aging process or to having cancer itself. Some were struggling with older relatives' cognitive loss with aging, and others even a degenerative dementia like Alzheimer's disease. Their concern was meaningful and was not an issue at the forefront when survival itself was the main goal. With the advances in breast cancer treatment, long-term survivorship increased. What seemed to be a minor intrusion into daily life loomed more prominently as the recovery continued. Other changes in the nervous system, such as neuropathy—the feeling of pins and needles or lack of perception, numbness in fingers or toes, or permanent sensory changes in hearing or taste—also accompanied the cognitive impairment.

Networking with fellow patients spread the word and even gave it a name—*chemobrain*—which was described by a bright professional woman who noticed she had to work harder at being a teacher and especially while studying for her master's degree. Allen Levine, a seasoned oncology social worker and then supervisor at Cancer*Care,* reported that patients in support groups and counseling sessions had been concerned and curious about this yet-to-be-acknowledged entity. Allen had also connected and introduced me to Dr. Claire Warga, a neuropsychologist at nearby New York University who had published *Menopause and the Mind.* Warga had encountered women who had no cancer in their 40s who had cognitive lapses and were worried they too were developing Alzheimer's dementia as well. Some women had recently been pregnant, but most, it turned out, experienced cognitive problems as the first insidious sign of the menopause to come, perimenopause. The cognitive changes sounded exactly like what we were hearing in the cancer treatment world. But Dr. Warga's patient group had no cancers and no chemotherapy. Amazingly parallel processes!

Right from the start, curious clinicians and patients had many questions. How much of a concern is chemobrain? Is it transient or enduring? What is the cause? How can we fix it? Compensate for it? Prevent it? Around that time, I was preparing a book chapter for the second edition of Dr. Jimmie Holland's book, *Psycho-Oncology,* on the central nervous system's effects of cancer treatment, providing me the opportunity for literature review and critical thinking. It became clear that brain effects of lifesaving chemotherapy were often not recorded or minimized. Reports from the medical literature or even the FDA did require package inserts that listed serious side effects (seizure, coma, death) but not the more subtle ones that may have shed some intellectual light on chemobrain. Subtle effects in long-term survivorship are of secondary importance until life can be extended by effective treatment.

A small but landmark study showed some expected but underreported effects of antinausea medicines during chemotherapy. It demonstrated the underreporting of seemingly minor symptoms as well as the need to combine medicines in support of a patient undergoing cancer treatment. Using one medicine to treat side effects in cancer treatment is an everyday procedure. Multiple medications are combined to combat nausea and vomiting. Bone marrow stimulators of red blood cells reduce the anemia that causes fatigue and the need for transfusion. Other marrow-stimulating factors increase one's resistance to infection, reducing the need for intravenous antibiotics and hospital admission. A common but off-label cancer pain management technique uses stimulant medicines to counteract the sedative effects of opioid narcotic pain medicines. Stimulants also treat attention deficit disorder and hyperactivity. Patients who took stimulant medicines in this way would kid around that they felt "sharper."

Colleagues began to refer to "chemobrain", and it was being discussed at clinical trials meetings. A group of investigators was brought together run the first known treatment trial of chemobrain. Such openness and acknowledgement encouraged patients and families to describe their experiences more candidly. Just a few years later, such information would be addressed in chat rooms and blogs online, replacing some of the conversation previously exchanged in infusion suites and radiation oncology waiting rooms.

The general trend of the lapses centered on certain tasks. Most common was the inability to remember information just heard or learned, such as hearing a telephone number and then not being able to recall it when phoning or forgetting someone's name after being introduced for the first time. Information learned long before was surprisingly preserved. As we all become more dependent on computers, and with the risk of comparing human learning to a computer operating system, consider this: the memory or hard drive was not affected; it was more akin to the "Save As" function that did not encode the information to the hard drive. Information, it seems, is not retained as it is entering our memory banks. Another skill with which patients described difficulty was multitasking, or the ability to do more than one activity at a time.

CONSULTATION IN A BOX: JUST FORGETFUL?

A poignant story was told by a prominent attorney who explained that, before chemotherapy for ovarian cancer, after a full day of work, she could cook dinner and supervise her child's homework while listening to the news on television, all at the same time. But her ability to concentrate and coordinate multiple tasks at once had suffered. Unable to do more than one task at a time, she was angry at herself for not being able to focus the way she had done in the past. Embarrassed and frightened that the managing partners in her firm would discover such difficulties and prevent her from going to trial in court, she refused to be interviewed by the media so that the judges in her courtroom would not realize the impairments she experienced. A writer who had been treated for testicular cancer recounted how he had begun to write much more slowly. He explained

continued

CONSULTATION IN A BOX: JUST FORGETFUL?

continued

he used to get inspiration for a twist in the plot or a character in his novels when he was not at his desk, and it would "disappear" if he didn't stop to write it down lest he forget it. Sheepishly, he even admitted that he at times lost the small piece of paper he would stick in his pocket. A colleague showed him a digital dictating machine small enough to attach to his key ring, and he used it during the day or in the middle of the night to keep his thoughts safe. A preacher treated for lung cancer reluctantly confessed that it took almost double the amount of time to produce his weekly sermons, which lacked the creativity his congregations expected of him and he expected of himself. He felt guilty even admitting so, as he was happy to be alive and did not want to seem unappreciative.

Many questions have yet to be answered. Further studies are now underway to do so. Is there something about having cancer, even localized cancer that has not spread to the brain, that causes cognitive impairment? Is it possible that many of us, as we age, do have some cognitive impairment that gets magnified by the cancer or its treatment? Is the decrease in estrogen or another hormone a major factor, paralleling Claire Warga's work? If it is the chemotherapy itself, which agents are the most implicated? Is it a combination of these factors and others? Recent neuropathological evidence reveals an actual change in the brain tissue, specifically in the glial cells that support the alignment of neurons (brain cells) that may help focus investigators on the exact causes and areas of the brain affected by chemotherapy.

Until quite recently, it was accepted that cancer may affect the body in a number of ways. It can spread close to where the tumor starts to grow (local extension), travel to nearby lymph nodes, or enter the bloodstream and travel to far-off organs. More current theories identify a fourth mechanism in which the cells give off proteins when they grow, and those proteins (called cytokines) travel all over the body and effect more generalized symptoms like fatigue and weight and appetite loss. It is possible that these cytokines cross the blood-brain barrier easily and can be part of the missing link to understand the mechanism of developing chemobrain. A model for such an effect is well accepted in a syndrome called limbic encephalitis, in which the limbic system in the brain becomes inflamed, causing cognitive and emotional changes the limbic system is thought to exert control over both emotions and memory. Such a model may have relevance here.

For now, the direction you need to take if you find cognitive impairment in yourself—or a loved one—is mostly practical. You should share this information with your cancer treatment providers. It is important to rule out cancer in the brain, as scary as that may seem. Effective treatments exist for some but not all cancers, and the situation may be treatable. Tips from the traumatic brain injury specialists such as being more routinized, writing lists, color-coding things, and using sticky notes can reduce the sources of frustration for everyone. Learning new skills, at least in theory, is supposed to reinforce the retention of information. Refer your oncology providers to the literature that does exist. Perhaps a trial of a stimulant can be helpful. Through Cancer*Care*'s educational efforts, printed materials are available online or from the agency directly. Through Cancer*Care*'s teleconference series, telephone-based educational seminars are available for both providers and patient/family audiences.

We will learn more about the causes of cognitive impairment soon, asking future patient generations to invest less of their quality of life to not only to survive, but also to thrive after diagnosis of cancer and its treatment.

WHEN DO I NEED AN EMERGENCY ROOM?

Each treatment team has its own threshold for when a patient needs an emergency room, but there are some areas that are common in virtually all practices.

Fever of 100.4 or Higher

We all learn to estimate if we have a fever by touching the forehead, with (hopefully) the back of one's hand. More accurate and safer is to use an electronic thermometer. Although devices are sold to take the temperature under an armpit or on the surface of the forehead, an oral reading, much preferred to a rectal reading, seems the most popularly recommended. Oral electronic thermometers often register in just seconds, avoiding the need to sit with one's mouth closed breathing through the nose for a lengthy period of time. Be sure not to use the thermometer within a few minutes of a cold or warm/hot drink or food.

High temperatures in cancer can be a sign of infection. Such infections, at a time when the body can't fight them off, need treatment long before they would without cancer or treatment. We regularly hear that in Western medicine, antibiotics are overprescribed as a takeaway from a rushed office visit. In primary care, that is very much so, but not here. Antibiotics are optimal sooner rather than later, once blood tests confirm an infection, or if someone appears to have one, are optimal. Rarely, fever is from the cancer itself, but only with proper testing can that be verified, and if so, the remedial plan changes. Whatever the cause, having a fever for just a few hours can cause a lot of fluids to be lost by sweating and through the breath, and that can lead to dehydration.

Shortness of Breath That Comes on All of a Sudden

Blood clots can start as a pain in the leg and travel to the lungs. Called a deep vein thrombosis, it is similar to what can happen when flying on a long plane flight in a cramped coach seat. Sudden leg pain and or shortness of breath needs quick attention, and an emergency room is often the only place that can do a scan and the blood work quickly. Anticoagulants may be necessary. Rarely, when the shortness of breath comes within a short period of time after chemotherapy with nausea and vomiting, an irregular heart beat, cloudy urine, and severe lethargy and/or pain in the joints, that can be the outward signs of a tumor lysis syndrome. Tumor lysis occurs when the cancer cells break down so rapidly they overwhelm the body's ability to dispose of them. But that comes on a lot more slowly than a blood clot.

Change in Level of Awareness That Comes on Abruptly, Not Related to Any Medication That Was Just Started or Stopped

Particularly in multiple myeloma, breast, prostate, or lung cancers that can easily affect the bones, once the bones release calcium quickly, it can affect the rest of the body, especially the brain and heart. This requires fluids and intravenous medications quickly and needs monitoring in the hospital.

Trouble Suddenly Moving Legs or Arms

If it is *not* just momentary or from compression (like sleeping on that side and having the area "fall asleep" from poor circulation or pressing in on a nerve), it needs attention. If cancer presses in on the spine, it can cause these symptoms and can be corrected. This needs an emergency exam and imaging.

Mental Confusion within Three Days of Stopping a Medication Abruptly

Withdrawal can occur from a variety of medications and can be addressed easily with immediate attention. It needs a review of all medications given during treatment and afterwards at home. Be candid about alcohol use, any over-the-counter medications or "recreational" drugs. Medical marijuana can contain impurities, especially in states where its sale is not controlled.

PEOPLE TELL ME HOW WELL I LOOK, BUT I FEEL AWFUL (AND WHY THAT MAKES ME ANGRY)

Though often offered as a compliment by someone who is well meaning but does not know what to say, patients often say how hearing you look well backfires. When you're feeling so ill and someone says, "you look well", it can be taken as simply superficial.

Many believe and experience just the opposite. The American Cancer Society joined with the National Cosmetology Association and the Personal Care Products Council to sponsor a program called "Look Good, Feel Better" at sites across the country. The program conducts seminars for women, teens, and men to help counteract the effects of cancer and its treatment. The idea that if you look healthy, you are treated as a healthy person has merit for many people, who appreciate the idea that self-care is part of the process of recovery.

What I Don't Want to Hear

What is said: "How are you?" What you think: "How can I be? I have cancer."
What is said: "You'll be fine." What you think: "How do you know?"

A very insightful patient, himself a therapist, explains it this way: People don't know what to say. They say something to put themselves at ease and hopefully put you at ease, but it works in reverse. "What people really want to say is, 'You look so tired and worried,' but know that such a statement is definitely impolite or insulting. So they go with an obvious, if poorly placed, compliment. What they really may mean is, 'I am relieved this illness has not affected me.' It's like somebody saying (in a non-cancer situation), 'You've lost weight.' But what they may be thinking is, 'How heavy you looked before.'"

Who Can Help Out at Home? Who Will Pay for It?

We used to care for each other at home because there was always someone at home (tending the crops on the farm or because only the husband/father worked outside of the home while the mother worked inside). People went to the hospital when they got sick, and they stayed there until they got well or didn't. No longer happens. Most people work outside of the home. Hospital stays grow shorter and shorter, and sometimes clock in at 23 hours to avoid being considered an admission, saving insurance carriers a full day's reimbursement. Having someone home convalescing means someone needs to be at home. But who?

Insurance for home care is limited. Most medical insurance has some home care benefits. The amount that is mandatory varies state by state, and beyond that minimum, as stipulated in the details of your policy. The language is at best confusing. There are different types of benefits, whose names may not expose all of the properties of the benefit.

Home Care

The vision that comes up is one of convalescing at home, getting better day by day, building up strength and resilience with restorative sleep, food, and good company. The vision is a bit idealistic. Families, friends, and the community at large are probably busy with their own jobs or school. Yet that is the mainstay of care. Insurance often helps with home care through a *certified home health agency* (CHHA). The insurance carriers defined the narrow circumstances that would cover visits to the home. Such services are often triggered by a discharge planner after a hospital stay or a call from your doctor's office. Much documentation needs to be done: what's wrong, what treatment is being given, what you have, and what you can't do.

Once the agency receives the referral, a nurse from the agency visits at your home, and that makes more sense than meeting you in the hospital if you are recently discharged. Meeting you in your home makes the most sense to assess safety. Is it a walk-up or one level? Are there any unsafe conditions—slippery rugs, for instance. Is someone within earshot at night? Once those basics are established, the nurse will identify any *skilled needs:* care of a drain left after surgery, intravenous medications, scars that need special dressings. With one of those conditions, a CHHA can also provide a home health aide (different job titles in different areas) who can help with personal care and light housekeeping (laundry, food preparation) for a few hours a day and for a few times a week. Help with things like taking a bath or a shower, organizing medications, preparing meals can be done in a time segment like that, but certain needs such as going to the bathroom, moving out of bed to a chair and back, or going to the bathroom cannot be limited to a scheduled visit and are ongoing needs. Certain supplies are included and are sent directly by a licensed provider of *durable medical equipment* included in the benefits, but perhaps not completely (the difference between the insurance company's payment and the charges are the *co-pays*). Catheters and surgical dressings are shipped directly to the patient's home, avoiding yet another trip to a pharmacy. Sometimes the equipment is purchased for one-time use (bedside commode), and sometimes it is rented (hospital bed).

The idea, at least theoretically, is that if someone can provide the specialized services on a fixed visit, then family and friends can do the daily care. That concept is where daily reality often conflicts with the vision the insurance companies have. The nurse who visits can *oversee* or *instruct* or *supervise* the home health aide or family members but is not there to do the tasks. That does offer a degree of quality control, but not constant presence. Few of us are aware of these limitations until we need to access them, and the universal reaction is that the services are so limited is rather universal. Home health aides undergo training and have a background check so they are *bonded* and covered under the agency's insurance policies. The agency also will supply a substitute if that home health aide is unable to get to work on a particular day, taking the burden off the patient and family to find a last-minute fill-in.

The hour-to-hour *custodial* needs that are not handled by the informal family-and-friends network often requires a *private hire aide* if the needs exceed what the insurance company allows based on their assessment of *medical necessity.* Often, the CHHA will have access to home health aides that can be hired outside of the insurance reimbursement. Some also have direct relationships to employment agencies that can connect you to private hire aides. Those aides may not have the same training or oversight as those whose hours are bundled with the skilled nursing needs. Although the cost varies from place to place, it is less expensive to have private hire aides. Some will even stay in your house and, with some time off for sleeping and other personal needs, be available to help with the day-to-day needs that your family cannot fulfill.

Most families have great concern that such needs are not temporary but ongoing, and the costs of 24/7 help at home add up quickly. Like child care costs, some families prefer to take the tasks upon themselves even if it means working less at their own paid employment since it is more costly than the salary they bring home after taxes. Some families have more than one individual who needs help at home, common with aging parents who need help simultaneously and whose care can safely be done by one private hire aide. Such an arrangement often means that it is the patient's and family's responsibility to hire, train, and supervise each aide and find a replacement for the aide's time off.

Creative solutions often work best in situations where you need help that extends beyond what your family and insurance can provide. Patients have felt it was the optimal time to "call in favors" from their extended community and have tapped church members or local fraternal organizations who amass a stream of volunteers who can each give a few hours. Working in shifts needs a good system and handing off, which can be set up with the help of the CHHA or a regular employment agency that refers home health aides who are directly paid by the patient and family. Nurses are well trained in handing off at the beginning and end of their shifts in hospitals. The same systems can work at home with adjustments.

It *does* take a village.

For some people who have anticipated this need, long-term care insurance can often reimburse for such custodial needs. Policies vary widely state by state and even within one company. Some are only accessible in certain states, not others. Services become eligible for reimbursement after a certain period of time, and only if the needs are significant. Some policies only reimburse a facility, and some only if the aides come via a CHHA. Others will pay for private hire aides or even pay a family member. Most policies have a lifetime cap on reimbursements.

■ *There are so many types of insurance: long-term care, disability, worker's compensation. Who covers what?*

Disability insurance helps replace income lost due to illness that arises during the time you are working. *Worker's compensation* insurance replaces income when the illness or injury arises directly from work on the job. *Long-term care* stretches beyond the time you are working and into retirement or a period of disability.

Depending on the state where you live, some benefits may be available during the first few weeks when you cannot work. The Social Security Administration's federal disability program offers benefits after six months of time in which you cannot work. Some employers and individuals take out additional policies before they are sick that supplement these programs. Long-term disability policies often exclude payments during the first few weeks or months but will pick up where the others left off.

Part II

The LEARN System

12 How Each Part of The LEARN System Can Guide the Healing Process

PRINCIPLES

There are some simple basic principles to help guide the LEARN System. They are easy to understand.

Having cancer takes effort, and much of it is spent on tasks imposed by others. Appointments for scans and other testing. Chemotherapy schedules, radiation therapy appointments, surgery dates, hospital admissions. All take time and effort. The schedule is determined by many factors: the type of cancer, where you are treated, and the modalities of treatment. There is certainly some choice of which to do, or when or in what order, but in a limited way. They are part of the process of having cancer and getting treatment. Since part of the burden of cancer is feeling so tired, why would a reasonable person want to add more tasks to do, not less? Isn't this time for the world to cut you some slack? Time to sleep a little later? Time to indulge in comfort foods? A daily nap in the middle of the afternoon? Leaving work a little early? Spending more time with the kids on something enjoyable after homework? A music break? Well yes, and no.

THE LEARN SYSTEM

A way of organizing the care from providers combined with the things that I must do to have the best quality of life and help the healing and recovery after a cancer diagnosis.

There are five components:

L Living

E Education

A Activity

R Rest

N Nutrition

Here are the basic principles that guide "My Recovery Plan". This introduction summarizes the background for what we do. It is establishes *why* the LEARN System is essential. The U.S. Constitution has the Preamble. Most books have a preface. Same idea.

THE BIRTH OF THE LEARN SYSTEM

Author's Note

Often times, knowing how something came about helps put it in context and make more sense. The LEARN System was born out of group-think. Innovative ideas frequently come as a result of working together and lots of discussion. In 2007, the New York Community Trust funded a project at Continuum Cancer Centers through Ronald Blum, MD, director of Cancer Centers and Programs, to develop and field test a Personal Health Record (PHR) as the centerpiece of a survivorship program for our head and neck cancer population. This patient group undergoes some of the highest intensity combined treatment of any cohort of patients, coordinating surgery, chemotherapy and radiation therapy. As a result of the high treatment demands of an *organ preserving* approach that safeguards swallowing, speaking and breathing, the recuperation needs are great involving many disciplines and providers. Large subsets of patients are either underserved, hard-to-reach, often minority or well-connected medical consumers who want a clear plan of course for their treatment and beyond. The New York Community Trust is an exemplary community foundation that pools contributions from donors to support projects with a direct impact on patients and families. I served as the clinical director of the program. In 2006 when the project was conceived, survivorship plans, a specific type of PHR we just starting to be used, mostly in breast cancer.

We debated about the contents: what information patients and community providers would need and want, and how to format it so that it was easy-to-use and correct, made us look at the pathway patients take at our cancer center in order to create a system. It could be generalized to the various types of settings where cancer treatment is provided. It made us think critically about which services this group needed at what time, and how to access resources both within our center and the community. A further extension became a teaching program for primary care providers so that the PHR could be easily accepted and put into use. Along with Elise Carper RN, NP, and Victoria Rosenwald, RN, MPH, two research assistants, Dimitri Yukvid and Erica Silen (aided by colleague Damien Francois), brought broad concepts and specific ideas into what emerged as a tangible document. To evaluate it and its acceptability, we worked with Marilyn Bookbinder, PhD, RN, a respected outcomes researcher in symptom management and palliative care to formally assess its effectiveness. The study itself was hard to complete because overburdened patients and families did not want to fill out more assessments for something that was *experimental* and had no seemingly immediate benefit to them. In our federally monitored medical research system, the informed consent process for this type of research has the same lengthy written consent forms as if one were to receive a yet-to-be-licensed chemotherapy drug. Such regulation deters participation in studies such as these. Of the patients who saw the merit and did agree, the majority found the PHR helpful and informative, in both its paper and electronic forms. In the meantime, other groups have forged ahead to develop and promote the use of survivorship plans, and in the intervening time, have published them on paper and electronically. The American Society of Clinical Oncology's patient resource site (http://www.cancer.net) has a selection of specialized forms using the same format. Journey Forward (http://www.journeyforward.org) has similar documents available through its website. LiveStrong—The Lance Armstrong Foundation has funded seminal programs in order to help guide survivorship. New formats will continually be improved and available.

The process of looking at the different components of care, figuring out who does what, and seeing how much of the work falls on to patients and families now that so much of cancer treatment is in the office rather than during a hospital admission all have contributed to the idea that survivorship plans do not begin only after treatment ends, but start at the time of diagnosis and carry forward. Deciding *when* to introduce each service helped crystallize the concept *of early and preventive intervention,* driving home the idea that early evaluation and information promoted a culture change and the principal impetus for the LEARN System. The basic components of the LEARN System are included in most survivorship plans, but the name itself is the creative brainchild of Elayne Feldstein, PhD, an English professor, marketer, educator, multiple cancer survivor, and good friend who has well-earned the title of *First Wordsmith*. With a pen, a few pieces of scrap paper, and a cup of coffee, she was able to combine the core issues into an acronym that had multiple meanings. Bravo to all who helped!

Until very recently, families and friends felt disenfranchised from influencing the physical symptoms of cancer or its treatment, except for weight loss. Concerned family members felt they were in their comfort zone to encourage, sometimes to the point of coercing patients to eat far beyond their capacities, often assuming that patients were "just depressed" (also felt to be in their domain of influence) without the understanding of the many factors that contribute to weight loss and mood changes in cancer. Using the LEARN System elevates each of the parameters to everyone's domain, incorporating the newest science with everyone's well-intentioned care and concern. The adoption of the electronic health record will make it much easier to access the source documents that contain the treatment information (such as: exactly how much radiation was received to what part of the body; the exact dosage of each chemotherapy drug). Until a national standard record is adopted, which is at least a few years away, such information is housed with each provider, and it will fall to both inter-provider communication with the patient and family acting as a courier to complete the PHR.

Basic Principles

- Cancer treatment is hard. I must keep focus on why I want to live through and beyond treatment to sustain me through those bad times.
- A certain amount of rest (not too much; not too little) is essential to repair the body and replenish the mind and soul.
- Eating well (the right foods in the right quantities) is vital to maintain bodily functions, safely withstand treatment, and reduce the recovery time as much as

possible. If I cannot eat in the traditional way, I need to get the calories in via an alternate route.

- Some regular activity based upon type of cancer, type and effectiveness of treatment and my general health maintains energy levels and prevents *deconditioning*.
- Knowledge about my cancer, the specific treatment plan, medications I take at home, appointments, and what I need to expect prepares me better and reduces uncertainty.
- Starting "My Recovery Plan" right away helps keep me and my family involved in the process, and directing the parts of the process that I can, and should influence.

■ *What is the proof that the LEARN System is effective?*

Outcome studies in cancer are often hard to conduct beyond proving survival or tumor progression. Quality of life and symptom management studies often require large groups to minimize individual differences. This scientific method of investigation works because it tests one component of care and leaves every other factor the same so that the specific effect of that one component can be teased out and measured. With five parts of the LEARN System, each part would need to be tested on its own, and finally all five together to be able to say with a high level of certainty that each of the five factors works together in a harmonious way, with good results. Each component has elements that are considered "best care" or have been tested. Having a clinical trial with one group involved in all five components and a second equivalent group— same age, gender, type of cancer, stage of cancer, and basic level of health would be difficult to find. Even if possible to identify at groups of cancer centers across the country, a large number of people would have to agree to participate, making recovery harder on the group that does not adopt the LEARN System. It was thought to be doubtful that any institutional review board would agree that a study is ethical if the treatment offered to either group is less than basic. But a progressive institution took on an evaluation of a different type of supportive care program with similar intent.

Recently, a group of investigators at Massachusetts General Hospital, one of the country's highly respected cancer centers, conducted such a landmark study in which 151 patients with late stage lung cancer were randomly assigned to receive "standard care" or "standard + early intervention palliative care." Those who had the additional care lived approximately three months longer and had improved quality of life. This is the first such study to show what had been previously thought to be common sense.

Since being inquisitive is one of the skills that helps us gather information about cancer and its treatment, the LEARN System should not be exempt. A summary of the best references is found in the companion manual for providers. There is a lot of information out there of varying quality.

Much of what is included in the LEARN System is good common sense. Some is intuitive within the framework of health maintenance that we routinely hear from our providers. Eat a well-balanced diet, the majority of which is plant based and high fiber. Minimize alcohol products, and avoid any tobacco-based product in any form. Move around as much as possible. Take naps. Stay involved. Keep mentally active. Learn as much about your cancer and its treatment as you can. Spend time figuring out what is *really important*. Enjoy the small things. Pause to look at the big picture.

Until recently, only a small minority of people actually set up their own recovery plan and didn't identify it as one. In general, people who exercised regularly, ate well and nurtured their minds and spirit routinely adapted their usual routine to a cancer treatment routine. Some did so easily, some less, due to the underlying feeling of having been "cheated," after having invested time, energy and money in living healthfully. The secret is that once the building blocks of a recovery plan are in place, and less of a change in routine is REALLY needed.

Most of us, however, do not live a life focused on healthy eating, exercise and contemplation. We are too busy with work, family and weaving the fabric of daily existence. When we find out about cancer, in general, we are stunned and start out overwhelmed and frightened. Who could think of a worse time to adopt a set of new habits? Or...who could think of a better time? Having a plan for recovery, "My Recovery Plan," from the time of diagnosis and on helps direct your time and energy so diagnosed patients and those in our circle focus time and energy on a specific goal: getting as well as possible. Restoration in the fullest sense of the word. Just when we need it the most, and feel the least like doing it.

Let's look at some parallel situations. At work the boss says you are taking on a new project. Everyone needs to do more, even if you are working close to the maximum. It is top priority. Some may walk away, feeling exploited. Some may be overwhelmed by the enormity of a new responsibility. But some will forge ahead into action. Stop. Look at the whole picture. Figure out why it's worth it. If it is, how can it be done? For a big task, divide it into pieces. Estimate how long each section will take. Figure out what supplies you need to accomplish your part of the work. Look at the calendar. Set small interim goals. Use technology as your friend. Begin to utilize a daily planner, cell phone, e-mails, Facebook, IMs, Twitter messages, or a blog. Technology can be a good friend. Plan on *not doing this alone.* Line up your team. That can be made of family, friends, or providers. No need to take a pledge like a sorority or fraternity, but close.

My Recovery Plan

"My Recovery Plan" involves the forethought and planning you have been practicing thus far. One of its main features is the LEARN System, which is a simple five-part system that incorporates each of the important components into a structure that is user-friendly from the first day and onward. There are five building blocks: *L*iving, *A*ctivity, *N*utrition, *R*est, *K*nowledge. To easily remember the parts, let's use the first initial of each part. Call it the LEARN System. *LEARN = Live, Education, Activity, Rest, Nutrition.* Elements of each of these five factors can be incorporated into daily life easily with a little effort. They may be all there already, but not necessarily cancer-focused. Many of the activities are double-duty in that they apply to general health maintenance, especially heart health, not just cancer.

p. 247
My Weekly
Recovery
Planner

But does it make sense to take on a new task when you are overloaded with tasks? Sensible question. You can use some help. This is the time. It is common for a pregnant woman to ask for help toward the middle of a pregnancy by naming a coach to practice breathing exercises and even be with the mommy-to-be at the very end of the pregnancy, at the delivery and for the first few days home. Often but not always this is a spouse. In the birth process in particular it is a good idea to bring the spouse into a featured role when in the past everything was so focused on the new mother, the expectant dad almost was left out.

It used to be the husband was relegated to the waiting room to pace and distribute cigars. Not the best use of his time. Now fast-forward 20 years. The term *pregnant* can be mentioned in public. Women tour the center where they will deliver, take childbirth classes and even learn breathing exercises *before* their due date. This is possible because there is ample time to prepare.

With cancer, there is usually no such prep time. There is often little advanced warning and less opportunity for pre-planning. But even so, it is possible or even probable that there is someone in your family or circle of friends may step up to help you. Whoever offers needs to be regularly available for a changing schedule over the course of a few months. It also helps, but is not absolutely essential, if your coach is a cancer survivor him or herself, or has experience supporting someone else through cancer treatment. Having personal or family experience with cancer shortens the learning process. Some coaches will actually attend appointments with you, and that's a great help, but often time consuming and so requires a very flexible work schedule. Early retiree friends, family members or work colleagues may be the most likely group to search. A progressive approach to childbirth involves a helper or a *doula,* an all-around assistant who is a layperson or a health professional who stays by you and knows what is outside of the expected so the midwife or obstetrician can be called. In parallel, at the end of life, doulas have been involved for centuries without that job title. Through recorded time, religious orders cared for the sick. In middle Europe, the fraternal *Bikur Cholim* did the same. Churches routinely had specialized orders, that defined their social meaning in taking care of the ill.

By extension of such a traditional concept, a doula or coach can be the first assistant for wellness and recovery. It makes historical sense, with a modern twist.

For example, someone may want to help but is not able to attend each appointment or treatment, This individual can be of the most assistance by working through the elements of the LEARN System in the initial discussions and help you set your tasks in each of the categories for the week. Reviewing, identifying, and writing down the week's completed tasks and accomplishments will be very helpful at the end of treatment to see how far you have been able to come, despite feeling tired.

Someone in your social circle is likely to agree to take on this job, which is not much different than being a family member, except for the more formal planning necessary. Other people in your circle who visit, go to the supermarket when you can't, drive you to your treatments and take you home are already doing the most time-consuming part of the job. Being a buddy in the LEARN System helps focus everyone's efforts, and helps them get a sense of accomplishment with you as the weeks go by. If your best candidate is not close by, many of the tasks, especially the discussions and goal-setting each week can be done electronically by e-mailing the week's worksheet back and forth to each other. It can be faxed. It can even be done over the telephone and each of you can record the same information to avoid having to get the page back and forth, since that way you'll both have the same information at hand.

If you have gone through your list and there is no one who can be a treatment buddy, ask at your treatment center if there are salaried staff or volunteers who act as *patient navigators.* The American Cancer Society (ACS) has trained volunteers to be navigators at many cancer centers around the country. They may be of help. Ask at your cancer treatment center, church or synagogue to see if there is a member who is a cancer survivor who may be willing to help. Or a few individuals, each of whom can help for a period of time. Almost all of us have been touched by cancer ourselves, or in our families, school, or workplaces. Many of us want to help if asked.

THE LEARN SYSTEM: LIVING

Living has earned the first place in "My Recovery Plan" because of its highest level of importance. Does that sound like an obvious fact? Well, it may not seem so at the time of diagnosis. Most of us, when we find out that we are facing cancer and life-threatening illness are automatically in "survival mode." We are focused on what we believe will be coming in the next few minutes, days or even weeks or months, worried about feeling sick, afraid we may die and feel fearful and isolated. This is to be expected, and not completely universal, but close to it.

During this time, the world will appear different. The fabric of daily life that would fill your days and nights, such as work, school, caring for your family, house repairs or even changing the oil in the car all seem trivial. The activities that used up a good deal of your energy are at this time, less important or unimportant.

In the midst of your worry, it would be logical to think that through a somewhat automatic and mysterious process, you identify your priorities quickly and focus on the things that are important in your lives: family, friends, faith, and the things that give us pleasure. Unfortunately, for most of us, these types of outlets suddenly become unreachable all of a sudden. Many people report that it hurts too much to do the things that they enjoy or find valuable and meaningful because they are a continuous reminder of what we may lose. Why be close with someone whom you may lose touch with? Rarely can anyone express these feelings, but they are there, and powerful.

So against these tides, it becomes first and foremost in the LEARN System in "My Recovery Plan" to set aside *at least* few minutes each week—and hopefully more, to participate in a meaningful activity involving some type of enjoyment or pleasure that reminds you of the time before cancer, and reinforces one of the main reasons that you want to survive. It helps keep those *long-term* goals front and center so that the *short-term quality of life investment* has purpose and meaning, and can seem worth it.

Of course, this *Living* activity needs to be something that is within your abilities and energy. It may be something as simple as making a phone call to a friend, relative or colleague and after responding to the obligatory, "Well how are you?" asking about something important to them or their loved ones. It may be even as mundane as reading the newspaper (not the cancer stories; they don't count here) or watching a newscast to see what is happening outside of the world of cancer and treatment. Or consider looking in on a frail neighbor and calling someone from church to discuss reactions to the past week's homily. The choices are almost endless. But doing something life-affirming every day will help both your present quality of life and ease your re-entry into the world when treatment is over. The exact time and commitment is up to the individual. But at least one life-affirming task is mandatory. Keeping track of the L component will provide a solid basis for a look-back at the end of treatment, like the cornerstone of a new building. Installing a cornerstone has its moment of ceremony, but it itself is not strong enough to hold up the building. Yet it is often inscribed, and it is that component that the public will visit; not the concrete, steel, bricks and wood that sustain the structure. The L is such a cornerstone.

You are not limited to one thing that gives a purpose to the burdens of treatment. Pick as many things as you believe to be genuine to you that you can manage. Yes, this requires some thought. This is the image, idea, person, concept that you want to think about when the going gets tough for that week. The things on your "L List" can change over time or may be enduring. There is no limit.

One school of thought that advocates living in the moment. Many of us rarely do that. We plan ahead, think ahead, and sometimes minimize our involvement in the present. Ironically, since so much of the LEARN System is built on an investment of energy today for a better tomorrow, the L component specifically forces a certain focus on today. There is a whole body of awareness, identified as *mindfulness,* which helps us focus on the present. It has been adapted for people with cancer in many ways. The adaptations are tools to use to help focus. Whether it be art work or some other creative venue, meditation or progressive relaxation CDs or tapes or group discussions at cancer centers, mindfulness channels some of our energies into the present so that the here-and-now is not skipped over. Divorced from spirituality or organized religion, there is a piece of mindfulness that is a part of most spiritual philosophies. For the purposes of the L component in "My Recovery Plan", mindfulness and the essence of today can be *coupled with* or kept *completely separate from* any standardized religious affiliation. Proceed whichever way is more acceptable to you. Or if not, follow your heart and your spirit, or even your early life training in organized religion if you experienced it to put mindfulness in a spiritual context. It is important to remember that mindfulness and living *in the now* does *not dwell* anywhere or with any one group. L is a human experience.

At times, newly diagnosed patients resent this suggestion. It can seem artificial, hokey or trite. Usually, after the initial shock, the L component makes sense. It may not be apparent at first, but it does.

The top section in the worksheet "My Weekly Recovery Planner Using the LEARN System" has a place to write your thoughts and feelings. This section covers the other LEARN variables as a roof arches over a home. Specify what you are doing or thinking in that box.

The
LEARN
System©

p. 247
My Weekly
Recovery
Planner

THE LEARN SYSTEM: EDUCATION; WHAT I NEED TO KNOW

My whole life has just changed: Yes…and no. Patients routinely say that things will "never be the same for me anymore." That has many meanings. They will not be free of worrying about cancer even if disease-free. It could mean, "I won't be so cavalier or so confident in the way I live about my life." Or "I won't take things for granted anymore." Entering this new world means learning a lot of new information and refining skills that you never thought you'd have. Cramming for a test is never easy. Living with cancer is not taking a test. It is a learned process. The LEARN System can help you by bringing the information you need and help you use the skills you have.

When looking at the experience of having cancer compared to another major health event, say a heart attack, the process of getting better is entirely different. The stereotypical response to having chest pain or a heart attack scare or actual heart attack is an immediate resolution of lifestyle change, since so much of the predisposing factors for heart disease are behavioral: "I'll start to eat better, right now—cut the salt and the fat. I will exercise every day. I will go back to the gym. I will take a yoga class to relieve stress. I will stop smoking. I've had my last drink." People are scared, but are not so debilitated. And the public health message so tied to things that are more under their control, patients commit to personal health reforms that make New Year's resolutions pale by comparison.

Most people facing a new cancer diagnosis, we are frightened and the work-up is extended (now just the first few hours for a heart attack) over days or weeks. The fright and the "busy-ness" of those initial days lead right into treatment, when the fatigue often starts. By the time the fright abates, so much day-to-day care often precludes making the time to take one of those proverbial steps back to observe what's going on. The idea of investing quality of life at least on the short term is mostly nonnegotiable. Here is an example of a typical chain of thought: "We want to live. Cancer can kill. We will do what we can to live and to put the cancer behind us". As Americans, we settled the West. We sent men to the moon. We—I can get through whatever it takes. Just getting by dominates our awareness, and getting by means holding together the things that involved us before we found out about the cancer. Family, work, school. Paying the bills. Getting the kids settled. Whatever makes up the fabric of my life. So if I was told that I might have some dry mouth, or have some lingering indigestion or some blunting of the nerve endings in my hands or my feet, it seems trivial. I want to live. At first it is hard to focus on getting better. It is a shock to be sick and have cancer! And these seemingly minimal side effects at the moment appear to be a small price to pay in order to live.

As time continues, and treatment morphs into healing and recovery, some of these seemingly trivial incursions on our quality of life become real. The fear is reduced (not gone) and the small—or not so small—side effects begin to loom larger and more disruptive in our lives.

CONSULTATION IN A BOX: A BITTER TASTE

BN, a high-powered attorney who frequently goes to court with his clients, prided himself in his good clear voice that he considers an asset to his career. He found out he had tongue cancer and learned of the proposed treatment He was enthusiastic about an *organ-sparing* approach to keep his voice. He greatly enjoys going to nice restaurants at home and while traveling. So eating and swallowing were also important functions to be preserved for his quality of life as well as to maintain his income and identity as a litigator.

BN struggled through initial radiation therapy and chemotherapy and surgery, then a lymph node dissection, even enrolling in a clinical trial to

continued

CONSULTATION IN A BOX: A BITTER TASTE

continued

minimize dry mouth that would likely accompany the maximal radiation therapy so that he could protect his throat.

Everything went well, and treatment was effective. With greater gusto and appreciation despite some lingering fatigue Mr. N returned to his law practice and to the many things that made up his life before the cancer was found. Eight years later, half in jest, he says that his ability to differentiate between superb and merely fine *fois gras* is not what it was before, and that being told he should not have the accompanying wine is a drag.

What seems trivial at first looms larger later on in the midst of survivorship. A woman with more of a spiritual approach to her cancer and survivorship jokes about the change in her "center of gravity" since she had her breast cancer, bilateral mastectomy. "Thank God," she says, "I *can have* a change in my center of gravity. I am glad to be alive." For others, the transition is not so simple.

Many people think, "My whole life has changed."

CONSULTATION IN A BOX: BELOW THE BELT

A young woman working as a fashion model is a famous presence in jeans and underwear ads. Hundreds of thousands have seen her lower abdomen stretched across billboards perhaps with a width of 15 feet or more. Her diagnosis of rectal cancer was certainly a professional liability. Hearing she would need abdominal surgery and likely have a colostomy, even temporarily, meant that jobs showing her pelvis more than life-size would be deferred. She did not come to a treatment decision easily, and traveled to every center of excellence for the treatment of rectal cancer that her Internet searches would discover and insurance would reimburse. She had to be certain that an abdominal scar at the least, or a colostomy at the most, would be unavoidable. It was unavoidable, and she reluctantly agreed but did not consent to a vascular access device (a *port* for intravenous access below her collarbone), but did get a long intravenous line into a vein in her arm since she had multiple admissions for dehydration. "I figured," she said, "that if I can't model briefs, I could switch to tee-shirts so my collarbone area was important too." Her strategy worked, and after her colostomy reversed, years later, she had a little more distance and time to think. "I can't believe that I put those choices first. I wanted to survive and I am glad I did. In modeling, you only have a short window of opportunity. I would have had to find something else anyway."

Questions I Want Answered

Some of the greatest challenges in cancer treatment today are the human ones. The ability to communicate nuance and uncertainty is something we teach in medical, nursing and social work schools. The skills can be taught and learned. As in surgery, there are certain predispositions that make the learning more effective and results better than minimal. Having the team approach lets each one use his or her best skills. The oncology subspecialist may not be the best at communicating, or can do so but not have the luxury of time. Whoever is in charge of the treatment team, whether it exists over a variety of private practices or is centralized in an accredited cancer program, needs to have the right people on the team. Would an owner of a baseball team have all pitchers? Same idea. So the postmodern role of the oncologist is to form the team, within the office or the community. Answering hard questions is sometimes the part that gets the least attention but is most valued by patients and families.

The following list of questions you might need to ask is comprehensive. It should be tailored and prioritized. Most providers—even those that value communication—can answer some on an initial consultation, since that is one of the main purposes of that visit. On follow-up visits, the most important ones need to be identified to be asked, with the idea that a few at a time is best. How many is a few? That depends on many factors.

What is cancer?

Why me?

How did I get it?

Why didn't I know about it sooner?

How do I find out what type of cancer it is and what treatment I need?

What is the stage and type?

Will this kill me?

How much time do I have?

Can it be cured? Controlled? Put into remission?

How will I feel?

Will I recover and be myself?

What will the treatment include?

Can I continue to work?

How can I arrange for a second opinion? (No offense, please, but this is serious and I need to know.)

Who can help with my kids? Will I need help at home?

What do I need to do during my treatment? Eating, exercise?

What will be affected by the cancer and by the treatments?

What about vitamins and supplements?

What are *clinical trials*?

What is important to me now?

What do I have to do to get better?

When will I feel OK again? Will I be the same?

Will the cancer come back?

Is it familial?

What do my family and friends need to know?

Will I be able to forget all of what is happening?

How long will I need follow-up care? What will it be?

Will I be OK?

What if nothing works?

What will happen if I get sicker?

Will you stick by me if treatment does not work?

How...and when will I die?

There are many similar situations in life when the questions are brewing, and there is not enough time to ask them all or get complete answers. Some of the questions do not have good answers as they rely on our abilities to predict the future. No one in any discipline or specialty has the skill to do so.

Acknowledging the questions is important. Answering what can be answered as time goes by is a good idea, but not for everyone. But you need to know just how much information—and what level—you need to know and can handle. Some of us are calmer and have an easier time putting one foot in front of the other without knowing the biomechanics of the foot, how shoes are made and understanding the complex nerve-muscle connections to make it happen. Having full knowledge is not how we all work best. We each know that about ourselves and the treatment team will not know that right away. For those of us who need less information, do not overload of follow someone else's formula. Someone among family and friends who make up our support networks may or likely will want to know the answers. The list can be a starting point for them as well.

■ How am I expected to feel?

That is a truly complicated question. No one goes about having cancer the same way. People do it in their own style. The unique characteristics that make us who we are do not change with cancer. Some people say they are "themselves but more so," feeling their usual way of coping more exaggerated.

CONSULTATION IN A BOX: A FAILURE AT BEING HAPPY

PP is one of those people who seems to "have it all," a 67-year-old man with a successful business, two wonderful kids, grandkids, and wife of 40 years. Mr. P is quiet and reserved, and not good at discussing his feelings without

continued

CONSULTATION IN A BOX: A FAILURE AT BEING HAPPY

continued

a lot of prompting. Mrs. P has never been comfortable with that, though always knew how to have a serious discussion with her husband when it was necessary. She learned to make an appointment and schedule a meeting with him. Throughout their marriage, this worked well.

Mr. P was recently diagnosed with prostate cancer, and after a variety of consultations, decided to have radiation therapy and androgen deprivation hormonal treatment. The cancer was limited to the prostate gland, with a Gleason score of 5 and a PSA (prostate specific antigen) reading of 9—all signs of a good prognosis. Although a surgical option was presented, Mr. and Mrs. P and his urologist agreed with the radiotherapy/hormone therapy option.

Surprisingly, Mrs. P knew no one with prostate cancer, though many women in their church and in their neighborhood had breast cancer. She attacked the Internet, and tried to read as much as possible about prostate cancer. She felt confident with the cancer center, doctor and treatment team. After a number of days, she even stopped thinking that her loving husband would die soon of cancer. She also read that "cancer develops as a result of stress" and she set out to take as much stress as possible out of their lives, easier to say than do. When she asked him how he was feeling, Mr. P gave his usual answer, "OK."

After a number of "OK" replies, she scheduled a meeting with him to find out a little more. At the meeting she asked him, "But how do you *really feel?*" His response was the same, "I'm fine. We have seen good doctors, will get the radiation therapy at a well-recognized cancer center, and it was caught early. What more is there to say?" Mrs. P wanted to hear that her husband was *happy* so that, consistent with her Internet readings, the treatments would be successful and that the cancer would not show up in his bones or his lung months or years later. She went about scheduling their free time to see all of their friends and relatives and planned a vacation to a lovely island resort two months after the radiation is to be completed. She searched their cable television menu and found two channels that show old situation comedies from the 1950s and 1960s and played them constantly on the television when he was home, laughing at each one and reminiscing about where they were when the shows were first aired. Their two children with their spouses and grandchildren began to visit on rotation, going to the movies (only comedies), miniature golf courses, to the video arcade at the mall, dinner theatres and any other activities with opportunity to laugh.

continued

CONSULTATION IN A BOX: A FAILURE AT BEING HAPPY

continued

Mr. P was exhausted two weeks into his radiation therapy, with the level of exhaustion far exceeding that attributable to the cancer or beginning treatment. The radiation oncologist checked his blood count in advance of the usual time, looking for anemia, an underfunctioning thyroid or even a low magnesium level. All were fine. Mrs. P said at the checkup visit that she "can't understand why this is happening as they are spending all of their free time keeping him happy" and related all they and done over the last few weeks. Mr. P, the oncologist and the nurse all started to smile. They asked her why she was campaigning to keep Mr. P happy, and she explained what she read online, and that if you don't keep happy, the cancer will recur, and the radiation won't work.

Mr. P took his wife's hand and tried to clarify if indeed what his wife read was correct. When the team explained what they knew about cancer and attitude, and how although the quality of his life was improved with all of the "fun" activities they were doing, he was spent. Mr. P said, "I guess I have failed. I am exhausted having my wife and my family make me happy. I am a failure at being happy." Everyone smiled and started to chuckle respectfully, out of relief and out of irony. All agreed that Mr. and Mrs. P could get back to their regular routine. The expected tiredness from the radiation therapy set in, on schedule as they cut back on their campaign to be happy. They did, though, enjoy the vacation after his treatment.

Think about Starting Some Record of This Experience

Yes—even more to do. But you will likely find it will be a very helpful reference in the early weeks after diagnosis. Such a record does not need to be elaborate, or can be as sophisticated as would like. A note a day on an index card, in a small notebook like a diary, photos of you and how you see others. The changes you are going through are striking. There are Journal pages in the worksheets for you to use. Copy as many as you need.

■ *Where can I get more and reliable information?*

There is a lot of bad information out there, as well as good information. It is sometimes hard to differentiate between the two. One helpful way is to consider information from reliable sources. Professional groups like the American Society of Clinical Oncology have much good material at http://www.cancer.net. Likewise, the ACS (at http://www.cancer.org) is often quoted. The ACS links to the American

CONSULTATION IN A BOX: TOO FEW WORDS

A 48-year-old man developed colon cancer, and although found at an early stage, it did require two surgeries, chemotherapy, and radiation therapy. He worked as a magazine editor, and was good with words. He hoped to work throughout his treatment, since much of what he did could be done at home, in the hospital, or a chair in the infusion suite as long as he could have his laptop with him. One of his colleagues was reviewing a book of Haiku poetry, a Japanese art form in which words are few and well chosen. He decided to pick one word a day that best reflected how he was feeling that day. He then formed a week's worth of words together. He hopes to self-publish it after his treatments are over.

College of Surgeons Commission in Cancer (http://www.facs.org/cancer) to find accredited facilities throughout the United States. Cancer*Care* is a social work–based agency that specializes in dealing with the nonmedical aspects of cancer for the individual patient and family network (http://www.cancercare.org). Many of the wonderful educational sessions are accessible by podcast after their initial broadcast. The National Cancer Institute (NCI) has comprehensive information on a variety of cancers, treatments, and the most up-to-date listing of clinical trials (http://www.cancer.gov).

Be wary of sites that want to sell products, especially those that offer a so-called cure. Cures for multiple chronic or life-threatening conditions should raise even more suspicion.

■ But this is a lot of work. *I didn't intend to get cancer. I never wanted to go to medical school. What do I really need to know?*

Yes, there is a lot of information here and out there. Not all of it applies to your situation. Some may never apply to you, some may later on.

In the recent past, perhaps until the 1960s, consumerism was not a part of our lives. In health care, there were fewer choices. In one of those perfect storm moments, medical care became an entitlement with the passage of federal Medicare legislation around the time of the technological boom when choice and consumerism collided in health care. A very traditional approach, still in vogue in many parts of the world, involves, "Whatever you say, doctor." No explanation necessary. Little chance to ask questions or expect answers. We got to be as inquisitive about our medical care as we are about the purchase of a car. Mix in the trend toward subspecialization, where life-saving treatment is been performed by providers whom we don't likely know. Garnish this situation with the information boom, making un-vetted information available as close as your Internet connection or local library. You need to find good information and information sources.

THE LEARN SYSTEM: ACTIVITY

Med School in a Box Seminar: Activity is Key from Diagnosis Onward

Any type of physical activity is *essential* during cancer treatment. Such a principle is so counterintuitive. Although it sounds backward, there is a tremendous amount of support for making activity a top priority during and after cancer treatment. Of course, there are certain precautions to take, but they are minor compared to the benefits.

The Downward Spiral

A downward spiral occurs when we eat less: there is a reduction in our energy, which in turn diminishes appetite, worsening fatigue. Such a pattern keeps going and going. It needs to be interrupted. The LEARN System changes the pattern from all sides. Living, Education, Activity, Rest, and Nutrition each and together specifically guard against the downward spiral. Working together, each part helps and encourages the other.

■ *But I get the rest part, not the activity part. Why?*

Recovery is better and faster. Small studies have resulted in suggestive evidence of improved survival. The qualifier *suggestive* is used because the studies need a longer period of time to mature. In the world of clinical research, a *mature* study is one in which the factor under investigation is measured after a time in which it will be thought to show its effects on the individual as a whole. Or as it is said, the whole is greater than the sum of its parts.

Activity itself is just being judged as effective in cancer control and prevention of recurrences. Prescribing activity *prematurely*—before the studies are complete—is recommended since it is helpful for other health maintenance, such as heart and lung function without deleterious side effects.

One of the contributory mechanisms of cancer-induced weight loss is a relative increase in circulating insulin levels. Insulin is made in the pancreas and balances blood sugars, to keep tissues working at peak capacity with the smallest energy investment. Diabetics have too little insulin, so blood sugar increases and causes damage to blood vessels and nerves throughout the body. Both are affected by high blood sugars. When someone does not have diabetes but has cancer, the blood sugars that can increase, which has an effect on cancer growth, an effect that is yet to be fully understood. It is likely contributory to cancer growth. Reducing these levels, theoretically, discourages growth. One of the best ways to control insulin levels is exercise. In addition to the heart and lung health benefits, activity makes sense all around.

Goals of Increased Activity

There are many reasons why activity and movement are extremely important during cancer treatments, especially early in the course of care. Simply put they are the following:

- Maintaining strength and function.
- Maintaining flexibility.
- Maintaining good heart function and lung capacity.
- Maintaining weight and body image.
- Maintaining energy.
- Maintaining good sleep.
- Minimizing the side effects of treatment.
- Promoting the best possible *quality of life*.
- Reducing the chance of recurrence or secondary cancers.

By keeping these functions at their best, you can maintain your quality of life during treatment. The real payoff is at the end of treatment and afterward. Having to work to regain lost muscle mass and flexibility takes a lot of extra effort. Such a loss is often called *general deconditioning*. Moderate to vigorous physical activity can also help prevent recurrence. Or make it possible to withstand the rigors of treatment with good quality of life in the physical, psychological, social, and spiritual areas.

■ *So why it is so hard to adopt a serious activity program during cancer treatment and afterward?*

Well, why is it so hard for anyone who is not facing cancer treatment? It is a lot of work, and takes a certain level of commitment and promise. It could be said that the time of a cancer diagnosis is the worst time to take on such a responsibility. Or ... it is the best time.

Patients who have a heart attack often have a moment of enlightenment when they find out they survived it. Many people vow to eat right or start to exercise. For most the promise passes like a New Year's Eve resolution or pleasing a higher power when experiencing a close brush with dying. Such a quick promise often is not sustained.

The arguments against adopting a more active life are many. "If I am going to die anyway, what's the difference? I am too tired. I am too busy. I am too angry." Too tired and too busy are too true. But what if treatment is effective? What if you are OK? Then you'll be in really bad shape. So let's figure out what you can do that is simple and basic that can be scheduled twice a day. For instance, try getting up and walking around for increasing time increments. Start with five minutes at a time. Invest in an inexpensive timer if your watch or phone doesn't have one. Increase the time by a few minutes each time, being careful to do only what you can do easily. If you cannot walk, change that to move around in a bed or a chair. You may need a formal physical medicine assessment so you can see what is safe and estimate your capacities.

The emphasis, at least at the beginning, is on stretching and avoiding weight loss by moving around to increase appetite and rest effectively. Muscle building comes later. You are not training for a competition.

Waiting Is the Worst Option

Motivation to be active is a concept that the medical community and public health officials have not perfected to the point of honing an effective message. The challenge in cancer is no more daunting. If it were a medication, it could be ordered on a prescription blank and with prior approval from the insurance carrier. Think of being active with the same level of importance and seriousness as anti-nausea medicine. It is not absolutely essential, but so important as part of the total treatment package.

Putting Activity Back into Activities of Daily Living

This is a concept that refers to the things we do every day, such as bathing, dressing, going to the toilet. Western society has mechanized much of what we did physically before. Take on household tasks and do them manually. It's a good start. If walking around your house becomes boring, branch out. Gradually. In an apartment, go out into the hallways. If that's not enough, every building has stairs. They may be fire stairs for an emergency, but they are generally accessible. Twice a day. Venture up or down and each day add a bit more. Too cold or hot outside? Many malls open before the stores open. They are generally at 68 degrees year-round. Go a little further each time. Wear comfortable shoes or sneakers. See if a neighbor already walks and will get you started.

Time to make it a bit more rigorous? Don't need to buy fancy equipment, though it may make it more challenging or fun. Fill two cleaned plastic milk bottles with water, half way. They should each weigh about four pounds. Hold one in each hand as you walk. Fill it further every few days. You can even drink the water if you're thirsty or it is hot out. Set out a short course and measure it with your car's odometer. Track your progress.

■ *Just home from the hospital? That couch or chair looks inviting, and it should be. But it will look more inviting after some activity.*

Exercise physiologists measure activity in units; metabolic equivalents of tasks, to be exact. That is the amount of energy the body spends to carry out the specified activity and is called a MET (Metabolic Equivalent of Task). More vigorous activities take more energy. A goal is to maintain about 18 METs a week at a minimum. It is a high goal. At the start, *any* activity is the first step to healing. The table opposite shows the amount of activity in common daily tasks.

■ *But I never exercised before. Where do I begin?*

But you walk around. Begin there. Use assistive devices that you have been using. Use a wheelchair that you can roll yourself? Good start. On bed rest? Have the visiting

Activity in METs (Metabolic Equivalent of Tasks)

Physical Activity	MET
Light Intensity Activities	< 3
sleeping	0.9
watching television	1.0
writing, desk work, typing	1.8
walking, less than 2.0 mph (3.2 km/h), level ground, strolling, very slow	2.0
Moderate Intensity Activities	3 to 6
bicycling, stationary, 50 watts, very light effort	3.0
calisthenics, home exercise, light or moderate effort, general	3.5
bicycling, <10 mph (16 km/h), leisure, to work or for pleasure	4.0
bicycling, stationary, 100 watts, light effort	5.5
Vigorous Intensity Activities	> 6
jogging, general	7.0
calisthenics (e.g., push-ups, sit-ups, pull-ups, jumping jacks), heavy, vigorous effort	8.0
running, jogging, in place	8.0
rope jumping	10.0

nurse or physical therapist demonstrate *range of motion* movements and do them twice a day, with help of your family and caregivers, then do them on your own.

■ *I'm a DIYer starting my own self-directed plan. What should I do?*

First ask the oncologist or oncology nurse if it is OK for you to start a program of increased physical activity. Describe the intensity (low, moving very slowly into the moderate range if possible). If you had recent surgery, the surgeon should weigh in on how long afterward he/she is comfortable with any plan. Particular points to discuss are the chance of any injury through bleeding if the platelet count is too low or the risk of a fracture of a bone at a spot where there is or may be weakened bones due to cancer. Ask about any limitations. Emphasize a slow, gradual start with the emphasis on walking and stretching. The routine can be simple. Warm up by moving around. Judge your pace properly. Don't overdo, which may be your natural tendency. Breathe deeply, using the full lungs and hydrate.

■ *I'm not a DIYer. Where can I turn?*

Can't do it yourself? Certified cancer centers have established relationships with either physical therapists, occupational therapists, speech and swallowing therapists and/or comprehensive rehabilitation centers. A formal referral may need to be made, depending on the insurance carrier's rules for your plan. There is an established track record and body of science that applies rehabilitation techniques from other diseases to cancer. Your insurance carrier may actually ask that a formal consultation by a specialist in physiatry be done. The insurance carrier's case management services may know or can find out. In some areas, insurance companies will refer patients with cancer for *specialty* care to traumatic brain injury (TBI) programs who may be the only local resources. Other policies will allow any prescribing cancer provider to authorize a consultation and treatment directly with the physical, occupational or speech/swallowing therapist who will begin with their own evaluation. An experienced physical therapist can set you up with a routine, show how to increase the length and intensity of the movements but will often say, "I'm not your personal trainer." However, you will learn techniques tailored to your situation, where you can move through some of the fatigue, as counterintuitive as that sounds. Physical therapy training involves a good deal of training in the science of body movement and its effect.

Your provider will offer the information for an *exercise prescription* that includes: reviewing any possible—even if only temporary—effects of cancer treatment (muscle or nerve damage), effects of certain chemotherapies on the heart, risk for fractures, specific movement of joints, and general medical history. Starting slowly is the best approach, especially when it comes to any activity that can build muscle.

Think of the rehab visits as an opportunity to learn what can be done at home as well as in the office with equipment. Different from a personal trainer, the physiatrist or physical/occupational/speech-swallowing therapist can instruct you to incorporate movement and milestones into your daily lives.

CONSULTATION IN A BOX: THE COUGH THAT WOULDN'T GO AWAY, THE FATIGUE THAT WOULD

A 48-year-old man developed a dry cough, and after a course of antibiotics, his primary care provider sent him for a chest X-ray that showed a single spot. Having been a smoker who stopped about 15 years ago, he was sent for a *spiral ultrafast CT scan,* which confirmed one small suspicious lesion. He was referred to lung surgeon, who believed that a biopsy could be done with a *fine needle under CT scan,* avoiding a larger procedure. The biopsy did show lung cancer. He came back 5 days later for the removal of the lesion via thoracoscope, a minimally invasive procedure, without any complications, so the hospital stay was short, too short for him to meet the physical medicine and rehabilitation team. A set of scans was done to make sure that the cancer was contained in the lung, and there was no sign of any cancer in any other organ, including the brain. On the road to healing well, the Tumor Board at the cancer center recommended combined chemotherapy and radiation therapy since it did spread to a close-by lymph node. The patient met both the medical oncologist and the radiation oncologist over the next few days. Treatment began

continued

CONSULTATION IN A BOX: THE COUGH THAT WOULDN'T GO AWAY, THE FATIGUE THAT WOULD

continued

within 10 days, enough time for additional blood work and urine tests to check his kidney function, and treatment planning for the radiation. Once he began treatment, the cough subsided, and breathing became easier. With starting treatment, as expected, he became very tired and took to the couch after getting home from his radiation therapy each day, already bored form watching way too much daytime television, not his usual routine. The lower end of his throat "was on fire," and it hurt to swallow, so his weight began to slide.

On the fourth day of radiation therapy, his radiation oncologist asked him, "how the physical therapy was going," and he guiltily admitted that he hadn't gone yet. A quick appointment was arranged and the evaluation showed he was in relatively good physical condition, but was getting *deconditioned* rather quickly, having had only a small surgery with the chemotherapy and radiation therapy starting after just a few days for recovery.

The physiatrist and all three oncology subspecialists agreed that although his type of cancer put him at risk for fractures, the scans were all fine and he could and should quickly proceed with physical therapy. The patient himself was a bit skeptical. "I'm so tired already I can barely drag myself in for the radiation. Chemo really knocks me out, and I am pooped." His family and trust in the advice he had gotten thus far convinced him to go along with the recommendation. He reluctantly came to radiation in his sneakers and workout clothes, and proceeded to physical therapy afterward. He started out on an exercise bike, and became winded after just five minutes. As he breathed in and out more heavily, he could not believe how much he had to focus on taking deep breaths. He reviewed some basic stretching exercises that he had used only after a not-frequent-enough basketball game or other sports. He was so tired on the way home, he fell asleep on the bus and almost missed his stop. Over the next few sessions, he did actually begin to feel stronger, and by the fifth one, actually looked forward to going. His breathing became more natural and less forced. His coughing subsided, and although his throat still hurt, he used more pain medicine and protective coatings given by the medical oncologist to swallow before he ate. His weight stabilized, and while he remained tired, the quality of the fatigue was different. He spent less time on the couch watching television, and more time upright reading and online. He even looked forward to eating, and the canned supplements became tolerable with some fresh fruit mixed in. His activity got more intense, slowly, and by

continued

> ## CONSULTATION IN A BOX: THE COUGH THAT WOULDN'T GO AWAY, THE FATIGUE THAT WOULD
>
> *continued*
>
> the end of his chemotherapy and radiation therapy, he remained tired. He said he could "pull myself up by those bootstraps" and realized that the push for more activity helped him "turn a corner."
>
> He continued to heal slowly, and learned which exercises he could do at home. About 5 weeks after his treatments finished, he started to feel even better, and by 10 weeks he was back at work. "I don't know if this would have happened without the physical therapy," he admitted, "and I really hated to go at first. But it really paid off."

THE LEARN SYSTEM: REST (AND SLEEP)

■ *Cancer-smart resting: Am I getting permission to rest? Wow!*

"Rest...I don't need a reminder to tell me to rest. This is something I already can do, and I do it well." Not given much attention or importance during cancer treatment, resting is a vital part of the recuperation process. It is almost expected after surgery. In polite company, it's often called a period of *convalescence.* But after chemotherapy or radiation therapy? Well, yes!

■ *Why is rest important to me?*

Effective resting helps maintain higher levels of activity at other times during the day. Making sure resting is effective takes a little effort. A lack of rest or sleep has a number of ill effects on the individual: reduced reaction time and judgment, poorer information processing, trouble with short-term memory, poorer performance in school or at work, reduced motivation and patience. Restorative rest and sleep tend to promote healing. "Restorative" means that at the end of the time period, or in the morning when waking for the day, having a feeling of being refreshed.

During cancer treatment, resting and sleep should be restorative.

■ *Cancer-smart sleeping: How much sleep and rest do we need?*

Sleep experts think adults need about seven to eight hours of sleep a day. Neither too much or too little is good. The changes that occur in sleep during cancer are not well studied. The usual sleep-wake cycle is changed by many of the routinely used medications during treatment. Particularly anti-nausea medicines and pain medicines promote a certain amount of sedation, and that interferes with falling or staying asleep. Corticosteroid mediation (such as dexamethasone or methylprednisone) can cause a type of hyper-alertness during the first few days of taking them. It is usually a comfort not to be so tired, but then becomes annoying after a few days.

■ *I see advertisements on television and in magazines for sleeping medications. Can they help?*

The television commercials promoting sleep medicines are not aimed at a cancer treatment audience. Using sedating medications regularly during cancer treatment can result in the medications lingering during the day, causing excess sedation and being *more tired.*

Much of the sleep changes have in the past been attributed solely to worrying. More modern theories actually connect sleep problems to the circulating cell proteins. Moderate to severe levels of depression or anxiety can be counteracted with careful use of antidepressants or anti-anxiety medications. Regular long-term use of sleep medicines can actually backfire. Sleeping medicines of the benzodiazepine family and those that are similar but technically members of different chemical families (zolpidem, or Ambien® or others; zaleplon, or Sonata® or others; eszopiclone, or Lunesta® and others; ramelteon, or Rozerem® and others) often cause tolerance, so you need more and more to get the same or even less of an effect. And dependence, with rebound insomnia if stopped abruptly or even not weaned slowly enough. If you keep the length of time to a few weeks or months only and for most people these medications are helpful. Using one every other night is of little advantage because the medications linger in the system. Staying off for six weeks or more helps renew their effectiveness, but the sleep during that period of time suffers. Although not part of the package insert labeling, many times using the sleep medications for three nights in a row can jump-start a good sleeping pattern and then will not be needed for a while. Three nights' use does not require a weaning period.

Over-the-counter sleep aids are often really diphenhydramine (Benadryl®, Tylenol PM®, Advil PM®, and others) are problematic for men with growing prostates, or even without prostate cancer, as they can slow down an already compromised urination.

Complicating the treatment of insomnia in the midst of cancer treatment even more is the common use of the benzodiazepines as anti-nausea medicines. Although one takes lorazepam (Ativan® and others), the benzodiazepine most often used for nausea during the day, it interfere with the usual brain function that promotes nighttime sleep and can make it harder to fall asleep at night without an additional dose.

Supplements such as kava-kava and valerian are not studied in cancer and can alter liver function, making the liver function tests rise and perhaps lead your treatment team to think that it is the chemotherapy and the impetus to reduce your dose erroneously. Melatonin, also sold as a supplement, has dubious use as a sleep aid, but is effective when adjusting between time zones in jet lag. That use makes it tempting to use for sleep, but may not be helpful.

■ *Can naps help?*

Naps are secret weapon against fatigue. Sleep experts believe that, without cancer, total nap time needs to be less than 60 minutes in 24 hours to avoid the body thinking it has already had part of its day's sleep, which would interfere with nighttime sleep. Thirty minutes may be less disruptive, but is less restorative. Best to set a timer or clock. Use a different one than the one used to wake up in the morning to keep the experiences separate in your memory.

"I really don't like to nap. What other activities count as *rest*"*?* Try relaxation exercises that can be found or purchased online, or use electronic helpers like white noise, water, or wave sounds. Perhaps a repetitive and automatic activity that has been previously mastered can be relaxing, like knitting. And of course meditation. Yoga could count for both rest and activity. In the quest for treatment and even prevention of jet lag, progressively changing the time going to bed and waking up, known as *phase shifting*, can be helpful when sleep comes on too early or late. Some cognitive-behavioral therapies can help structure such a plan, and provide other tools, such as progressive relaxation or even medical hypnosis. Expressing frustrations and fears via creative writing, sometimes called *emotive-expressive writing* may help as a constructive outlet. Understanding the distress of having cancer, undergoing treatment and the uncertainty of the future can be placed into perspective with focused counseling.

Every certified cancer center and most office-based oncology practices have trusted behavioral health professionals for referral. The use of anti-anxiety and antidepressant medications often should involve a psychiatrist with special training in cancer to optimize the doses and anticipate potential interactions. The American Psychosocial Oncology Society (http://www.apos-society.org) may be able to suggest referrals in your area.

■ *Instead of sedating medicines at night, how about stimulant medicines during the daytime?*

There is some success in using stimulant medicines during the early portions of the day. Two newer medications have been tested in clinical trials. *Dex*-methylphenidate (or Focalin® and others) is a more purified version of methylphenidate (Ritalin® and others), and modafinil (Provigil®) can help add energy and alertness if properly monitored. Caffeinated drinks may even be a good daytime energizer for *early* in the day. With each of the medications listed, being irritable, jumpy, and *wired* or having a sense of palpitations is a sign to cut back on stimulants.

The
LEARN
System©

■ *Can I trust what I read on the Internet?*

Sometimes, not always.
Use the list of Trusted Internet Sites in the Resources section.

p. 338
Trusted
Internet Sites

■ *How come my treatment team is not giving me the information they want me to have?*

There are multiple obstacles to providing all of this information at the oncologists' office. Time is a significant factor during follow-up visits as it is for every provider. Even with dedicated time and interest, the information keeps changing.

THE LEARN SYSTEM: NUTRITION

Just the mention of the word *nutrition* conjures up extreme positive and negative reactions for us all.

When we feel sick and frightened, and worry about our future, what it will be like and how long it will be, food and nutrition are very low on our priority list. "What's the difference?" some of us say. "I feel too sick to eat." For many that is so, and for some, especially those with breast or prostate cancer with connections to changes in hormones, changes in appetite and even pregnancy-type cravings dominate your days and nights. With your new changed relationship to food, those special family/friend events where food is front and center seem more remote as it is harder to participate fully and as you once did. You are tempted to say, "No, not today. Thank you anyway" and step away. That robs you of the social part. Without exception, food is the glue of almost all social situations: holidays, family gatherings, parties, celebrations. If you are less interested and not able to eat, you may be self-excluded from vital social interaction. Yes, during chemotherapy the smells are disturbing, sometimes even the blandest ones. Yes, seeing people indulge can be repulsive when it is hard to hold down Gatorade. Generations of patients report that as disturbing as these situations can be, it's worse to be in the next room or in an upstairs bedroom isolated and not participating. The social part—so much of an antidote to the feeling of like you are struggling alone against cancer—is lost.

■ *Why can't I just eat right?*

That's a complicated issue. Looking at what you should be eating before, during, and after cancer, there is little difference to what you hear all the time. From your primary care providers, television medical news, your first grade teacher and the *mandatory* health classes most of us had in high school, it's a consistent message from everyone. Heart attack prevention strategies and many other professional societies echo the same message. Our optimal modern diet should be made up of mostly plant-based foods with whole grain carbohydrates, fruits and vegetables of many deep colors, nuts, beans and low-fat dairy foods, less generous portions of meats and minimal amounts of fats and sweets, which should be mono-unsaturated oils and unprocessed sweeteners. Everybody tells us the same thing. So why don't you get it?

There are many theories, some more credible than others.

Cost: Such a diet is much more expensive than one whose main ingredient is made of processed flour, sugar, and salt.

Access: Availability and shelf life makes the less healthy foods easier to ship, store and sell. Access varies greatly in inner city and rural areas.

Work: Unprocessed foods are harder to make quickly and require more care to maintain safe temperatures without spoiling. With virtually everyone in the family outside of the home during the day, the ease of preparation of less healthy foods becomes attractive.

Culture: We are surrounded by advertising for foods that may taste or look good or are convenient but provide poor nutrition. It is big business. Food stylists use glue, shellac, and many hardware store products to make the food attractive in a photo shoot. Including a combination of fat, salt and sugar in the same food can make anything taste appetizing. Coupling a pumped-up and perfect food image with food that is bad for you has deleterious health effects. It has been said that if there were a good profit margin in whole grain products, fruits and vegetables, we would be a healthier society. Fancy marketing has unfortunately shown to be powerful and persuasive opponent to good eating.

Prevention of original cancer: There is a significant pool of data that strongly suggests reducing tobacco exposure, maintaining a healthy weight, being physically active, and eating a healthy diet can help prevent cancer. Somewhat beyond the scope of this book, it may not be just coincidence that the advice is the basis for what we need to follow during cancer treatment. Due to the difficulties in isolating each of these factors in clinical research, each factor can be tested for a specific group with studies looking at diet and exercise very difficult to conduct as well.

A Cancer-Smart Meal Plan—Not a Diet: What Should I Be Eating?

The
LEARN
System©

p. 266
What I Am
Supposed to
Be Eating

A number of recipes from two respected oncology nutritionists are printed in the worksheets. These provide variety from the usual easier to prepare healthy foods. Depending on your food budget, culinary expertise, energy level and willingness of those close to you to help, smells tastes and the type and textures of food you can swallow make it difficult to suggest one meal plan for the many variables in cancer treatment.

Many patients have made good suggestions to others, and there are a myriad cookbooks aimed at the cancer treatment community. Some cancer centers produce their own self-published versions as fund-raisers for community outreach.

Breakfast (first meal of the day): *If chewing or swallowing is limited,* consider thick, smooth foods rather than thin ones and avoid small pieces. Yogurt smoothies with active culture yogurt (advantage over ice-cream) may be made appealing and fiber rich with any fresh fruit of the season blenderized into them. (Berries are ideal, but expensive. Frozen berries that are unsweetened retain much of the flavor fiber and vitamins in contrast to other frozen products. They meet the *deep color* standard. They also contain a good dose of fiber.) Commercially prepared supplements are fine but can get boring when you are drinking the same flavor day in and day out. The same berries or seasonal fruits can be added to them. Sometimes the sweetness is less than appealing during chemotherapy. Instead of ordering a month's supply through your pharmacy plan if they are reimbursed (some are not), try one can from the pharmacy's stock and see what sits best. An alternative for breakfast-type foods can be hot cereals. Why hot and not cold cereals? Cold cereals generally have a high sugar content, though the manufacturers are rising to the occasion and reducing sugar content or balancing them out with higher fiber content. Hot cereals are generally softer to swallow, with fewer sharp edges. Cold cereals with a favorable fiber profile and low sugar can certainly be heated with warm milk and softened, carefully on the cooktop or in the microwave. Whole wheat and combination grain cereals are ideal. Other choices for breakfast involve egg substitutes, which are almost completely egg whites (the healthier part of the egg), or purists can make their own with the whites of the eggs separated from the cholesterol containing yolks. In some parts of the country, the amount of cholesterol is lessened by the introduction of omega-3 fatty acids. Scrambled or even poached eggs slide down when lubricated with a monounsaturated oil flavored with a bit of butter. Soy-based faux sausage can be crumbled for a breakfast that can approach a restaurant-style offering, and when finely chopped can be mixed with the eggs to avoid scratching the throat or esophagus.

Such a focus on breakfast comes from a pattern known to oncology providers for years. People often say that they are hungriest in the morning, which is likely due to being without food at night and having the reserve energy after some rest to swallow and process foods. Such a morning hunger may then be the physiological result of a *relative hypoglycemia* (since no food has raised the blood sugar during the night) or may be the simple result of the idea of facing a new day with some optimism. Or both. Some cultures eat breakfast foods that the typical North American diet considers for later in the day; during treatment that is an artificial distinction. Bean-based foods, often with rice (make it whole grain) can be an alternative to breakfast food boredom. While traveling for business or pleasure, you may consider eating the local foods instead of those you are used to. This is a voyage too, so go to it.

Lunch/dinner and throughout the day with trouble chewing and/or swallowing: Soups are the mainstay of food choices, but not just the usual ones. Virtually any nutritionally solid meal can be made into a soup. The source of protein should be varied between plant and some animal-based products to get the variety of amino acids. Called *essential amino acids,* they are important protein building blocks that the body cannot make. Find your inner chef or someone who can cook for or with you. Since the concept of *blenderizing* foods can make anything seem unappealing, calling it a soup or a stew and it is a lot more appealing.

Weight Loss in Cancer

"If he'd just eat a little more…" Reducing weight loss during cancer: Weight change happens to almost everyone during cancer. It can be life-threatening. Sometimes, weight loss is the presenting symptom that brings someone to the doctor for a checkup in the first place. Once the presence of cancer is confirmed, weight loss is experienced by up to 80 percent of patients. (Weight gain with cancers connected to hormones, such as breast or prostate cancer generally occurs early in treatment; severe weight loss with breast or prostate cancer needs the same attention as with other types of cancer.)

One of the clearest ways to think about the relationship with cancer and weight loss is to compare it to earning saving or spending money: income, savings, and spending need to be in balance in order to avoid bankruptcy. It's the same idea about weight, in order to live well.

"Why do we lose weight with cancer?" is a commonly asked question. The overly simplistic view is that we are upset, and frightened, deterring us from a pleasurable experience like eating, so we eat less. The implication of that idea is that if we just *buck up* and try harder, we can regain the weight. Apart from being simplistic, such a theory implies that if we just had more willpower and a better attitude, we would not have lost the weight to begin with, or may not have even gotten the cancer. Extremely incorrect conclusions.

Weight loss with cancer happens for a number of reasons. Not all apply to everyone, but most apply to the majority.

The Cancer Itself

Growing cancer uses much energy in the form of calories. The energy is needed for the cancer to grow. It is theorized that the cancer cells can siphon off energy first, before healthy cells. Hundreds or thousands of calories can be needed. Then, how can cancer affect the body? It can grow in the area where it started, enter the lymph nodes (a waste refuse system for tissues), or enter the blood supply to go to areas far from the original tumor. Cell proteins released by growing cancer cells circulate throughout the body, and those proteins can enter healthy cells and put them in overdrive, expending extra calories. This is cancer-*induced* weight loss.

Weight Loss Associated with Cancer

Many factors and events account for this part of the weight loss.

General Anesthesia: This slows down or stops the large intestine from working. No food during those few days until the bowels start up again.

Chemotherapy/Radiation Therapy: Dry mouth and changes in taste or smell make eating less enjoyable and harder. Irritation to the mouth during both therapies or even yeast infections make it less pleasant, harder to eat, swallow.

Follow the Path of the Food and There Is a Reason Not to Eat at Each Point: No smell to excite the digestive system, little to no saliva to help taste and swallow, taste buds turned off, mouth sores, pain in mouth, too tired to chew and swallow, food feels like it gets stuck on the way down to the stomach, stomach cramps, sometimes painful gas collections, nausea, lower abdominal cramps, diarrhea, or constipation. Too tired for frequent bowel movements. Pain that discourages most activity. Poor sleep that diminishes daytime energy.

Eating Well Is a Lot of Work: Shopping, getting the groceries home, unpacking, cooking, cleaning up after cooking, and eating all need energy and attention.

Whole foods must be eaten by mouth. A variety of commercially made food supplements (not to be confused with vitamins and herbs, also called supplements) are made for various types of special needs: diabetic, lactose or casein intolerant, and gluten free are just a few examples. When that is not possible technology can bypass chewing-eating-swallowing with feeding tubes. The thought or mention of a feeding tube makes everyone grunt, but if it is needed, it can be a lifesaver. A tube placed through the abdominal wall with the help of a scope is an outpatient procedure requiring little to no anesthesia. Whole foods can often be put in a blender or food processor and be made thin enough to use in a feeding tube. Many commercially prepared supplements can be put right into the stomach or intestines where the process of digestion can extract the nutrients. These tubes can be an unpleasant but necessary lifeline. An optimal amount of *good calories* is ideal, minimizing those from simple sugars, which are *empty* calories. Monitoring the supply is essential. All cancer centers and most private practice settings have a nutritionist or registered dietician on site or available by referral who can help identify the foods with more good calories than bad and mesh those requirements with food preferences and personal dietary preferences.

Just maintaining bodily functions is specifically called *resting energy.* A fine balance between calories taken in and exercise needs accounts for the energy we use at all times (resting energy). Calories are of course spent with any activity as well. Apart from dietary adjustments, there is not much one can do to lower the resting energy used. So to minimize this energy loss, we need to fool the body. Some medications can help the body save such energy and the medications used are the same that help maximize calories saved, so separate agents are unnecessary.

Saving is the key area. Having the body retain calories as *lean body mass* (muscle) is the main idea of the story. Water adds pounds; fat has calories but does not supply the strength, just the heft. Muscle is what you need.

So how do we save lean body mass? It's a rather simple multipart approach:

As much as possible of the food eaten need to be made from *good calories:*

- Whole grain, slow-digesting carbohydrates (rather than sugars that break down quickly).
- Lots of proteins from a variety of sources that include *essential* amino acids.
- Essential amino acids are protein building blocks that the body cannot make, so they must be eaten.
- Supplements that literally fool the body by diverting the calories away from supporting resting energy and directing them toward building lean body mass.
- Fruits and vegetables of many and deep colors, the more varied the better.
- "Good" monounsaturated and polyunsaturated fats that do many helpful things, such as help absorb all of the other foods, counteract dryness from many medications and even maintain bowel function by keeping the surface of the stool slippery.

■ *This sounds pretty varied. What's left out?*

Sugared foods made with cane sugar or high fructose corn syrup (recently renamed *corn sugar*), carbohydrates with white or enriched flour, fats from animal-based sources. Doesn't sound like too much, but many of the foods that we consider comfort foods are loaded up with these ingredients, with significant doses of salt that keep them tasty.

Is *cheating* allowable? Well yes, to a point. It can be debated if these foods are really hazardous, but in small quantities, as a treat, they are considered *acceptable.* Virtually any cardiologist will give you the same list.

■ *How can the nutritionist or dietician help?*

A lot. Taking these basic principles and turning them into practical and enjoyable meals that coordinate with cancer treatment needs specialized guidance. Figuring out the optimal amount of calories and how to find them from the healthy sources is an important task. Each cancer center of private oncologist's office should have someone in their community that they work with and trust. Caution is key. Diets that claim to avoid cancer are not what's going to be helpful. Be suspicious of advice that omits major groups of foods. Be equally leery of anyone who wants to sell you their specially made product claiming it is the "only one" out there, or it is all you need to take in. This is a vulnerable time, and believing such claims is attractive.

There are points to clarify, with little hard information to back them up: *What about organic fruits and vegetables?* Is it better to introduce a small amount of dirt, or a small amount of chemicals when my resistance is low and it is harder to fight off infection? *Must I limit my animal protein sources to free-range meats and poultry or wild (nonfarmed) fish sources?* Though all are rather controversial questions during cancer treatment, though there may be good reasons to act on the side of prevention. An experienced oncology nutritionist or dietician will help you apply the information to your own particular circumstances.

■ *Shouldn't these dietary changes themselves be sufficient? Why do I need other supplements?*

Another very significant point. Expanding the selection of foods within the guidelines itself, however, may not be enough to forestall weight loss. Replacing the many thousands of calories, one needs to support the body is likely *not possible* with dietary changes alone. But any medications used to alter metabolism and divert the calories to building lean body mass during treatment cannot work unless good quality calories are introduced into the body.

■ *The mention of a feeding tube is scary and seems like a radical step. I love to eat. Why can't I just put all my effort into eating what I need to and forget the feeding tube?*

Sounds promising, but not always possible. If there is any sort of blockage between the mouth and the rectum, a feeding tube of some type is essential. For head and neck cancers, lung, esophageal or stomach cancers, the inflammation to these areas or yeast infections may make it too painful to swallow for days at a time.

■ *I need more information about feeding tubes before I agree. What should I know?*

There are many types of feeding tubes. One type, used in emergency situations, is placed through the nose and into the stomach. That is the type of tube used only in an emergency. Feeding tubes are small, latex tubes that are placed directly in the stomach (or even upper part of the intestines) and bypass the mouth, esophagus and part of the stomach through a small hole in the abdominal wall. A tube placed in the stomach is known as a PEG (percutaneous enteral gastrostomy). A PEJ (percutaneous enteral jejunostomy) is placed in the intestines. They are recommended in different situations, depending on the type of cancer. The tube is placed by a gastroenterologist using a gastroscope or an interventional radiologist under imaging. Generally, it is an outpatient procedure with local anesthesia and minimal recovery. The tube is fixed into place with a few stitches. In almost all circumstances, it is a temporary solution to maintain caloric intake. What is confusing and often causes a negative reaction is that similar tubes are used in the frail elderly who have not had made their wishes known in advance about their use, and families agonize over a relative without food or fluid at the end of life. It is a very different situation from the start of cancer treatment, yet the residual fear is that the beginning of cancer treatment is "end of life" and that once the tube goes in it will be permanent. Such an association causes a more negative reaction than should be applicable.

■ *Once I have it, what do I need to do to maintain it?*

The nurse or dietician from the practice where it is placed should demonstrate using a syringe and water to keep the tube open and clean. Blenderized homemade foods or commercially manufactured products can be put in with a large syringe, or even a pump to use overnight or that fits in a fanny pack that can provide nutrition over 24 hours. Refer to the worksheets for further information about feeding tubes (pp.312-313).

■ *I've heard that I can be fed intravenously and that can avoid a feeding tube. Is that a better alternative for me?*

Total parenteral nutrition (TPN) or peripheral parenteral nutrition (PPN; *parenteral* means "avoiding the mouth") are very purified formulae of nutrition that go right in through tubing larger than a regular intravenous line. Both need close monitoring with daily blood tests and are often started in the hospital, while continued at home with high-tech home care services. The amount of potassium, sodium, and other substances needs to be supplied within a narrow range, causing the need for tight monitoring through regular blood tests, daily when the system is started, and then every few days thereafter. TPN or PPN is an extremely rich source of nutrition, so concentrated that it becomes the perfect growth medium for bacteria. The major obstacle preventing routine use is the likelihood of infection, which can easily spread throughout the body at a time when resistance is low due to cancer and its treatment. Some erroneously believe that its high cost is a deterrent to its use, but likelihood of infection is really the main factor.

TPN and PPN do have definite and important uses in cancer treatment, where the benefit outweighs the risk of infection. In situations where there is a specific goal, such as before a surgery to remove an isolated metastatic spot on the lung, liver, bone or even brain, TPN or PPN helps put the body into "fighting" mode to withstand the surgery and recovery. When TPN or PPN is offered, the specific goal and endpoint need to be clear in everyone's thinking so that the burdens of TPN or PPN are worth the benefits.

■ *So let's assume I can eat and swallow. What should I be eating and how much?*

Here's where the nutritionist or dietician can be of initial help. She or he will need to know: What's your height and weight? Has your weight changed? Have you been *trying* to lose or gain weight? From this information your body mass index (BMI) can be easily computed and pattern of weight change established. *Unintended* weight loss is problematic if it exceeds 10 percent of body weight. With 10 percent unintended weight loss, the goal is to juggle a number of factors: general food preferences, access to groceries, ability to shop, clean, ability to cook, and access to kitchen equipment. Knowing if someone can help is essential. With low energy and little facility to cook, family and friends who want to be of help become key, even on a rotating schedule so that each one has an assigned day to provide the right food.

Eating adequate quantities of such foods is a challenge, when experiencing background nausea and fatigue. This is not a culinary experience. The calories—good calories—are essential. So if it takes a long time to eat breakfast, capitalize on it. It's usually the time of day the body wants—or will allow—a bulk of calories at once. Go for it!

Sounds like too much? What about a really well-prepared fruit smoothie with additional protein supplement? Fresh fruit, seasonal fruit, even some hidden vegetables.

■ *What about snacks?*

Snacks are a good way to sneak in some calories. Have the smoothie you didn't have for breakfast that day, or one of a different flavor. Fruit, yogurt, ice cream, or a handful of nuts. Add peanut, cashew, or almond butter, or protein powder to boost its influence.

Later in the day: high protein hummus or tofu-based snacks. Whole wheat bread dipped in olive oil? Try nut butter on something whole grain. Peanuts are good, but it can be made of any shelled nut: cashew, walnut, or a mixture of various types. Watch the salt in many shelled, nut products. Adults as younger children have peanut allergies, but it is way less common. You will certainly know that before cancer treatment starts.

■ *What are some lunch and dinner suggestions?*

Think soups of different bases: chicken, fish vegetable. Loaded with proteins and vegetables. Check out the recipes at the back of the book.

Eating is not an optional activity; it fuels the body during treatment and gives you the building blocks to repair. The first few days after chemotherapy are a hard time to stick with principles. Take in what you can, especially fluids, and then add the foods back in as the nausea subsides. If you're on the $5HT_3$ blocker nausea medicines—ondansetron (Zofran®), granisetron (Kytril®), dolasetron (Anzemet®), palonosetron (Aloxi®) with or without aprepitant (Emend®)—the first three to five days may be OK (eat the higher quantities as able), but the following days may leave you with a more subtle, background feeling of nausea, so eating on those days may actually be impeded.

■ *What if I'm doing everything outlined, but my weight is barely budging? Or what if I have lost a lot of weight from having cancer?*

Then food alone is not enough. As a general rule, supplements can make a significant difference if used properly. Two general groups of supplements are known to be helpful.

The ones that are helpful are *omega-3 fatty acids,* also known as "fish oils" or "marine oils." They come in a variety of forms. Prescription strength Lovaza® (omega-3 fish oil esters, approved to reduce very high triglyceride levels, a form of fat the body retains that can predispose someone to heart disease; used to be called Omacor®)

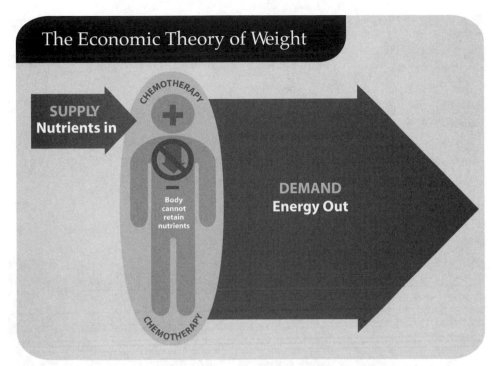

Obstacles to maintaining weight: The energy demands on the body during chemotherapy far exceed the amount of calories a person can comfortably consume in a day. Plus, chemotherapy can inhibit the body's ability to retain nutrients.

comes in capsules and can be taken with food. Omega-3 fatty acids are commonly found in salmon, mackerel, or sardines. Omega-3s help maintain weight by preventing proteins from growing cancer cells from entering healthy cells and speed up their operation. Over-the-counter omega-3s come in different products with varying levels of purity. There are two main subtypes of omega-3s, eicosapentanoic acid (EPA) and docosahexanoic acid (DHA), that help the most with the most effective preparations having the majority as EPA. They also come in liquid supplements that can be added to other foods. The capsules can easily be cut and the contents put in any food with some fat already in it or used on the peasant-style whole wheat bread mixed in with olive oil, sometimes referred to as the *ideal couple,* helping both weight loss and constipation. The more purified products have the remnants of the fish smell and taste removed.

Protein supplements that are usually sold in health food stores are marketed to guys who want to bulk up at the gym. Not the best for cancer-induced weight loss, this type of product is generally too heavily concentrated with one protein, often creatine. Although inadequate studies have been done on single amino acids, a mixture of proteins is probably easier on the kidneys, and during treatment that is important because the kidneys will be handling enough extra work. Adding protein powder to anything possible that is not heated or frozen, such as yogurt or smoothie drinks will help boost their value to the body. Whey protein is a better-tolerated alternative. Keep in mind

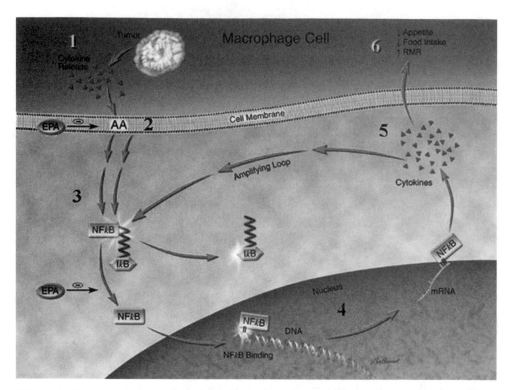

Slide 12.1. This illustration shows graphically how a cancer cell goes into *overdrive*. The large cancer cell absorbs the *cytokine* unless the EPA (eicosapentanoic acid, an important omega-3 fatty acid fish oil) binds the *AA* (*arachadonic acid*) in the cell wall. If the cytokine enters, then the cell soaks up calories in overdrive. Copyright Abbott Laboratories. Reprinted with permission.

that as a *supplement* it is an add-on, an addition to meals and shakes but do not substitute for proteins from many food sources. They are *in addition* to the many types of proteins needed to maintain ideal body weight.

Two types of proteins in particular have been tested. Carnitine (*not creatine* or the sound-alike blood test of kidney function *creatinine*) has been shown to blunt cancer-related fatigue at doses between 1,000 and 3,000 mg per day. What has been shown effective in small, well-done studies is a mixture of three essential amino acids: glycine, arginine, and β-hydroxy butyric acid. In studies of patients with pancreatic cancer or head and neck cancer, these amino acids have been shown to stop the weight loss and even help in weight gain.

These individual amino acid supplements can be purchased separately or can be bought premixed in a commercially available product, Juven®, a flavored product that is most effective in twice a day dosing.

Other medications that can help stabilize or gain weight are megestrol acetate (Megace®), one of the female hormones responsible for the monthly menstrual cycle and to support pregnancy. Megestrol has been tested in men and does not cause any feminizing changes in voice or breast development. Megestrol acetate helps weight gain, but it is a gain of fat or water retention rather than lean body muscle so it is

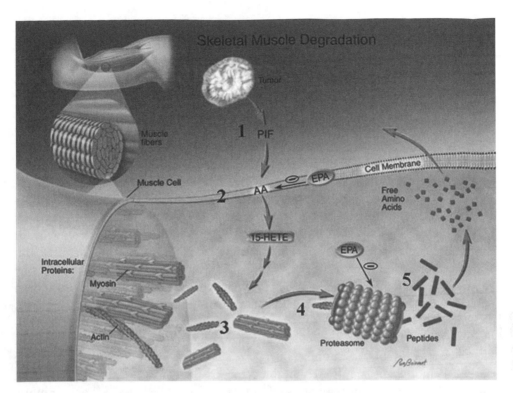

Slide 12.2. In a skeletal muscle (muscles you can control and that are responsible for movement and supporting the body's weight), the cytokines will similarly enter the muscle, increasing its need for calories, causing weight loss unless opposed by the EPA fish oils that bind the AA so that the cytokines cannot enter the muscle cells. Copyright Abbott Laboratories. Reprinted with permission.

suboptimal. It also helps increase appetite, though odd food cravings were a concern in trials. Odd cravings are common at the start of chemotherapy, a mechanism also not understood. Megestrol acetate is available in a liquid so that the whole day's dose can be taken at once. In a small minority of patients, it can encourage blood clot formation, so it needs to be monitored.

■ *What are the other medicines available to stimulate appetite?*

A very *legal* version of marijuana is available in capsule form to treat certain types of glaucoma (increased pressure in the eyes) or nausea/vomiting from chemotherapy. It has been tested in HIV/AIDS more than cancer, but is commonly used in cancer. It is called dronabinol and is marketed as Marinol® (and nabilone as Cesamet®). Its formula has been designed to give the least "high" while causing the most "munchies." Dronabinol although effective most often results in an increase in fat or fluid retention, so it is helpful in addition to the omega-3s or the amino acid mixture. A commonly asked question involved the use of smoked marijuana, which unfortunately does not make sense. Introducing possible bacteria at a time when resistance is low is not a good idea, and is often irritating to the lungs or esophagus, a condition which can be misidentified as pneumonia by providers not knowing about the self-prescribed, inhaled marijuana. Then there is the legal issue, which varies from state to state and is always controversial. For those of us who challenged our kids or have been scolded by our parents about smoking pot recreationally, it becomes even more controversial. Politics aside, claims that smoked pot may be more effective are hard to substantiate as one crop is not the same as others. Very savvy patients and families half-jokingly ask about baking marijuana brownies in a 350-degree oven, with the idea that heat may knock off the bacteria. It is safer, but not as safe as the purified product.

Still other prescription medications have a limited track record in increasing weight. Cyproheptadine (Periactin®) is an antihistamine often used for kids who get a paradoxical agitation from diphenhydramine (Benadryl®), which despite its sedating properties, is often used for appetite stimulation. It is questionable if the amount of appetite stimulation is worth the sedation. Thalidomide, used as a treatment for multiple myeloma but with severe side effects in pregnancy, such as holding back arm and hand formation in a fetus has also been used as a weight gain agent, perhaps by suppressing the same cytokines, as omega-3s or megestrol. Melatonin has also been described to have an appetite stimulating effect with questionable value.

Commonly used medications are *steroids,* are actually from *two* different drug families which have both been used in cancer weight maintenance. First, corticosteroids, like those used in arthritis, asthma, allergic reactions, or as an anti-nausea medicine during chemotherapy, are also responsible for at least a temporary weight gain during cancer. Unfortunately, the temporary effect wears thin in a few weeks. Long-term use of steroids can have significant side effects on bone health, mood, and reduced ability to fight off infection. Steroids do at least for the first days of use, give a kind of euphoria to some, making it a commonly prescribed item with limited usefulness. The weight gain from steroids is likely limited to water and fat as well.

A second type of steroid, like those used illegally in bodybuilding, is *legally* available for use in cancer-induced weight loss. Marketed in the United States as oxandrolone (Oxandrin®), it can increase lean body mass and weight. For some, in anything but small quantities, it causes unusual hunger resulting in overeating and a fatigued version of " 'roid rage." It is not generally used except for selected people where the side effects of the other appetite or weight stimulants are not worth the risk of weight loss. It can be of great help to selected patients.

The importance of maintaining weight is extremely high, and the work involved for patients and families to increase the quantity and quality of the calories as well as use supplements is vital and underemphasized.

■ *What about soy?*

The information is spotty. Concentrated soy products can reduce prostate specific antigen (PSA) levels in men with advancing prostate cancer the same way that estrogen does. Most believe that a little soy is fine, just as is an occasional tofu burger, soy sauce on foods, or cup of miso soup. The body does recognize soy *isoflavones* as estrogen, and it has the potential to promote breast cancer growth or suppress PSA. It is prudent to minimize soy intake, not avoid soy completely until more is known. Soy is

MED SCHOOL IN A BOX: WEIGHT GAIN IN CANCER

Why do I gain weight while having cancer? There are a few causes of weight gain with cancer. It is important for your provider to make sure that the weight gain is not fluid retention. Fluid can collect in many places: hands and feet, abdomen around the stomach and intestines, or even near the lungs or heart are somewhat common. Once your treatment team figure out the weight gain is not extra fluid, the most likely reasons are the changes in hormones connected to breast or prostate cancer and its treatment.

Hormones often encourage the growth of either breast or prostate cancers. In breast cancer, that is probably estrogen and progesterone. With prostate cancer, it is testosterone. All of these hormones regulate sexual function and the secondary gender characteristics: voice or muscle mass, and even hair growth. Let's look at them separately for now.

In most breast cancer, it is felt that one of the major effects of chemotherapy is to reduce production of estrogen and progesterone, which can often encourage the cancer to grow. Women just starting on their initial chemotherapy often experience sudden hot flashes accompanied by muscle and joint aches, acne-like pimples, and feeling that they cannot remember names or handle multiple tasks at once. As we currently understand it, these are signs of menopause that come on suddenly and seemingly out of place. This is almost like a quick onset version of menopause that women go through with natural aging, but not gradually. It is actually just the opposite of what most women describe about their menarche, the time when the menstrual period starts and breasts begin to grow. During that time, it can seem that the girls in the class are smarter, stronger, and more mature than the boys born in the same month and year. Despite breast development, many girls become leaner while developing fat around the hips.

That biological phenomenon is nowhere more striking than when ovarian control of estrogen and progesterone is suddenly stopped either surgically or from breast cancer chemotherapy. The hot flashes are the most obvious, and less often are the other functions assessed. It is usually a total package and is unnerving. Women talk about suddenly "feeling old," attributing to the weight gain, stiffness of their joints, muscle pain when moving around, hot flashes, and the cognitive impairment. A logical suggestion would be simply to replace the estrogen, but that is risky, and likely to encourage a recurrence more quickly, or even prompt metastatic disease.

So without natural estrogen or replacement in pills, weight gain is a usual and expected part of estrogen loss. The best we have available at this time is to be careful from the very beginning time of diagnosis and avoid eating foods that will put the pounds on. That news, hard for

continued

MED SCHOOL IN A BOX: WEIGHT GAIN IN CANCER

continued

anyone to hear even when feeling well is ill-timed when at the time breast cancer is discovered, especially if chemotherapy begins quickly. Being expectedly upset, the tendency is to reach for comfort foods which take different forms in different cultures, except for their striking commonalities. Comfort foods are usually sweet and/or salty, and starchy. These foods especially add weight at a time when we are most likely to cut corners on exercise, if regular exercise was part of the past regimen. The weight that is gained, as when menopause is from usual aging, seems even harder to lose.

For women who do not receive chemotherapy but have breast surgery followed by radiation therapy, it is uncommon to experience the same degree of hormonal changes directly from the radiotherapy. But often, soon after radiation therapy, additional hormonal treatments with or without chemotherapy is started in order to suppress any estrogen left. Those anti-estrogens or estrogen blockers do reduce the amount of estrogen made and circulated in the body, priming the system for weight gain, which is not really a side effect of the medication, as it is often attributed.

a good source of protein from a plant source without saturated fats. It is helpful in the healing process as a good quality protein source.

■ *OK, so what do I need to do* right away *to avoid estrogen suppression weight gain?*

The basic LEARN formula meets these needs perfectly. The general guidelines are the same: a diet based mostly in vegetables and fruits of many deep colors and whole grain foods. Protein sources from grains, nuts and dairy, egg products, fish, and lean poultry with less reliance on fattier meats should stabilize the weight. If following these guidelines is insufficient, watching portion size is needed. It is hard to apply the usual principle of extra exercise to the point where more necessary calories are expended than taken in during chemotherapy or radiation therapy.

■ *But I have prostate cancer. How does this all apply to me?*

The changes that happen with prostate cancer mirror exactly what happens with breast cancer. From a technical point of view, the hormone is testosterone, not estrogen and progesterone, but the effects are pretty much the same, with different timing. Men's development is not marked with such an obvious life event as the menstrual flow to mark the change from puberty through aging with its intensity and frequency. Testosterone makes men stronger and smarter, but the peak comes a later age than estrogen does in women. The peak comes in the late teenage years, and into our 20s, with a loss of stamina, muscles mass and an edge starting into the 30s and 40s and beyond, but at a very slow pace. It really isn't that noticeable until the 40s, and hair loss is often the first visible sign. Some impotence often follows, hence the big business in drugs for *erectile dysfunction*.

When prostate cancer is treated with hormone blockers, chemotherapy or surgery, a rapid decline in testosterone causes a similar effect in men that is seen in women with breast cancer. What is surprising with a fast testosterone decline is the presence of *hot flashes* that we usually attribute only to women in menopause. The experience is pretty much the same, feeling hot then cold within a few minutes and often breaking out into a sweat. Most men are astounded, and the adjustment to it is a sensitive point that has some men question their masculinity.

The weight gain pattern follows in a similar way. Weight may often be creeping up anyway after 40, and later, but the abrupt reduction in testosterone has a similar effect as estrogen suppression in women. The advice is also boringly the same: early intervention having fewer to no high comfort, high carbohydrate foods at a time when they are most craved, and following the hard-line dietary guidelines: rich in deep colored fruits and vegetables and whole grains, protein sources that minimize red meats, with few sweetened foods or animal-based oils.

Among is the most poignant moments in cancer centers around the world is observing a husband being treated for prostate cancer while his wife is being treated for breast cancer at the same time, both sitting in the waiting room and both having both hot flashes at practically the same moment.

■ *I am at two months after my chemotherapy or radiation therapy. This hormonal treatment will last for years. What can I do now?*

It's never too late; it's just more work and effort. No one really wants to hear it, but there is little alternative.

Obstacles and How I Can Overcome Them

■ *My sense of taste is "not right." What can I do?*

Taste buds are specialized nerve endings in the mouth and throat and most concentrated on the tongue. They are frequently affected by cancer or its treatment. Tastes are blends of five basic flavors: bitter, acid, sweet, umami, and salty. They each turn off and back on at different times during and after treatment, making sweet foods taste bitter or creating any other possible mismatch. Eating certain foods and not others, or having very intensely flavored foods can sometimes help. Using non-alcohol-based breath sprays or mouthwacshes can help. The effect is virtually always temporary.

During treatment, the fungus that normally lives in the mouth and upper digestive tract can begin to grow more rapidly than usual, classically leaving a *bad taste* in the

The
LEARN
System©

p. 266
What I Am
Supposed to
Be Eating

mouth, or even showing up as white patches that float in saliva or sputum. These look surprisingly like cottage cheese curds. This condition is usually easily treated, so if candida or *thrush* is a cause of the bad taste, something can be done about it.

◼ *I have too little saliva. What can I do?*

A dry mouth is listed as a side effect of many drugs used during cancer treatment. Radiation to the mouth can also slow down saliva production. There are a number of different products to try. Over-the-counter products like Biotene® come in a variety of forms: gels, liquids, mouthwash, toothpaste, sprays, or gum. Potassium iodide has been used for years to increase saliva during the mumps. Although it is a time-tested remedy, it is somewhat risky, as it can throw off the body's salt balance and thyroid function. There are a number of commercially made brands of artificial saliva. Pilocarpine is a prescription item that increases salivation, but can change the heart rhythm, so caution is advised. With a small leakproof spray bottle, an inexpensive homemade mouth spray can be made from water (tap or filtered, depending on your supply), a few drops of glycerin United States Pharmacopeia (USP) (in pharmacies for internal use, not in craft stores, which is not USP-rated), and a some grated lemon peel or other flavoring. If you add one of the alcohol-based flavorings such as those used in baking, use as little as possible. The glycerin keeps the water on the surface of the mouth and the throat longer than spraying plain water only.

◼ *I have too much saliva. What can I do?*

Many medications have a drying effect. Over-the-counter phenylepherine or other decongestant, old fashioned diphenhydramine (Benadryl®) is more drying than any of the nonsedating antihistamines. Many prescription drugs can also help, and you may be able to capitalize on their drying, a common side effect, which would be helpful when there is too much saliva. Those that contain a *belladonna alkaloid* such as Donnatal® or hyosciamine, both used for irritable bowel, are particularly good. Pain medicines or anything that is constipating can also help, though using pain medicine as a drying agent is generally not the best idea unless there is no other response to any of the other medications. A prescription item cevimeline (Evoxac®) can also help.

Over the counter guaifenesin (Mucinex® and others) thins thick secretions and is often preferred to a drying agent since comfort is the goal. Often trying one at a time is necessary to see which approach helps the most.

◼ *It hurts to chew. Any suggestions?*

Blenders and food processors can make most foods smooth and easy as well as safe to swallow without chewing. Almost always, thicker liquids are easier than thinner liquids. The idea of blenderized anything is not a food prep technique that most people would find appealing. But as a preferred alternative to commercially prepared supplements, almost any food can be made tasty. Often it means intensifying the flavor with extra nonsalt seasoning. It will take some trial and error to adapt your favorite recipes to approximate the taste of its non-blenderized version.

■ *I have cancer of the esophagus, head and neck, or stomach. I am told I need a feeding tube. Is there an alternative?*

Although it seems excessive, having the feeding tube can be lifesaving during treatment for certain types of cancer. If it is too hard or painful to chew or swallow, it will be close to impossible to get even the minimum number of calories into the body. Ask your oncology treatment team for guidance. Generally speaking, a feeding tube should be recommended for any cancer to be treated that is located between the tip of the nose and the stomach—mouth, throat, esophagus, gastric cancers. If you're losing more than the 10 percent of your ideal body weight, a feeding tube may be suggested no matter where the cancer started, so that you can replace the calories before your body notices the effects of poor nutritional intake.

■ *For the first time in my life, I am very constipated. What can I do?*

As soon pain medicines are started, stool softeners should be started preventively. Stool softeners are not laxatives. Docusate (Colace® and others) draw water into the stool, which makes it more pliable and makes you strain less. Docusate with fluid and fiber should be prescribed with the first dose of pain medicines, though often neglected or comes as an afterthought. Fiber to *bulk up* the stool also helps, but sometimes feeling full on fiber means you don't want to eat. Adding some unsaturated fat to the diet also helps keep the stool more *slippery* on the outside. A tablespoon of olive oil (or canola oil) with the beginning of lunch and dinner can help, but careful not to aspirate it (feeling like the oil is going into the lungs by coughing or talking while swallowing). Dipping some whole grain bread in the oil as in an upscale restaurant makes aspiration less likely. Glycerin suppositories help in the same way, but in just a few minutes.

Once constipation occurs of if the softeners and oil are not strong enough, there are a series of laxatives. The basic principle is to start with the least noxious ones and progress only as needed in a step-wise format (see the Constipation Ladder). Glycerine suppositories moistened with warm water then inserted into the rectum are often helpful as local lubrication. For non-diabetics, pitted prunes or prune juice are gentle stimulants. They actually irritate inside of the intestines that the body wants to expel the stool. Cascara is an inexpensive similar product. Mixed with docusate, it is known as Peri-Colace®. Senna also is popular, in tea or in capsules, as it has the reputation of being *natural.* Bisacodyl (Dulcolax® and others) comes in tablets that work in about six to eight hours, but in suppository form can help more quickly, in 15 minutes to one hour. Milk of magnesia is a time-honored standby as long as you have good kidney function. When mixed with cascara, it is sometimes referred to as a "black and white," homage to the soda fountain drink of the same name. Lactulose is a man-made sugar that also irritates inside of the intestines. Diabetics may find their blood sugars rise from lactulose. Over-the-counter Miralax (polyethylene glycol) acts by adding a soluble heavy substance to push the stool along through the intestines. Go-Lytely® has the same active ingredient but comes with salts and is made to be taken with a lot of water to replace the salts and fluids that leave the body when you clean out for

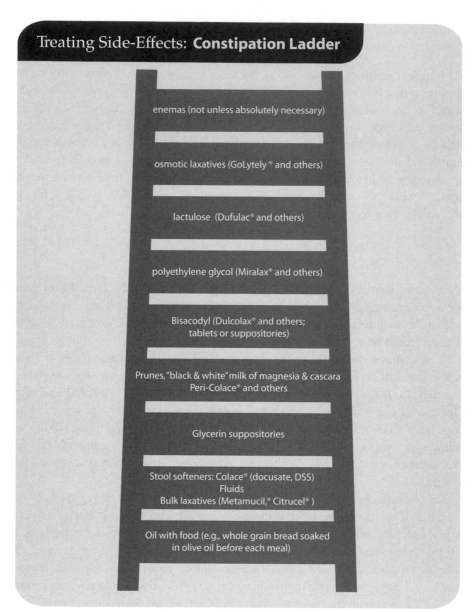

Treating Side-Effects: **Constipation Ladder**

enemas (not unless absolutely necessary)

osmotic laxatives (GoLytely ® and others)

lactulose (Dufulac® and others)

polyethylene glycol (Miralax® and others)

Bisacodyl (Dulcolax® and others;
tablets or suppositories)

Prunes,"black & white"milk of magnesia & cascara
Peri-Colace® and others

Glycerin suppositories

Stool softeners: Colace® (docusate, DSS)
Fluids
Bulk laxatives (Metamucil,® Citrucel®)

Oil with food (e.g., whole grain bread soaked
in olive oil before each meal)

Start at bottom of ladder, increasing dose if necessary. When maximum dose is reached, move to the treatment option one step up on the ladder. Continue up the ladder as each maximum dose and desired effect is achieved.

a procedure. Often used as a preparation for colonoscopies, it should only be used in smaller quantities a few times a day for help with opioid-induced constipation and to maintain good bowel movements. It needs to be refrigerated once dissolved in water to stay fresh. Use the colorless flavor packets that come with the gallon mixing bottle to vary the taste glass by glass.

Enemas or manual disempaction by a heath care provider are the last resorts as these procedures can be too irritating or even cause bleeding or infection. If none of these works, hospital admission is needed to administer very strong quantities of laxatives that are given in combination with intravenous fluids to prevent dehydration. Rehydration at that point may be the only alternative, and one that should be a rare intervention.

■ *Can't I take care of all this with my vitamins?*

This is an extremely controversial area. Vitamins are *helper* substances that cannot replace good quality and a good quantity of calories. Without vitamins, the body cannot process many of the foods we eat, but vitamins do not substitute for the foods. Vitamins are not nutritious in and of themselves. Some of us would like to think that a pill can take care of everything.

Vitamins fall into two basic categories: fat soluble and water soluble. The fat-soluble ones (vitamins A, D, E, and K) can build up in the body and be stored to toxic levels, so the amounts taken needs to be close to what is considered "correct," which may be more than the USDA minimum requirements. The water soluble vitamins (the sub-types of vitamin B and C) are only toxic at extremely high doses, and the body can most often dispose in the urine what it can't use.

Some alternative theories about cancer support the idea that if cancer is an *inflammatory condition* (which it is), then avoiding the inflammation with *antioxidant* vitamins can prevent cancer or keep it under control, or even prevent a recurrence or relapse. These theories make it seem as if taking antioxidant vitamins (vitamins C, E, and A) is helpful during cancer treatment as they can also prevent the chemotherapy or radiation therapy from damaging healthy cells. Others feel that taking antioxidants at high doses during treatment can also dilute the effects of chemotherapy and radiation on active or dormant cancer cells. Part of the appeal of the vitamin and antioxidant group comes from political advocates, portraying inexpensive and easy to obtain substances as being denied proper testing or merit as they are not profitable to a pharmaceutical industry looking for good profits. Some of the claims are theoretical in a laboratory but not in live patients, so critical judgment is essential.

For now, the sensible approach is to limit vitamin intake, unless differently instructed by the cancer treatment team, to a good quality multivitamin during treatment and then perhaps afterward, the oncology dietician or nutritionist may have some more individualized suggestions.

There have been some studies of a super-potent vitamin A for cancer prevention and to prevent recurrences, so the potential to harness these compounds after testing in good clinical trials exists but is not there yet.

■ *I hate to cook: What about food in cans or boxes?*

Studies that examine the merits of homemade food versus commercially prepared food cannot be conducted due to the variability in home food preparation. It is sensible to think that well-prepared homemade foods can be customized to individual preferences, and the choice of ingredients can be left to the cook. Controlling the amount of saturated fats, sugars, and salt in restaurant-made foods is hard to do as well. But any calories are better than none at all if the scale shows weight loss. People in remote areas have purchased foods prepared by commercial kitchens that follow dietary guidelines and can be shipped overnight express, but that is an expensive service.

■ *I'm not a chemist: Who can help?*

The skills to put together an ideal diet exceed what we all learned in school. Dieticians and nutritionists who have extra experience in oncology should be available in hospitals on site or by community referral through any treatment center approved by the American College of Surgeons Commission on Cancer or at an NCI-approved comprehensive cancer center. Oncology nurses and social workers excel at networking, as do office managers in private oncology practices. So you can ask them for a proper referral in your area. Look online at http://www.oncologynutrition.org or http://www.cdrnet.org/certifications/spec/oncology. The American Dietetic Association offers specialty certification to dieticians and nutritionists who complete postgraduate training and examinations, and the organization can help locate one of the certified members.

Under Medicare reimbursement guidelines, nutritionist services are reimbursed for patients who have diabetes or end-stage kidney disease, not cancer. Medicare fee schedules often drive reimbursements for private insurance carriers. Nutritionists or dieticians who work in collaboration with a physician, advance practice nurse, or physician's assistant can sometimes provide services that qualify for reimbursement. Some private insurance plans will even consider nutrition services under their complementary medicine benefits. It is important to read your policy information carefully or call your insurance carrier to verify the stipulations of coverage.

Part III

Make Your Plan and LEARN It

13 New Challenges

■ *No one understands my pharmacy plan: What are formularies, co-pays, and "donut hole" gaps in benefits?*

This is a quickly changing environment. Pharmacy plans come from many sources, such as private insurance, employer-sponsored plans, Medicare, and Medicaid. Each plan has its own rules, and plans vary even within insurance companies based upon the negotiated clauses in each policy. Knowing the rules helps you avoid much aggravation, many trips back and forth to the pharmacy, and endless calls to your insurance provider.

Prescription drugs, when new to the marketplace, are made by one pharmaceutical company and sold under one brand name in the United States. Although the drug is assigned a *generic* name, it is only sold by brand, which controls the pricing of the medication. After a period of about 12 years, when the patent expires, a drug can be produced by the same or other manufacturer and sold under the generic name. In a generic drug, the active ingredient is the same, with the generic drug having an equal dose, strength, route of administration, safety, effectiveness, and intended use. Generic drug producers can change the size, color, shape, and coating on the tablet or capsule as long as the active ingredient is unaffected. These characteristics can be changed periodically, so a generic drug from a certain manufacturer can look different when the prescription is renewed, but those changes should not affect its effectiveness.

It is a good idea to write down both the brand name and generic name of your medications, the dose, and the number of times a day you take it. Carry this information with you. When a prescription is refilled at the pharmacy or by mail, it is best to compare the new label with the name, dose, and usage on your list to catch infrequent but possible pharmacy errors. The Institute of Medicine investigated drug errors in their report *To Err is Human,* concluding that many can be avoided using better systems and double-checking the prescription. It is a good idea for all of us to check whatever prescriptions we get in person or through a mail-order pharmacy service. That same list can update all of our providers and be available should an emergency arise.

At times, some medications with *different generic names* are very similar to another one that may already be available in generic form, a *therapeutic equivalent,* and your plan may ask the prescriber to substitute one for the other. Most times, that is perfectly fine, but in a small number of instances, the effects are not the same. Your pharmacist and provider can agree if a therapeutic equivalent is right in each situation. The request may come because the prescription plan has a *preferred price* for one medication due to sales volume, and it can reduce costs for you and your plan.

With the intent of making the system more user-friendly, the pharmacy providers have grouped medications into *tiers* based on costs, and the insurance coverage for each tier may be different. If a medication is not on the approved list (often known as the *formulary*), there may be no coverage at all, a significant co-pay, or coverage only with *prior approval.* Getting such prior approvals is almost always frustrating and time consuming for providers and pharmacists. To protect privacy, callers need to identify themselves and patients with many points of information, requiring a degree of preparation for each call. Waiting times vary between providers, time of day, day of week, or proximity to a holiday and can be lengthy. Once the caller and patient are identified, often a series of questions follows from a pregenerated computerized list. These questions need to be answered thoughtfully in order to speak with the pharmacist or to qualify to have a form faxed so that a higher level of medical information can be transmitted to the provider to see if the situation meets the criteria for an *override.* Generally speaking, there is a short turnaround time of a few days, and emergency requests are handled differently company by company. At times, the medicine in question is being used for an *off-label indication,* a use that was not FDA approved, and the provider will not budge. Other times, there is some professional discretion that can be negotiated between provider and pharmacist. If there is approval on the phone or by fax, sometimes the prescription can only be filled if the approval number is written on the actual paper prescription or computer-generated order. If approved, the override may only be approved for a certain number of months when the process needs to be repeated. Such a system discourages providers from prescribing outside of the formulary, but since each pharmacy, carrier and contract has different rules that are constantly updated, it is virtually impossible for the provider to keep up with the lists and rules for every patient at each visit. Health care reform may or may not streamline this process.

A *step program* is not a plan to teach line dancing, but a way that the prescription insurance plan reserves the cost of the newer and more expensive drugs (*not* necessarily the most effective) to be dispensed only after the older, less expensive ones are used. Authorization often requires similar paperwork from—or a phone conversation with—your provider to verify a poor response to the agents on the lower steps in order to move to a higher step. Some plans, modeled after Medicare Part D Drug Plans have a *donut hole.* Costs are reimbursed at the beginning of the year until an interim maximum is reached, then are uncovered for a certain dollar amount of medications dispensed, then are covered more generously after that threshold is reached.

QUESTIONS I WANT ANSWERED

■ *I thought my pain could be controlled: What can I do?*

Pain is universally the most reported symptom during cancer. Cancer becomes painful when it expands near or in a bone or a nerve. Inflamed tissues from radiation therapy or chemotherapy can also be painful.

Pain can be treated with a variety of pharmacological and nondrug modalities. Although cancer pain can be variable, from mild to moderate to severe, it responds best when all the available remedies are used. Two basic properties of the pain, how *strong* the pain is and the *type* of pain, help determine what pain management techniques are needed.

Pain Measurement

Pain needs to be measured when you present for treatment. You should be asked at each oncology subspecialist visit to rate the *quantity* or the *level* (*strength*) of your pain on a scale of 0 to 10 (0 = no pain; 10 = worst pain imaginable). The *type* of pain will also determine what should be done. There are a few basic questions:

Does it stay in one place or travel around? Does it vary at different times of the day? Does anything make it better or worse (movement, position)? Is it possible to describe it in words like "stabbing" or "burning" (or any other)? This information, in medspeak shorthand, is the *PQRST* of pain (*P* = what *p*rovokes it, *Q* = *q*uality, *R* = *r*adiates, *S* = *s*everity, *T* = *t*ime).

MED SCHOOL IN A BOX: CANCER PAIN MANAGEMENT

Cancer pain is treated with a variety of medications. There is a logical progression from one to another, adding or subtracting and mixing medications of various families. It is not a random choice. Two very important principles of pain management are to (1) to try each medication to the maximal tolerated dose before changing to something else and (2) to take the doses at times that reflect how long the medication lasts, not randomly (at least at the start, to find the *minimal effective dosage*).

The initial choice of intervention is based on the quantity of pain. Since pain is traditionally measured on a scale of 0 to 10, the subgroups are as follows:

0–3: mild pain

4–6: moderate pain

7 or above: severe pain

For mild pain, often at the beginning or after treatment, acetaminophen is often the medicine used first. It is a good pain reliever for mild pain and also lowers fever, and does not act as an anti-inflammatory at all. Acetominophen is often used first because it does not make the platelets slippery, an important factor during surgery, radiation, and chemotherapy. Platelets are cells in the blood that are part of a complex mechanism that allows the blood to clot. Aspirin and non-steroidal anti-inflammatory drugs such as ibuprofen (Motrin® and others) and naproxen sodium (Aleve® and others) make the platelets less sticky and for that reason are recommended to protect against small clots that can lodge in the narrow arteries around the heart and cause a heart attack. Chemotherapy and radiation therapy can reduce the number of platelets, that are important to clotting during and after surgery. Since sticky platelets are so important, anything to make them less sticky or less effective is not used. For inflammatory pain *after treatment,* ibuprofen or naproxen are good choices.

Acetaminophen works effectively every four hours or so. To get the most relief from the least medicine, it is better to take a smaller dose every three to four hours than wait for the pain to get strong and take larger doses every 6 or 8 hours. In the pain

The
LEARN
System©

p. 251
Important
Blood
Tests

treatment world, that is called "staying ahead of the pain." Taking a half-tablet every 3–4 hours means you use just as much as a whole tablet every 6–8 hours and probably get more relief without gaps in the middle when the pain returns. Acetaminophen is marketed as Tylenol® in the United States, but many other brands of pain relievers and chain-store in-house brands contain it as well. It is digested in large part by the liver, and as a result, taking full doses for a long period of time can make the liver work harder (measurable by *increased liver enzymes* or *increased liver function tests* on comprehensive blood chemistries, a standard test; see worksheet with common blood tests and the normal values). Since most other drugs, including chemotherapy, are digested by the liver, keeping this system at its peak performance is important, so the maximal amount of acetaminophen should be 2,000 mg/day. That works into about six regular strength tablets or caplets or the equivalent liquid, with each dose about 325 mg, or four extra strength doses in 24 hours, with each one being 500 mg. Although the package insert or label information may say up to 4,000 mg/day, that has been recently questioned and really only holds for use of a few days at a time. Newer *long-acting* arthritis-formula preparations may stretch the time it's effective, but it still needs to add up to 2,000 mg/24 hours or less.

Cancer pain often lasts longer than a few days, so the packaging advice that would work for just a few days' use has to be adapted to its special circumstance.

If the acetaminophen dose is at maximum or pain is getting worse, the next change is usually to add or substitute an opioid agent, also called *opiates* or *narcotic pain medications.*

The opioid analgesics are extremely useful and safe tools against cancer pain when used properly. For those who would like to understand *how* they work: opioid medications reduce the transmission of pain from certain pain receptors all over the body, and at the same time, they calm the part of the brain where the transmission of the pain message is received. Their secondary effect is to provide a few hours of *feeling good,* known as *euphoria.* This combination of sedation and euphoria makes these medicines so attractive for overuse. Not so curiously, patients with cancer pain, even those who have had substance abuse problems before they developed cancer, do not describe feeling high or euphoric, just out of pain when the pain is bad. As the pain is controlled with a response to cancer treatment, the euphoriant and sedating effect returns.

Without having used many opioids in the past, reaching this point is meaningful to the individual as well as his or her caretakers. It is a confusing decision for those patients who have used opioids significantly in the past, whether prescribed or procured illegally.

Opioid medications, like people, come in families, where certain attributes are more likely shared. In general there are three families: codeine, morphine, and methadone families. Most of us tend to think of codeine as the weakest family. This opioid is commonly given for moderate pain after small illnesses or procedures, like dental work. Some states that tightly control opioid prescriptions with special forms or code numbers keep a few types of codeine less regulated so it is available to the public in emergencies. Codeines come in a variety of subtypes, natural, semisynthetic, and synthetic. The differences between them are mostly personal. Some people do better with one of them than the other. "Better" means more relief with fewer side effects. It is not just a term in the competitive marketplace that sustains the many forms of codeine sold.

TYPES OF PAIN MEDICINES

For mild pain:

acetaminophen (Tylenol® and others)

aspirin *

nonsteroidal anti-inflammatory medications *

ibuprofen (Motrin® and others)

naproxen sodium (Aleve®, Naprosyn®, and others)

diclofenac (Flector® and others)

meloxicam (Mobic® and others)

For moderate pain:

codeine family

oxycodone (Percocet® and others; long-acting OxyContin®)

hydrocodone (Vicodan®, Vicoprofen®, and others)

codeine (Tylenol #2, #3, or #4®)

For severe pain:

morphine (morphine sulfate; MS Contin®, Avinza®, and others)

fentanyl (Duragesic®, Actiq®, Onsolis®, and others)

hydromorphone (Dilaudid® and others)

methadone (Dolophine® and others)

Helper (adjuvant) medications: especially effective in nerve-ending pain (neuropathy), nerve damage pain; strengthen the opioids (above).

amitriptyline (Elavil® and others)

nortriptyline (Pamelor® and others)

gabapentin (Neurontin® and others)

pregabalin (Lyrica® and others)

corticosteroids

methylprednisone (Prednisone® and others)

dexamethasone (Decadron® and others)

* Use with care during chemotherapy and radiation therapy to avoid changes in blood clotting.

Side effects commonplace with codeine drugs are most commonly some cognitive slowing (tired, hard to focus or remember things, feeling that thoughts are slowed down), sedation, nausea, and a *group* of side effects that commonly appears together: constipation, blurry vision, and urinary hesitancy. They are to be expected and only rarely serious, with the proper simple precautions taken.

Most forms of codeine (known as Tylenol #2,#3, or #4® and others when mixed with acetaminophen), hydrocodone (known as Vicodin® and others; Vicoprofen® when mixed with ibuprofen), oxycodone (known as Percocet® and others when mixed with acetaminophen; Percodan® and others when mixed with aspirin) are available, and these are most often the starting points to treat mild pain that is responds poorly to acetaminophen alone or to treat moderate pain. They offer relief for about 3–4 hours at a time, wearing off after that. Optimally, for maximum relief any short-acting codeine preparation needs to be used at the least effective dose given every 3–4 hours at first, following a plan that *stays ahead of the pain.* It is necessary to take initial doses of codeine in this way for the first few days to establish exactly how much is needed for pain relief. This means being *on the clock* for those first few days, but is important way to find the least effective dose. Even a half or quarter of a tablet every 3–4 hours can make a big difference, more than one tablet every 8 or 12 hours. If regular dosing is helpful, changing to a long-acting version in this family (oxycodone—extended release, marketed as OxyContin® and others) can be given twice a day with a dose adjustment for moving to a longer acting agent.

From a patient/family education point of view, we have just hit a brick wall. Most of us read in the media about abuse of OxyContin, particularly when it is ground down and ingested in a way that was not intended by the manufacturer, so we think of it as a drug of abuse, and that is often an obstacle for most people who need legitimate pain relief. Taking a pill just two times a day instead of every 3–4 hours is a distinct quality of life advantage, but just hearing the name of the drug brings up many fears. Safe and thoughtful prescribing practices bundle the prescription with a written summary of instructions, including this explanation and the expected warnings about driving and using machinery when first starting the medications until it is clear that the drowsiness and cognitive impairment do not impede safety. With the first dose, constipation should be anticipated and counteracted with stool softeners (see Constipation Ladder on p.136).

The most effective dose is the smallest that suppresses the pain or makes it bearable, balanced against side effects. The dose can be further minimized with the use of helper medications, also known as *adjuvants.* Acetaminophen here is a common addition, as are other medications depending on the quality of the pain. There is no maximum dose of codeine. The dose is judged on the basis of effectiveness balanced against side effects.

Fears, real and exaggerated, need to be addressed with these drugs. Everyone who takes opioid analgesics (pain medicines) develops both *tolerance* and *dependence. Tolerance* is when you need more drug for the same effect as time goes by. It is predictable and happens with other drugs, but not as scary. *Dependence* means that even if the pain is well treated, it is extremely important *not* to stop the medicines abruptly to avoid withdrawal symptoms (nausea, shaking, sweating, or a rebound of pain). Stopping the use of opioid pain medicines is easily done by tapering down slowly, to avoid withdrawal. Medical guidance can be quite helpful if needed. Stopping an opioid should not be sudden.

The question about *addiction* is one that is worrisome for most every patient and family, and a serious concern of many providers. Addiction occurs when a drug is used by someone to feel euphoric or sedated to drown out bad feelings (anger, frustration) rather than for pain relief. With addiction, medication is often procured illegally either through nontraditional sales (buying on the street, or via a friend), misrepresenting to providers in order to get unnecessary or duplicative prescriptions, or selling or trading pain medications. There is some overlap between substances in that someone with previous experience overusing alcohol may also over-use opioids, for example. For people who have had a personal background of substance abuse or a close blood relative with substance abuse, caution should be high on the part of all prescribers to watch for any unusual pattern of usage. The majority of patients without substance abuse before their cancer can safely and with little worry use opioid pain relievers. Most of the time, patients are so over careful that they underdose themselves after negotiating clear parameters with providers, and the challenge is to optimize the dose to balance pain relief with worry.

If the codeine family at proper dosages is either ineffective or only partly effective, an *opioid rotation,* or switch to another family of opioids, should be considered. Another effective, but misunderstood family of pain medicines is the *morphine family.* The reactions to suggesting morphine are almost universal. They are most often negative reactions like, "(S)he must think I'm dying to give me morphine" or "I'm no addict." In the 1960s and earlier, heroin bought on the street was often erroneously called morphine, giving it—even today—a connotation of illegal use for addictive purposes. The idea that morphine is used to kill patients with end-stage cancer is also street myth, reinforced by film and television, where with a wink and a knowing smile, the dosage of an intravenous morphine infusion is elevated to suppress respiration so that a suffering patient or family member will be relieved of an extended period of dying. Such a phenomenon is truly limited to fiction in almost all circumstances. Most patients who have such advanced disease have been on opioid medication for some time, so a sudden increase is likely to do little except make someone drowsy, constipated, retain urine, or all of these effects together.

Morphine, ironically, may be the least expensive and best-tolerated opioid, except for the public relations and educational obstacles. Any opioid is metabolized (digested) into morphine in the body, so it takes less wear and tear to extract pain control on the part of the liver and kidneys if the end product is administered from the start. It comes in tablets to swallow; immediate release tablets that dissolve in the mouth; or liquid that can be swallowed in food or by itself, and can be put into a feeding tube, or even put under the tongue for quick absorption. As with codeine, the short-acting version lasts 3–4 hours, and then once the needed dosage is established, it can and most often should be converted into a long-acting preparation that can be taken once, twice, or three times a day for convenience and to stay ahead of the pain. Similar attention needs to be paid to avoid constipation and ease bowel movements. The limitation of long-acting morphine (MS Contin® and others) is that if crushed or split, the long-acting coating is interrupted and a lot gets absorbed quickly, defeating the purpose of the long-acting product.

Technology has actually provided an alternative to crushing or splitting the pills or capsules with the advent of the transdermal delivery system. Also called the *patch,* it actually contains *fentanyl,* an ultra-short-acting version of morphine that can be administered via the skin. It lasts for about 72 hours (three days) and works best when placed over muscle or fat, not directly on a bony area. It is a short-acting medication in a long-acting dispenser to get the 72 hours of relief. Fentanyl (Duragesic® and others) takes about 12 hours to seep in through the skin to the bloodstream where it is circulated, so when starting or stopping, a temporary dosage of a shorter-acting preparation needs to be available for the first 12–18 hours when the patch is applied initially. The fentanyl also is marketed in a transmucosal delivery system on a so-called lollipop stick, which is used in the mouth so it dissolves and gets directly into the bloodstream (Actiq® and others), and a very small patch, that is applied to the inside of the mouth for quick relief (Onsolis® in the United States). This small patch can be used in conjunction with the long-acting patches to better estimate the minimum effective dosage needed and use for *breakthrough* pain that comes on unexpectedly while on a regimen of long-acting pain medicines.

If the stigma of using morphine itself is not enough, an alternative is even more problematic from an informational standpoint. Apart from long-acting morphines or codeines, an alternative not commonly addressed in public is the use of *methadone* as an effective long-acting opioid. Unlike the other agents, it is neither the coating nor the delivery system that makes methadone long acting, but it is a property of the substance itself. Due to the stigma from use in methadone maintenance programs for substance abuse, the fear that methadone needs to be obtained in liquid form at a specialized clinic is untrue. Methadone used as a long-acting pain reliever is obtained by prescription in local pharmacies that stock it as they do the rest of the opioids, in a safe environment and following state-based guidelines for inventory and dispensing. It is the only real alternative when a long-acting opioid is needed and the co-pays or deductibles in the pharmacy benefit make it unaffordable.

Adjuvant (helper) medications should be embraced, not avoided. Helper medications beyond acetaminophen can significantly reduce the total amount of opioid medicines used. However, their use makes the daily pill schedule more complicated and adds additional costs of co-pays to even the most generous pharmacy coverage. Apart from organizing more pills (or liquids), since the adjuvants are mostly in other stigmatized drug categories, it takes more learning. Many people say, "Enough pills" when adding yet another to the daily regimen, but here the extra effort pays off. Sometimes off-label anticonvulsants (drugs suppressing seizures in epilepsy) or antidepressants are extremely helpful additions, *not because the cancer brings on seizures or depression,* but because some of the chemistry overlaps. Pain signals use some of the same neurotransmitters as those important in epilepsy or depression. The stigma is unwarranted, but still needs mention. Lidocaine patches (like the familiar Novocain® that dentists use for local anesthesia; Lidoderm® and others) can be helpful when used for 12-hour periods directly over the area of the pain. If that area is in the exact same spot where you're receiving radiation, be sure that the patch is not on during the treatment time. Lidocaine patches need to be placed directly over the painful area, exactly the opposite instructions that come with fentanyl transdermal patches, which are applied over muscular areas anywhere, a point of great confusion.

Topical aspirin has questionable use in cancer pain but has been helpful to patients with feeding tubes that have been in place for a while where scar tissue develops right under the skin.

Non-pharmacological ways of reducing pain also effectively reduce the reliance on prescription pain medications, but it is very unlikely that they will replace

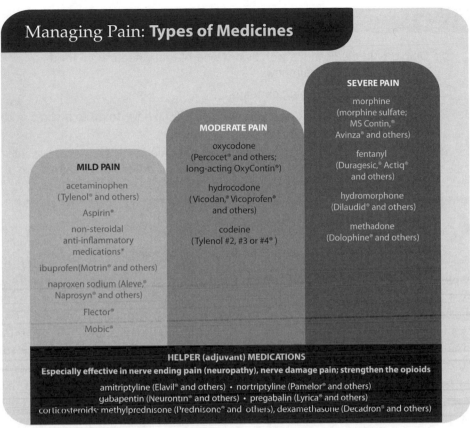

Managing Pain: **Types of Medicines**

SEVERE PAIN

morphine
(morphine sulfate;
MS Contin,®
Avinza® and others)

fentanyl
(Duragesic,® Actiq®
and others)

hydromorphone
(Dilaudid® and others)

methadone
(Dolophine® and others)

MODERATE PAIN

oxycodone
(Percocet® and others;
long-acting OxyContin®)

hydrocodone
(Vicodan,® Vicoprofen®
and others)

codeine
(Tylenol #2, #3 or #4®)

MILD PAIN

acetaminophen
(Tylenol® and others)

Aspirin*

non-steroidal
anti-inflammatory
medications*

ibuprofen(Motrin® and others)

naproxen sodium (Aleve,®
Naprosyn® and others)

Flector®

Mobic®

HELPER (adjuvant) MEDICATIONS
Especially effective in nerve ending pain (neuropathy), nerve damage pain; strengthen the opioids

amitriptyline (Elavil® and others) • nortriptyline (Pamelor® and others)
gabapentin (Neurontin® and others) • pregabalin (Lyrica® and others)
corticosteroids: methylprednisone (Prednisone® and others), dexamethasone (Decadron® and others)

*Use with care during chemotherapy and radiation therapy to avoid changes in blood clotting.

them entirely. Examples include massage, yoga, meditation, progressive relaxation (sometimes referred to as hypnosis), Reiki, tai chi, and hot or cold packs (careful— not too hot or too cold, especially for *neuropathic pain,* where the nerve endings are less sensitive). There is an ever-growing body of evidence to point to the usefulness of the non-pharmacological modalities in pain relief, but because they are complementary treatments, often they are not taken as seriously as they should be taken.

Neuropathic pain itself can come from the cancer or treatment, or it can be complicated by preexisting medical problems. It is a different kind of pain where the nerve travels along the nerve tract from the pain sensors in the hands, feet, or even nose, ears, nipples, penis, or vagina. When trying to assign descriptive words, most often it is *burning, pins and needles, hot and cold,* or *numb.* Neuropathic pain is a side effect of many medicines used in cancer: the taxanes (paclitaxel or Taxol®; docetaxel or Taxotere®); 5 FU; cis-, carbo-, or oxali-platinuim; vincristine; vinblastine; and vinorelbine (Navelbine® and others). It is generally temporary and reversible. The numb kind responds to medications the least, but they can still help. Rarely, when surgery cuts nerve fibers, neuropathic pain can occur, such as after the removal of a toe, leg, or breast.

MYTHS ABOUT PAIN MEDICINES

1. Opioid pain medications won't work when I really need them if I take them for moderate pain now.
2. Morphine is just for dying patients.
3. Methadone is for addicts; if you prescribe it, I'll have to go to a clinic and stand in line with a cup.
4. I will become addicted. (Addiction is when someone misrepresents their level of pain, tries to get extra prescriptions, or refills from multiple providers or buys the medicines illegally).

■ *Once I start opioid medications, will I ever get off them?*

When managed properly and with a good response to treatment, coming off the opioids safely and without withdrawal is usual. There are some practical guidelines. First, discuss with your provider first and develop a schedule together. In general, the shorter time you are on an opioid, the shorter the taper. Reduce the total daily dose by a few milligrams per day every three to five days. Three days seems to be the minimum for short-acting opioids. Longer-acting opioids, or a longer time on the medication, calls for slower tapering. Although it is counterintuitive, the last few doses are the hardest. Tapering from 60 mg/day of morphine to 15 mg/day is much easier than tapering from 10 mg/day to zero. It is best to stay on the long end of the three-to-five-day interval for the last bit or even increase the interval between changes to seven days. Mild diarrhea is truly the absence of constipation and can be easily controlled with a few doses of loperamide (Imodium and others; in tablets or liquid).

■ *I am a dog lover. It would help me a lot to bring my dog to chemotherapy. I think it will reduce my pain.*

Yes and no. Your dog may not be the best to visit you during chemotherapy. As well behaved as you swear your pup is, a number of agencies across the country train dogs just for such medical purposes and make them available to patients at cancer centers across the country. The Good Dog Foundation, a New York–based organization, supplies dogs and volunteers, *animal-assisted visitors,* to study the exact effects during chemotherapy and radiation therapy. Similar agencies dot the country. The hope is that the canine visitors promote a positive impact on quality of life, decrease the number of missed or late appointments, and reduce the need for nausea or pain medications. Rules regarding visits by pets (and young children) to health care settings have been relaxed nationwide, though this varies between states or counties. If you ask that your own pet be allowed to visit you, make sure that the dog's paws are cleaned to the health code specifications and it is trained to behave well in such circumstances.

■ *Who does what?*

To say that having cancer is a "time of change" is an understatement, but nowhere is that more evident than at home. Such changes affect everyone in the family. The patient is no longer doing what he or she did before. That could be less, or more. For some families, everyone pitches in without a master plan. Other families take a more organized approach, dividing responsibilities for as long as necessary. Most patients appreciate the help and resent it at the same time because they realize that they are adding burdens to those they love. Working within energy or post-operative limitations, getting things done around the house can (and should) be bona fide activities in the LEARN System. Those of us who have few relatives around must rely on our extended circle of family, friends, volunteers, and paid staff via home care.

I NEVER EXPECTED TO BE BIONIC: CARE FOR PORTS, PEGs, AND TRACHES

Yes, bionics are a part of most patients' cancer treatment experience. There are many types of devices used in cancer treatment, and some endure through "My Recovery Plan". *Tracheostomies* (or *traches*) are tubes put into the windpipe through the neck to help avoid any obstruction in the mouth or nose. When they are put in during an emergency, the location or handiwork may be less than ideal. But when one is part of the plan, surgeons can better prepare patients about what to expect and have the opportunity to make it look better. Some patients graduate from the machines attached to the tracheostomy and then, after a while, can sustain themselves on the air that moves through the hole, which eventually *granulates* and then closes up.

Percutanous endoscopic gastrostomy tubes (or PEGs) are placed through the abdominal wall directly into the stomach or upper part of the intestines. If there is a blockage or the cancer or its treatment has prevented the usual action of the mouth or esophagus, it bypasses those affected areas. PEGs need to be kept clean. They are held in by a surgical stitch so they don't pull out so easily. All fluids or foods that are smooth enough to fit through the tube can be put in with a large syringe; overnight feed can be put in by a pump; or feedings over the course of the day and night can be put in with an ambulatory pump that can last for up to a days. Most oral medications can be put through the feeding tube as well. Care must be taken to keep the entry point to the abdominal wall clean. PEGs are literally lifesavers during care. They are unfortunately associated with much struggle, particularly when they are advised for frail elderly patients who may or may not have cancer because local state laws insist that patients, even those who are seriously ill, must have one put in if they don't have an advance directive or written documentation. Caring for a PEG is not as daunting as it may seem—see the "Enteral Nutrition (Tube Feeding)" worksheet at the end of the book.

The LEARN System© / p. 312 Enteral Nutrition (Tube Feeding)

Even if you think that you don't need a feeding tube, really listen to the staff to benefit from their experience. A feeding tube may not be able to be placed once the chemotherapy and radiation therapy start because there may be an increased risk of bleeding or infection. Even if you only put through some water each day, that will keep it functioning until it is needed. Rarely does someone need to use their PEG permanently. Most patients can eat enough after treatment is over and recovery is progressing. As they begin to get more calories in through eating, the PEG is used less and less.

Caring for the tube and using it is much easier than it seems at first.

■ *I guess a* port *is not where the ship is docked. What is this type of port?*

If you are going to have the type of chemotherapy that requires intravenous administration for more than a few times, a *port* will likely be recommended. Slang for a *venous access device,* a port is like a long intravenous line that feeds deep into a vein. The catheter that is placed is designed to be there for weeks or months. Because of its long dwell time, it is placed under sterile conditions, using gloves, skin washing, and in a sterile place, turning placement into a surgical event. Many venous access devices are two way, in that fluids, chemotherapy, even certain feedings can be given through them, and certain blood tests can also be drawn through them. Those are blood tests that are not affected by the bit of anticoagulant put in the port to keep it clear. Many of these devices are installed below the skin under the collarbone, but some are external tubes through the skin of the abdomen. Some types used more for home antibiotic or fluid administration for a few short weeks can be placed in the forearm.

If you do have such a device, you'll need to verify if it needs to be *flushed* between scheduled uses. If you cannot do it yourself, a family member may help or a nurse from a *high-tech* home care service will flush it at home (or even at work), or you may need to visit your treatment center to have it done there. The type of device you have, your insurance coverage, and your ability to learn how to flush your port (or if a family member can be taught) will determine how the maintenance will take place.

If your port is to be accessed by a staff member, politely confirm that he or she is specially trained to do so or *certified.* If your port is below the skin under the collarbone, a special bent needle should be the only type used to access it. Learning how to use that type of needle is the reason for the special training and certification.

MY GRADUATION: HAZING IS NOT JUST
FOR FRATERNITIES AND SORORITIES

Virtually everyone has one of these *hazing* experiences. It seems odd, but it happens. After treatment, and usually after you're feeling significantly better, something develops: a cough, a bout of diarrhea or constipation, a pain flare, or trouble urinating. There may be a good reason for it to have happened. But the fear that it is a recurrence washes over you and can put you in a tailspin. That it may likely be totally innocent and separate and *not* due to cancer does not occur to you at that moment. Only fear.

When that happens—and it likely will—follow "The Rules." Is it a true emergency? (See the diagram). Do you need to call an MD or RN on your treatment team? If not, don't jump to conclusions…it is not cancer until proven otherwise.

Learn "The Rules." Rule 1: If it comes and goes, it's not likely cancer. Rule 2: If it comes and stays, it needs to be checked. Rule 3: Follow Rules 1 and 2. Rule 4: Re-read Rules 1 and 2.

Everyone goes through it; it's a rite of passage. Acknowledge it as a bittersweet experience and one big step through the process of healing.

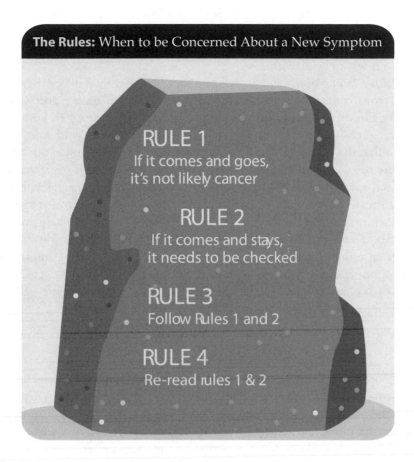

The Rules: When to be Concerned About a New Symptom

RULE 1
If it comes and goes,
it's not likely cancer

RULE 2
If it comes and stays,
it needs to be checked

RULE 3
Follow Rules 1 and 2

RULE 4
Re-read rules 1 & 2

Cancer Central: Everyone Needs to Tell Me His or Her Cancer Stories

Everyone "knows" someone who's had cancer—even if not your type; someone treated by the "head of the department"—even if they are not; someone who knows someone who knows someone else. Why do people do this? They may believe it gives them extra credit to not get cancer themselves. Perhaps they honestly want to be helpful but do not know how. Solution: Say, "Thank you. I appreciate your idea/concern/help. I'll think about it. I'll ask my doctor or nurse. I'll talk about it with my family. I'll look it up on the Internet."

The 24-Hour News Cycle and My Cancer

Before living in our wired world, there were many barriers to family, friends, coworkers, or neighbors who wanted to ask you how you were doing. They could knock on the door, send a greeting card, and hope for a reply or call. Now with a host of electronic media, e-mail, instant messaging, social media sites, and cell phones in our pockets, we are connected 24/7. Telling the story and giving the details cannot only become a burden but can also make things seem worse. When something bad happens in the world and continual news flashes pop up on our computer screens or on the radio in the car every 22 minutes, the constant updates make the event seem even worse than it was to begin with.

Technology can be our friend as well as a foe. Put together a list of the e-mail addresses of your concerned friends and family, and post an *update* ever so often to provide the information without repetition for you or your caretaker. Post the information on a social website. For those less well connected, change your voice mail periodically so that the caller can hear the information when calling in to your telephone. And be sure to say, "Thank you for asking." Callers get their *extra credit* that way.

Two electronic "friends" are already available to you. The American Cancer Society (ACS) features a *CaringBridge* on their website that sets up a system for you to communicate with those people who care (so much). The ACS also can help you connect with *Circle of Sharing* that uses an existing Microsoft HealthVault® software. DIYers stick with an e-mail group that they set up themselves for routine information. A writer-educator friend sends out consecutively numbered "Medical Update #X" to her circle of sharing, with a rundown of what has happened since the last e-mail and the next steps in her treatment.

■ *How do I know what to do next?*

Who coordinates the care? Start by asking your oncologist and oncology nurse. The Institute of Medicine report *From Cancer Patient to Survivor—Lost in Transition* has called attention to this previously overlooked need. There is little agreement about even the minimum testing or which services are necessary after cancer treatment and beyond. Traditionally, the period of time right after treatment has been an unofficial *rest period* without much other scrutiny until recently. By following the LEARN System all the way through treatment, you have a solid head start. The basic elements of "My Recovery Planner" using the LEARN System already have you being active, eating optimally, resting, and doing something every day that is pleasurable or meaningful.

Some of the most elegant work, in both timing and content, has been done by a variety of disparate groups: The National Cancer Institute's Office of Cancer Survivorship, the Journey Forward Consortium, American Society of Clinical Oncology, the ACS, and grantees of the Lance Armstrong Foundation have advocated that treatment centers develop survivorship plans that can be referenced by patients and providers alike. Though many have been published for breast cancer, few have been produced for other cancers. There is no standardized form but indeed a great first step has been taken. The ideal survivorship plans must include the things you need to know as well as the things you need to do (sound familiar?) as well as the things that providers must do. One main controversy remains: how many follow-up imaging studies need to be done and when. The idea that there is a so-called right time to do follow-up studies and what those studies should be is debated all of the time. Practitioners need to balance the potential good that can come from identifying a recurrence early and the risk of additional radiation exposure or risk of surgical biopsies of the suspicious spots.

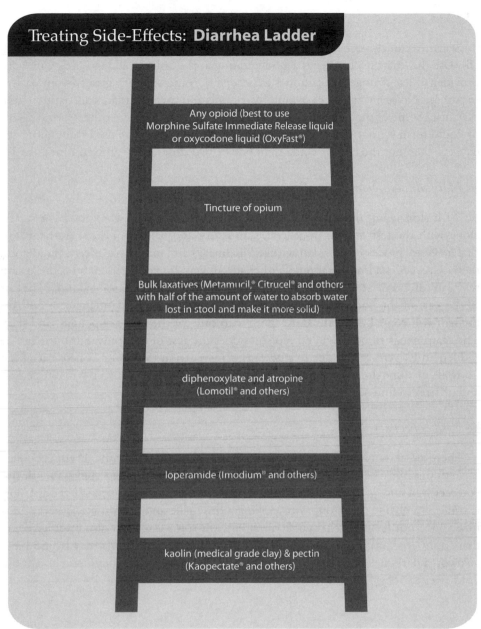

Treating Side-Effects: **Diarrhea Ladder**

Any opioid (best to use
Morphine Sulfate Immediate Release liquid
or oxycodone liquid (OxyFast®)

Tincture of opium

Bulk laxatives (Metamucil,® Citrucel® and others
with half of the amount of water to absorb water
lost in stool and make it more solid)

diphenoxylate and atropine
(Lomotil® and others)

loperamide (Imodium® and others)

kaolin (medical grade clay) & pectin
(Kaopectate® and others)

Start at bottom of ladder, increasing dose if necessary. When maximum dose is reached, move to the treatment option one step up on the ladder. Continue up the ladder as each maximum dose is reached.

Other items are particular to certain cancers or treatments. For example, it is common for the thyroid to slow down when tissues are radiated near the thyroid in the treatment of lung or esophageal cancers. Diarrhea is common, at least temporarily, after radiation to the pelvis.

■ *I have diarrhea, not constipation. Suggestions?*

Diarrhea can also occur with some chemotherapies, particularly 5-FU (5 fluoroura-cil). Use the Diarrhea Ladder as a guide, staring at the bottom and working with your provider to use stronger medications as needed. Dosing can vary greatly from patient to patient. No one wants to over-bind their stools and then alternate constiaption with diarrhea. Some of the agents such as loperamide (Imodium® and others) are available in liquid form so that small amounts, even a few drops at a time used throughout the day can even out the bowels better than one or two doses a day at fixed times.

■ *Maintain skin, hair, and nail care*

With skin being the largest and most visible organ in the whole body, it suffers along with the rest of you. In general, skin is dry and nails are brittle. Aquafor® or Biafene® are processed petrolatum (like Vaseline®) and moisturize nicely. If radiation therapy precedes administration of either adriamycin, doxorubcin, or a taxane, a skin reaction can occur at the site of the former radiation (called *radiation recall*). Hair loss to the part of the body that is under the radiation site can be permanent or perhaps the hair will come back thinner. Keep up with care for the hair, scalp, nails, and skin. The scalp needs to be clean and moist, as does the rest of the body. Sunburn can be sudden and severe, partly due to a *photosensitive* reaction to the sun. There have been no trials of minoxidil (Rogaine® and others) or finasteride (Proscar® or Propecia® and others) to find any special niche after cancer.

■ *Neither here nor there*

There are certainly pluses and minuses during this period of time. If you have sick leave or disability benefits and are not working, there's have unexpected time off. But you feel well enough to do enter into enjoyable activities. Treatment-related hair loss is still quite obvious, so along with looking a little pale and the fatigue, others recognize you're not feeling well. People often cut you some slack but also often give you that funny look, as if you are imminently dying. But some people may be kind and give you a parking spot, a seat on the bus, or a place in line. Use judgment; accept but don't overuse. Say, "Thank you."

14 Medical Problems I Had Before Become More Complicated

MEDICAL PROBLEMS I HAD BEFORE CANCER JUST GOT MORE COMPLICATED

True. As the survivor population grows, we are getting more experience managing the effects of cancer and its treatment on preexisting illnesses that we had before the cancer, even those not connected to it at all. Continuing medical education programs for primary care providers in this growing area are uncommon. Providers who see many older patients often have the experience to recognize when there is an overlapping issue that needs more attention. Is there an internal medicine or family medicine consultant who has experience with cancer survivors in your area? Can the palliative care service help? Palliative care is truly for symptom control, not just in the last days of life. Often misunderstood by patients, families and colleagues, in some settings the symptom management specialists who see patients all the way through their treatment and even as long term survivors are palliative care specialists.

Some of the situations that may get care from overlapping providers include:

MEDICAL CONDITIONS THAT NEED NEW ATTENTION AFTER CANCER

Diabetes (especially type I: insulin-dependent type)

Heart Disease

Ulcer Disease

Preexisting Pain Problems

Diabetes

The usual pattern of blood sugars can be thrown off by a number of cancer-related or treatment-related circumstances. Corticosteroids can raise blood sugars for even a few weeks after they are administered. Gastroparesis (slowing of food through the stomach and intestines) often gets worse after chemotherapy and rarely gets much attention. Any preexisting peripheral neuropathy is intensified by neuropathy from chemotherapy.

Heart Health

Certain chemotherapies, particularly the anthracyclines like adriamycin (doxorubicin), can affect the heart muscle and need monitoring after treatment is over. Medications

CONSULTATION IN A BOX: SLOW TO DIGEST

A 32-year-old man had been diagnosed with a neuroblastoma at his 13th birthday and was treated with high-dose chemotherapy and radiation therapy. Though his family was frightened he might lose his cognitive abilities (always in the top 10 in his class), he made it through without any discernable loss of his thinking or studying abilities and continued to do well in school, getting his graduate degree. His digestion, however, continued to be slow, causing burping, stomach rumbling, and the feeling of fullness after a large meal. Without the prior cancer treatment, he and his family would have thought he had a sensitive stomach or irritable bowel, but a low level of gastrointestinal slowing was diagnosed after imaging and functional testing. All were relieved he did not have cognitive impairments, of course, despite the annoying left-over effects of treatment.

CONSULTATION IN A BOX: BLOOD SUGARS IN FLUX

A 48-year-old man was diagnosed with lung cancer after enrolling in a clinical trial to test the use of spiral low-dose CT scans to diagnose early stage lung cancer. He had also been diagnosed with diabetes as a teenager, but with *tight control,* his blood sugars remained good with a proper diet and exercise. His endocrinologist was pleasantly surprised when the man he was able to go off insulin and back to oral diabetes medications. The CT found he had a small lesion, which was fully removed in surgery. During the surgery, biopsies of the lymph nodes were done, and two nodes had traces of cancer. So he was advised to take chemotherapy including paclitaxel. The premedication with dexamethasone (Decadron) to avoid both nausea and swelling worked well but sent his blood sugars into the high 300s (should be between 80 and 120 mg). Extra doses of insulin (called *coverage*) brought his blood sugars back into a good range within days.

that were prescribed to lower your blood pressure before treatment may have been discontinued during treatment may need to be reevaluated. Lipid levels can take weeks or months to return to the pretreatment pattern and can be affected during a period of hormonal treatments for breast or prostate cancer.

Ulcer Disease

With their particular affinity for stomach lining (gastric tissue), chemotherapy and corticosteroids can work to irritate these quite a bit. If you are predisposed to gastritis, peptic ulcers, or esophagitis (or have stretches in the esophagus from heredity, weight, or alcohol use, sometimes called a *Barrett's esophagus*), be sure your providers know that so you can be given adequate protective medications. This often involves mixing one medication from each class, starting one at a time and then adding on the next type to control the symptom without overmedicating: proton pump inhibitors such as rabeprozole (Aceiphex® and others), omeprazole (Nexium® and others), omperazole (Prilosec®, Zegerid®, and others), lansoprazole (Prevacid® and others), and pantoprazole (Protonix® and others); histamine-2 blockers like cimetidine (Tagamet® and others), ranitine (Zantac® and others), and famotidine (Pepcid® and others); protective coating agents like sucralfate (Carafate® and others); and antacids (aluminum and magnesium hydroxide or carbonate salts, Gaviscon®, Maalox® Mylanta®, and others). Since many of these medications are sold without prescription, ask for guidance from one of your providers as to which to start first, how to add a second or third agent, or to evaluate when more testing needs to be done.

Preexisting Pain Syndromes

These conditions may get worse after cancer treatment. Neuropathy may intensify. Any prior accident that has mostly healed, even from years before, can worsen, even temporarily. Intervention needs to be tailored to the limitations imposed by the cancer treatment. Ask for advice from one of your providers.

CONSULTATION IN A BOX: CAR ACCIDENT OR RADIATION?

A 50-year-old engineer was treated for Hodgkin's lymphoma at age 22 with chemotherapy and radiation therapy, which included his upper chest. Four years later, he was in a car accident and injured his neck, right in the same area as the radiation. Luckily, he recovered from the accident without pain and a lot of good physical therapy. In his 40s, he developed a relapse of the lymphoma, and during treatment, his neck pain flared up, with more pain than he had remembered after the accident. Careful imaging studies did show that there was no lymphoma found in the bone marrow of that area. He responded well to chemotherapy again but was left with chronic neck pain needing nerve blocks, physical therapy, and pain medications.

Following "The Rules" becomes ever important in this type of a situation.

CONSULTATION IN A BOX: JOINT EFFORT

A 68-year-old woman was treated for early stage breast cancer with a lumpectomy, radiation therapy, and an aromatase-inhibitor estrogen-blocking medicine, to take for five years. She had developed mild to moderate osteoarthritic from her 50s and on, which left her with mild morning stiffness that was made tolerable by regular exercise and over-the-counter glucosamine with chondroitin sulfate from the big-box store. The breast cancer treatment made the arthritis more severe as she began the aromatase inhibitor. For the first time since the arthritis started, she needed occasional over-the-counter naproxen sodium (Aleve) to diminish the stiffness and inflammation, which she kept to three times a week maximum. Although the flare-up was worrisome, she continued her activities and travel.

15 Hormones and Hormone Blockade

Hormones are chemical messengers that flow through the body. They need to be in balance, since their effects are so wide reaching. Because hormones are coordinated through the hypothalamus and pituitary gland in the brain, they each affect the other. Such interdependence means that they all have to stay in close balance.

Hormones are rising in importance during cancer in two major areas. Growth of two of the most common cancers, breast and prostate, is encouraged by hormones. These same hormones, testosterone in prostate cancer and estrogen and progesterone in breast cancer, may also affect energy, mood, and cognitive function in many other cancers as well. Since these are fairly new findings still in the process of in evolution, there are no standards to monitor hormonal function during treatment (except in the better established links to breast and prostate cancer).

HORMONES AND YOU

Testosterone

Testosterone is the main hormone in men that controls sexual function. The characteristics associated with men—hairy and oily skin, muscle development, and a deep voice—are all related to hormone surges early in the teenage years. The amount of testosterone peaks in late teenage and early adult years and then slowly declines. The decline is not as dramatic as in women with estrogen. There are significant changes that do occur, and since the term *men*opause is already used for women, the term to describe this phenomenon in men is *andropause.* Androgens are the hormone family to which testosterone belongs. Andropause generally involves a decrease in energy levels, muscle mass, sexual desire, and function. Hair patterns change, with less growth on the top of the head and more on the arms and chest. Some cognitive decline is thought to accompany andropause, and certainly some hot flashes occur, though much more subtle than in women. If we think of the many changes men go through as teenagers *in reverse,* it is easy to see how important testosterone is to every man's general health. From an early age, men also produce a small amount of estrogen.

While testosterone is present in younger men in higher levels, it overpowers the small amount of estrogen that men make in their adrenal glands. The effects of that little bit of estrogen become more noticeable when the estrogen is not overshadowed by the testosterone. Although we are learning more and more about the physical effects of waning levels of testosterone, as we are living longer the societal significance of these changes in a frail elderly population is yet to be explored as we are living longer.

In cancers that are not related to testosterone (all except prostate, male breast cancer, and testicular cancer in which hormones are routinely replaced), we are just beginning to learn about the consequences in daily life of the reduced testosterone. In the general population, about a third of males younger than 45 years old have low testosterone levels. In cancer survivors during and after treatment, about double that amount, or two-thirds of men, have low testosterone levels. It is believed from what we know now that the reduction in testosterone is responsible for some of the fatigue, deconditioning, cognitive impairment and sexual dysfunction during cancer treatment. The implications of these findings is now under study, and at some point in the future, testosterone replacement may be found both safe and effective to maintain strength and stamina during cancer treatment.

In prostate cancer, the lack of testosterone is more dramatic, since the reduction happens more quickly due to pelvic radiation or hormone suppressing medications to discourage prostate cancer growth. Instead of having a slow decline, men who have hormonal treatments for prostate cancer lose their testosterone (and their physical and mental edge) over a few weeks. Hot flashes related to the testosterone loss are common for this group and are at times disabling. Medications can reduce testosterone's actions in two ways. One group stops its production in the testicle by blocking the brain's stimulation; this group includes leuprolide (Lupron®, Eligard®), goserelin (Zoladex®), triptorelin (Trelstar®), histrelin (Vantas®), and degarelix (Firmagon®).

A second useful type of hormone suppressor works to protect cells from the small amount of testosterone from the adrenal glands. These *antitestosterones* reduce testosterone's effect in any tissues. These include bicalutamide (Casodex®), flutamide, and nilutamide (Nilandron®). These drugs typically are given along with an LH-RH (luteinizing hormone–releasing hormone) agonist or given before taking an LH-RH agonist. The term "agonist" refers to a chemical that promotes the body to produce a certain hormone or hormone precursor.

Men who have an *orchiectomy* (surgical removal of the testicles) experience the same changes over a short period of time as well. Before the safety of replacing the testosterone to natural (physiological) levels is assessed, the LEARN System can and should be used to conserve lean body mass. This is especially important to maintain optimal cholesterol and triglyceride levels for heart health. Using testosterone gel, patches, or implantable pellets that last three to six months after prostate cancer is controversial, as it is not known if it would encourage a recurrence. The hot flashes can range from minimally bothersome to very uncomfortable. There are a number of things to try. Off-label use of a number of prescription medications is reasonably effective with the proper instruction. Upon learning that these medications are approved to treat seizures or depression, many patients and families react to the stigma of the conditions they were originally licensed to treat, despite many studies showing their effectiveness and tolerability. Clinical trials have been completed on paroxetine (Paxil®), venlafaxine (Effexor®), and gabapentin (Neurontin®). Acupuncture and relaxation training exercises may also be of help. These treatments can either stop the flashes completely or minimize the number or intensity so that they are more bearable and less embarrassing.

Estrogen

Much of what has been learned about estrogen has been applied to testosterone. It has been long accepted that estrogen without the opposing effects of progesterone encourages the growth of many types of breast cancer. It is part of the standard testing on biopsies of breast tissue to look for estrogen and progesterone receptors on the cell's surface. Much of the treatment for breast cancer reduces the amount of estrogen made or used in the body in a variety of ways.

The politics of estrogen has been a large part of the picture. In the late 1950s and 1960s, routine *hysterectomy* and *oophorectomy* (removal of the uterus and ovaries) were perceived as a solution against fibroids and the need for repeated, smaller procedures for menopausal women. However, some perceived these as genderist and unfair impositions on women's choice, since most gynecologists were male and menopause is not necessarily an illness. With oral contraception and women's individual empowerment in their health care, many rejected the common recommendation for hysterectomy and oophorectomy. Experiencing more menstrual periods, using hormone replacement therapy in menopause or the older oral contraceptives increased the risk of breast cancer. The oral contraceptives that were first used in 1960 had formulations with much stronger doses of estrogen than what is used today. It is believed that those high doses or extra menstrual cycles without hysterectomies contributed to the increased risk and incidence of breast cancer today.

This historical information underscores why it is generally not safe to use estrogen to offset the symptoms that breast cancer treatment brings on by reducing estrogen level to a bare minimum. By extension, whether estrogen comes from a factory—or from a plant—from a theoretical point of view, it cannot be used to reverse the symptoms. That includes, until we have further experience, black cohosh and concentrated soy supplements. These are worrisome because they have been shown, as prescription estrogens can, to reduce the PSA (prostate-specific antigen) test in men with prostate cancer. So it is projected that they can have the same estrogen-like effect in women, risking a recurrence. Although sold without prescription as supplements, their safety for patient use after having breast cancer is dubious.

Whether either estrogen or progesterone can safely be taken with monitoring so that the proper levels for one's age can be maintained is of interest and be confirmed through future clinical trials.

HORMONE REPLACEMENT AFTER CANCER

For certain cancers, hormone replacement is advisable and routine. In testicular cancer when both testicles are removed, replacement testosterone and other hormones that are in balance with testosterone (such as thyroid hormone, thyroid hormone, various types of cortisone) should be considered if necessary, in consultation with the oncologist and a consulting endocrinologist. If only one of the two testicles is removed, the remaining testicle usually produces enough testosterone without needing replacement. (Some men may opt for a testicular implant that weighs down the scrotum avoiding embarrassment but it does not restore production of testosterone or sperm.)

Estrogen or estrogen-progesterone replacement used to be commonplace after treatment for ovarian cancer, but more recently with better responses to multimodal treatment, there is fear about its relationship to an increase in recurrence, so replacement is no longer standard practice.

Cross-gender use of hormones is becoming more commonplace in very specific circumstances. There is some use of estrogen in men with prostate cancer to suppress testosterone (especially diethylstilbestrol [DES]), which had been associated with clear cell cervical cancer in daughters of women given DES during pregnancy. Testosterone has been used in an off-label way for women who have had breast cancer whose sexual desire and function has been severely affected by treatment. There was a reticence to give breast cancer survivors testosterone to improve sexual satisfaction as the body converts at least a small amount of it to estrogen. It is believed that anastrazole (Arimidex® and others) blocks the conversion of testosterone back to estrogen; it is thought to be safe but needs to be tested as well.

ESTROGEN BLOCKERS

With breast cancer treatment focused on reducing estrogen to prevent recurrences, families of hormone blockers are often recommended in place of or in addition to surgery, chemotherapy and radiation therapy. These include tamoxifen (Nolvadex ® and others), anastrzole, Femara ® and others). These medications work by suppressing estrogen production or blocking the entry into cells on the cell membrane's receptors.

There are advantages and disadvantages to each of these drugs and new information is continually discovered, so the choice, order of use, and length of time prescribed changes continuously. Some minimize bone loss, others do not. Some are used to prevent a second breast cancer from developing as well as minimizing the chance of a recurrence. Some are associated with more hot flashes than others. This is an area that requires good discussion with your oncologist to clarify what is best for you.

Complicating matters even further are the application of estrogen blockers in women who do not have breast cancer but are at high risk for it with a strong family history and confirmation that they carry a genetic predisposition. One of your oncology sub-specialists may recommend a visit to a genetic counselor as you finish your treatment to review your family history in detail. Certain patterns of cancer in the family bring up the feasibility of genetic testing for patients and some close relatives.

Thyroid Hormone

Radiation treatments to the head and neck, lungs, or chest can suppress the action of the thyroid gland and result in symptoms that may have been prevented by early screening blood tests: fatigue, tremor, constipation, or serious depression. Such effects may only be evident months after the treatment is over. A basic screening blood test can be done by any of your providers. It is commonplace to be tired after cancer treatment, so the fatigue associated with low thyroid function can be easily misconstrued. So, having your thyroid checked if you have any of the symptoms may be quite a smart idea.

There is not yet an accepted standard of monitoring after cancer treatment that applies to all cancers, so therefore this is an important point of discussion with your providers.

16 I'm Not Spiritual: Am I in Trouble?

Spirituality has been long a neglected dimension in medical care. This makes sense in the context of the separation of church and state as a political principle in many countries with advanced medical care. The idea that spirituality is a personal and private entity separate from medical care underscores the political precept. It has been reinforced, until very recently, with the total lack of discussion of spirituality in medicine or nursing. As medicine and nursing became more pluralistic reflecting the various ethnicities making up our society, there was even less incentive to embrace any potential religious dynamic in medical care. The glaring exception has been end-of-life care where pastoral counseling is a core component of hospice care and the cliché of many a medical drama when someone whispers "get the priest" or "last rites." Spirituality was often relegated to such acts of final *reconciliation*.

I'M NOT SPIRITUAL: HOW CAN A CHAPLAIN (OR PASTORAL CARE PROVIDER) HELP?

Not limited to "strictly religious" issues

Modeled after Uniformed Services Chaplains ("There are no atheists in foxholes.")

Frame discussions of general importance:

"Why me?"

Cancer as a moral failure or weakness of character

Meaning of life

Burdens of care on family and friends

Missed opportunities in life and due to illness

Military medicine, especially during combat, also has included chaplaincy services on the front lines to cope with the impending losses to maintain morale. A common saying grew out of such pastoral care: "There are no atheists in foxholes," referring to the ground holes in which soldiers take cover during battle. Community-based parish priests or rabbis often visit the sick in hospitals or at home but were not traditionally part of the hospital culture outside of courtesy sickbed visits for parishioners and end-of-life visits. Surprisingly, the rise of faith-based groups founding some of our most prestigious medical centers and medical schools did not bring spirituality into the mainstream.

A bit in advance of, and in parallel to, stressing wellness in our medical care system, an interest in spirituality as a healing art and science has leapt out of its traditional role at end of life and is now recognized as an important component of the total care of patients with both life-threatening and chronic health conditions. Access to pastoral care is a standard of the American College of Surgeons Commission on Cancer when it accredits cancer programs nationally. Likewise, the Joint Commission on Accreditation of Hospitals asks that each hospital have access to pastoral care services internally or in the community for accreditation. The Association for Clinical Pastoral Education Inc. is a national organization that standardizes and accredits programs and providers in hospitals and schools.

Such interesting history has evolved quickly to the point where some patients (and even staff) see themselves at a disadvantage unless they incorporate spirituality in healing.

In cancer treatment, pastoral care is not just about religion and certainly is not limited to end-of-life care. You don't have to participate in formal religious rituals to have everyday concerns about how cancer will affect you and your family. There is overlap between counseling done by individuals in medicine, social work, psychology, nursing, or other disciplines, especially in this area. Feeling stigmatized at having cancer, questioning that cancer is a weakness of moral character, and questioning the meaning and purpose of life are universal.

Pastoral care chaplains probably have the most experience helping sort out answers to these questions all the way through treatment.

CONSULTATION IN A BOX: SUNDAY THE PRIEST WAS BUSY

A 98-year-old woman was admitted to the hospital after feeling very tired and found to be anemic. Imaging showed a growth in her colon, and indeed the biopsies done at surgery showed that it was malignant. No lymph nodes were involved, and the imaging studies could not identify any spread. Her prognosis was excellent.

She herself had not had much experience with hospitals or surgeries. Her post-operative pain was difficult to control due to her sensitivity to pain medicines, causing hallucinations as they relieved the pain.

Before sunrise early on a Sunday morning, she thought she saw a priest in her room which frightened her, assuming she was sicker than she was told and he was there to bestow Last Rites. As the daytime nursing shift settled in, she demanded that her nurse get a priest to confirm her "vision," but all but one of the hospital chaplains were busy conducting Sunday services. Due to her insistence, the available Chaplain On-Call, a Rabbi rushed to her room to see how she could help.

"Who are you?" asked the patient in distress. The Rabbi calmly explained that the Catholic and Christian ministers were busy with their congregations, and that she could call them in when done, but wondered what she could do until then.

"I don't think you'll understand," the patient said. "My training," the Rabbi returned, "has prepared me for many kinds of fear, not just the Jewish kind. Can you tell me what happened?"

continued

CONSULTATION IN A BOX: SUNDAY THE PRIEST WAS BUSY

continued

The patient, a bit incredulous, explained her early morning vision, and reiterated her doubts.

"The nurses told me your surgery went well, and that the cancer was very small. Nothing else was found anywhere. One of the nurses overheard the surgeon tell you it was his opinion that the cancer would not bother you before something else did. I think you saw your fear in the room this morning, not a priest. The Lord has not given up on you."

The patient smiled and started to cry. "I'm embarrassed for not giving you a fair chance. You know exactly what I am going through, and what to do. After I am out of the hospital, I am going to ask my daughter to take me to services at your temple one Saturday morning. I may need help explaining this to her, though. She'll worry that I am turning my back on the church after 97 years of going to mass."

They both laughed.

This case demonstrates the utility of spirituality in cancer care and the value of hospital-based services. Overlap between religions and the universal condition is stressed that overrides the technical differences in faith systems.

If your local minister is uncomfortable or not familiar with the texture of cancer treatment, your hospital or cancer center will be able to help connect you with someone who is more comfortable exploring this dimension of care with you. For more information, visit the website of the Association of Clinical Pastoral Education (http://www.acpe.edu) or Healthcare Chaplaincy Inc. (http://www.healthcare chaplaincy.org).

17 Finding My Way Back Is Not What I Thought but Is Possible

Many patients never thought about what it would be like to get better. They were so focused on not having the chance to get better that the recovery part never occurred to them, and they couldn't think about what it would feel like. Some could only prepare for the worst, not the best.

A diagnosis of cancer is frightening. Patients are so burdened when they "hear the word" and then about the treatment that they never get around to thinking about what it would be like to get better. Whether out of superstition, exhaustion, or both, early affirmation of the work to be done in survivorship helps open the possibility for the future.

■ *I just thought that I'd get better on my own. No one warned me it would be like this. How come?*

The answer has a few dimensions. In the cancer treatment world, it is pretty much accepted that most people absorb about 40 percent of the information given at the time of first consult. The process of recovery was likely mentioned, but it was too remote to consider if survival was the most important thing addressed. Fully detailed discussion may have even been minimized for fear that it would provide too much information too soon. The process might sound so burdensome that you would not give it a chance or be more than could be absorbed at that moment.

■ *As time goes by, for the most part I am feeling better, but I find myself getting angry that I'm not fully better and not feeling better fast enough. Some things are just plain annoying, and I try not to think about them. Why can't I be more grateful?*

What would have been considered minor things when you thought you would not survive treatment are now annoyances and seem like impediments to a good life. The exact incursions on daily life vary by age, type of cancer and treatment received. Certain odors, itchy skin, having to find a bathroom quickly, needing to scope out a handrail walking down steps or a tired feeling that unpredictably comes on in waves are the types of situations that patients describe. Unfair—but many make peace and allow these impairments to be part of their lives and work with or around them.

■ *Whom can I turn to? Who understands?*

Here is where a community of veteran patients makes a contribution to healing that no one else can. A survivorship group in person near where you live, on the telephone, or online can help bring together those who have been equally frustrated at

CONSULTATION IN A BOX: A NEW DESIGN

A 58-year-old woman who works as a dress and hat designer developed ovarian cancer, discovered when she had pain on her right side and went to her primary care doctor. Luckily, the cancer was limited to the ovary. She underwent quite a bit of treatment: removal of both ovaries; intravenous chemotherapy with paclitaxel, carboplatinum, and bevacizumab; and then peritoneal washings of paclitaxel through an intraperitoneal stent. She recovered slowly and well, though she was left with persistent peripheral neuropathy. At first she was relieved to be alive and to have survived the cancer and the treatment, and she was proud to be able to go back to work after a seventh-month absence. She followed the LEARN System, which got her back to her yoga class and maintained her weight during treatment. She avoided hospitalizations completely after the initial surgery.

What she did not adjust to so easily was the neuropathy. Working "like my grandmother taught me," she did not rely on a seamstress to make her sample dresses and hats but did so herself with the help of only one assistant. Her hand-sewing skills were impaired. Despite exercises and multiple medication trials, the feeling of pins and needles in her hands were less intense, but her sewing was "not as exact as it used to be." "It no longer hurts to use such a small needle and thread," she would say in exasperation, "but it just does not look as pretty—or crisp—as it once did." She needed to rely on others to do the handiwork, which disappointed her until she discovered that she could sketch the stitches on a computer screen for someone to follow. "It's OK," she said, "that I learned computer-assisted design. But my grandmother would certainly not approve."

the end of their treatment and those who have found creative solutions. Many patients scoff at the idea of a support group, assuming they are not joiners. These tricks, coping mechanisms, and shared experiences that other survivors can give you can be extremely valuable. So don't count yourself out.

Alternatively, individual counseling is particularly helpful for this type of a stumbling block. Such counseling, which is targeted at cancer survivorship, is available locally through a number of sources. Oncologists of any subspecialty, or their oncology nurse or office manager depending on the setting, will know clinicians in your area that they have referred other patients to with a satisfactory result. The approved cancer center or program will also have counselors on site or can provide a referral. Some will even be in your insurance plan network. A local chapter of the American Cancer Society will also be helpful about knowing who is in your community. If such services are not available locally, reach out to CancerCare, the national organization whose mission is to provide counseling and even some financial assistance for individuals with cancer and their families (http://www.cancercare.org or 1-800-813-HOPE). The American Psychosocial Oncology Society helpline (http://

www.apos-society.org or 1-866-276-7443) can also locate services close to home. The Wellness Community (http://www.thewellnesscommunity.org), also a nonprofit group, has centers in various cities, as does Gilda's Club (http://www.gildasclub.org), named in memory of Gilda Radner of "Saturday Night Live," except that the centers are called clubhouses.

Using the electronic medium to its fullest, the American Cancer Society has duplicated the discussion points from their live, in-person series *I Can Cope* and put them online at http://www.cancer.org/Treatment/SupportProgramsServices/Programs/Participateina-CancerEducationClass/ICanCopeOnline/index. If you live too far from a center that features *I Can Cope* or feel too tired to travel, this online resource is a great option.

◼ *I can't believe my sexual desire has changed so much. Is this forever?*

No, the amount of fatigue, hormonal changes, psychological distress, social disharmony, and general fear often places sex way down on the priority list—for now. You will experience reawakening of your sexual function slowly as treatment ends. For now, try to continue to be intimate with anyone you are close to already, even if it omits sex. If you can, bring it up with your partner. Your partner likely does not want to burden you. Just spending some intimate time together when possible doing intimate things is the key to bridge your relationship until both your desire and function return. Depending on the type of cancer you have and the treatment you are starting, some of the intimate moments may seem ridiculous or impossible. You may not want your partner to see you with a _____ or without a _____, or with a tube from your _____ (you can fill in what reflects your situation). Hugging, snuggling (if possible without causing pain), or just spending time together close by each other watching a movie or listening to music can be restorative. Your spouse or partner has been through a bevy of feelings along with you. He or she has not been the focus of attention. They have experienced your cancer diagnosis vicariously, living it through your experiences. Their estimation of your suffering may be even more profound than expected since it is magnified by their frustration that they can't take your cancer away.

In parallel to the information and services available for the identified patient are a myriad of resources for family members and close friends. Each of the organizations in the resources list has specially tailored programs for those whose lives have been changed by someone they love with cancer. Use them!

With the additional time burdens of caretaking, online and telephone services are more accessible to caretakers than those offered in person.

◼ *Where can I get more and reliable information?*

American Cancer Society (ACS)
National Cancer Institute (NCI)
Cancer*Care*
American College of Cancer Survivors (ACoS)

See the list of Trusted Internet Sites at the end of the Resources section at the back of the book.

The LEARN System©

p. 338
Trusted Internet Sites

Part IV

The First Three Months after Treatment

18 Living beyond Cancer—
The First Three Months

You've reached a milestone. If you think about how you felt right after treatment, you're now a world away. So why don't you feel 100 percent better? Well, it's still too soon. If you've had a lot of chemotherapy, radiation therapy, or both together, and a surgery thrown in, you're still healing. Knowing that the passage of time will bring further healing remains a frustration if you'd like to feel better right away. Through the LEARN System, you are speeding up the process, but it is not instantaneous. That's not always easy to say or admit in public, but it's probably true. You're asking yourself, "What if I still have cancer (*residual*) or what if I am having a relapse or recurrence? Has all of this effort, suffering, fright been for nothing?" Well, perhaps...but not likely. When patients are asked about their reaction when residual cancer, a recurrence, or a relapse is found, responses are about 50/50. Some people say, "I feel cheated. I was able to endure the last few months with the idea that I could be cured, be done with all of this and get on with my life. I don't know if I can muster up that hopefulness again." Others say just the opposite. "Look, I'm alive. I want to stay that way. I'll do whatever I have to. I know what to do. I know how to handle the side effects. If I have to work at getting better for a longer period of time, I will do it." Two completely different responses, with a range in between—are you surprised?

SEE HOW FAR I HAVE COME

You will see that that as the weeks go by, your worksheet entries change. Moving on from immediate concerns, the scope of your content will likely show that you are looking beyond the immediate day-to-day concerns about day-to-day symptoms and looking at longer-term ideas. As you are feeling better, but not back to how you felt before the initial diagnosis, you can see some light at the end of the proverbial tunnel.

ADJUSTMENTS TO THE LEARN SYSTEM

Here's where things get very individual and personal. What concerns you now very much depends upon who you are, how you spend your time, and how much control you have over your immediate future. Make sure to think about what needs work *now*. Universal concerns are almost always about appearance and reentry into the world of people who have not had cancer treatment.

Living

Think about what concerns you the most now, like feeling better and sustaining a remission. Try to figure out the things you *can do* within the limitations of your energy to get back to whatever gives meaning to your life. You may or may not be working or be back at school yet. You may or may not need less help around the house. What has helped sustain you, and how is that helping now? Have you read a memorable book or magazine article you would not have gotten to otherwise? Have family members or friends surprised you by helping more than you could have imagined, even if it was as simple as a phone call or an e-mail? Have your children been a little less self-involved than they have before?

The *L* function of the LEARN System now becomes one of planning for a future of uncertainty. You may be saying to yourself, "How is that possible?" It is. This type of planning requires you to make two simultaneous plans: one if you will need monitoring and more treatment, and one in which you will need monitoring but not more treatment. That is a hard process, since your plans affect many people: your family and friends, your co-workers, the other parents in the car pool, and whomever you join forces with to carry out your daily tasks. But for the moment, turn off the music or television and your cell phone. Think of what your life will be like in three months or six months from now.

Education

The main skill you are relying on is patience. You are still not sure how enduring your response to treatment is, even with optimistic initial reports. But of course, you want to be as hopeful as possible. What practical things do you need to know or do now? This is the time to review the bills you have left in the pile and make sure that your insurance is keeping up with the charges you have incurred. Do the same for any household expenses. You probably postponed some of the regularly scheduled aspects of daily life, and depending upon where you live and the time of the year, it would be a good idea to make sure that none of these practical things escape you. Remember to have your car inspected, your annual servicing of heating and cooling systems, and your income taxes filed. Was there a family conference with your kids' teachers that you were unable to attend? Look through whatever system you use to track things: your checking account register, cancelled checks, last year's credit card statements, your budget book, or last year's calendar, if it is still on the wall or on your telephone or computer. Use whatever sources of information you can find. You may be asking yourself, how is this *educational*? Balancing the demands of daily life and cancer treatment is a highly coordinated dance. Whether you have a long-term remission or still face more treatment, learning how to establish this type of equilibrium will help you in the future. Since you may not working or back at school during the first few weeks of this period, now is the time to master a bit of juggling. As mundane as all of these regular life details seem, it is also helpful in moving yourself out of the cancer world slowly by dipping your toe (then your foot) in the waters of everyday life.

Activity

However far you have come in daily activity is a true bonus up until now. Without the LEARN System, his is the point you would have gotten to when someone would suggest that you start to become more active and try to gain/lose weight. Now, keep it up, push a little more, but not to the point of overwhelming fatigue. This is likely the time to get the physical medicine and rehabilitation consult, the physical therapy appointment, or the personal trainer with clearance from your treatment team. Varying your routine will get you more physiological "bang for your buck." As the seasons change, so do your activities. So the weather itself may push a variation of the activities you will engage in.

Rest

Still very important! You are likely not resting more, but the quality of rest will improve a bit. If you're not back to work, schedule rest as part of your day, at your low point when you feel the most tired. If you're a *morning person* or a *night owl,* that is not likely to change. Use your power nap to recharge.

If you are back at work, most employers will try to make a reasonable accommodation for you to have a quiet place for a short power nap. In an economic downturn, it is more expensive to retrain new people than keep the experienced employees. Make a request for a quiet place if you do not have an office with a closable door. A colleague who had cancer or who had an important person in his or her life with cancer will probably be a good ally. It is the few workplaces that do not accommodate such a request that make the news, not the many that accommodate such special needs to retain valued employees.

Nutrition

Pay serious attention now. What is your weight in relation to your *ideal body weight?* Look at both the number of calories you are taking in by mouth or tube, as well as the sources. A follow-up visit to the nutritionist will be helpful. Although the principles are still the same, your taste buds are waking up, and eating is more pleasurable, helping vary your diet. If one of the basic flavors read by the taste buds (bitter, acid, sweet, salty or umami)) is overactive, that taste should be toned down in your food (if it's *salty,* be careful to avoid inherently salty foods, and don't add additional salt to anything for now). If the *bitter* taste is overpowering, add extra sweetener (honey or *stevia* rather than table sugar).

The LEARN System©

p. 266
What I Am
Supposed to
Be Eating

Since this is the time that you're starting to eat more again, it's the ideal opportunity to weed out the foods that may be implicated in recurrence or relapse and introduce the ones that can be protective. Despite less than definite (but promising) evidence for the helpfulness of such a diet change, each of the suggestions is consistent with what we should do for *heart health* to minimize the risk of heart attack and stroke.

If you have a PEG (percutaneous enteral gastrostomy) or PEJ (percutaneous endoscopic jejunostomy) and are at the point where you are transitioning back to oral nutrition, this is time consuming and requires effort. Actually, the basic idea is *the same as if you are still below your ideal body weight.* Your digestive system has been underutilized for a few weeks or months, and it needs to be reconditioned. Start with thick, small portions and increase a little at a time. Adjust the taste to compensate for the group of taste buds that have not yet returned (bitter, acid, sweet, salty, umami) by using extra seasonings in that category to overcompensate. Use the recipes in the worksheets as a jumping off point. Try smoothies loaded with fresh fruit (not juice, which lacks the fiber) and soups with protein and vegetable sources as the main ingredients. Vary the ingredients so there is more variety. Tofu (no joke) is a tasteless extra protein source that takes on the flavors of what it is added to (caution for breast cancer patients to avoid too much soy).

MED SCHOOL IN A BOX: BEST FOODS FOR HEART HEALTH AND CANCER

When you're at the point where you're eating to return to or maintain your ideal body weight, these guidelines will be helpful when choosing ingredients.

What to Include

1. Folic acid (vitamin B9) from foods rather than a supplement; peanuts are a good food source. Peanut butter is a great way to add peanuts to a dish, as long as the first ingredient is peanuts. Label reading is essential. Many national brands are mainly corn syrup (or similar) with peanut flavoring.
    Breakfast foods: fortified whole grain cereals, oranges, melons, strawberries (frozen second best for nutritional quality and fiber)
    Lunch/dinner/snacks: asparagus, eggs, chicken, liver, beans, sunflower seeds, green leafy vegetables (spinach)

2. Tomato products (cooked and concentrated instead of fresh tomatoes to maximize *lycopene* content) such as juice, sauce, paste

3. Green tea contains catechins, strong antioxidants (iced or hot depending on the climate where you live).

4. Grapes (especially purple or red which contain resveratrol and lycopene)

5. Water

6. Beans

7. Cabbage family vegetables: cauliflower, broccoli, kale, brussels sprouts, bok choy

8. Dark, leafy vegetables: dark lettuces, spinach, kale, chicory, chard

9. Garlic

10. Spices: turmeric and curcumin

11. Berries: strawberries, raspberries, blackberries, blueberries (contain anthocyanins that give red color, ellagic acid, and pterostilbene)

continued

> ## MED SCHOOL IN A BOX: BEST FOODS FOR HEART HEALTH AND CANCER
>
> *continued*
>
> **What to Avoid**
>
> 1. Alcohol
> 2. Cured meats (hot dogs, delicatessen-style meats that are smoked or preserved to last without refrigeration)
> 3. *Saturated* (animal) fats
> 4. Minimize fried foods.
> 5. Minimize grilled or broiled foods that are charred or burned on the outside.
>
> Yes, it may be more expensive and need more preparatory work. Yes, it is healthier.

COMMON HEALTH PROBLEMS AND EXPERIENCES

The follow-up that you need, such as office visits, blood work, or imaging really depends on what type of cancer you had and what treatment you got. You may want to ask someone on the treatment team to help block out what will be expected for the next few months, so you can best plan, using your personal health records to organize the information. Attach a calendar to the back or a list of what is due and when. Worry about a recurrence or relapse often peaks now as you inch closer to feeling like yourself and are quietly afraid that feeling well won't last. Those around you do not always appreciate that the worries about the future affect your decision making about many activities, even such an everyday decision such as replacing your cell phone.

> ## CONSULTATION IN A BOX: WHAT I THINK IS NOT WHAT I SAY
>
> A 26-year-old woman who had been treated for Hodgkin's disease finished treatment about three months ago. She still gets easily winded, owing to both her chemotherapy and radiation treatments. She is getting better, but not as quickly as her impatience would like. Because others have trouble hearing her on her old cell phone with the moderate level of her shortness of breath, she has decided to replace her cell phone and is standing in the store looking at different models, getting a hard sell from the salesperson.
>
> *continued*

CONSULTATION IN A BOX: WHAT I THINK IS NOT WHAT I SAY

continued

She tries to be pleasant and smiles when possible, but everything the saleswoman says brings up an internal answer that is different than what she winds up saying to be polite. For example:

Salesperson says: "Great haircut. Your hair is so cool short." Patient thinks: "You don't know that I was completely bald six weeks ago."

Salesperson says: "Are you going to take out the insurance? It is $4.99 a month for the next 24 months. If your phone is lost or stolen after that, it will be replaced after that for free." Patient thinks to herself: "If I live that long."

Salesperson says: "Your rollover minutes are yours for life." Patient thinks: "Whose life? You may be making a really good deal for your company."

THINGS THAT MATTER NOW: PUTTING THE TREATMENT BEHIND ME

With good initial reports, you're in the process of feeling better but not quite back to yourself. You had hoped to really feel better than you currently do, and that can disappoint you even more. Your hope to put the initial treatment behind you is more advanced than the speed at which the body can repair.

This is the first time where all of your efforts thus far using the LEARN System and starting "My Recovery Plan" early starts to visibly pay off. How you ask (this is all a lot of work, and I want to make sure it's worth it)? Without the benefit of a clinical trial, it is hard to say this with statistical significance, though years of experience demonstrate that by having followed the precepts of the LEARN System, you are feeling better, faster than without all of your efforts. Your progress, specifically how fast or accurately you can move or get things done, is better than it was, even though some remnants of your treatment remain.

Journaling or Creating

This is not for everyone, but something to seriously consider. The purpose of having someone else help with the busy work of "My Recovery Plan" with you was to save precious energy. You should have more energy now. Journaling or having some other type of record can help you, years in the future, make some sense out of the illness and your evolution during treatment. Journaling sounds formal, but it does not need to be elaborate. A daily quote onto an audio recorder or photos could will help show where you've come from and how. If you did start some ongoing recording of your experiences from the time of diagnosis, now is the time to take a few quiet minutes and review it. See how far you have come. There are Journal pages in the worksheets for you to use. Copy as many as you need.

19 How People Treat Me

"People still don't treat me like they used to. Either they think I'm contagious or I am going to break. Sometimes they talk about me being heroic and describe me as being "brave" or "strong." That's OK for a while, but it's a burden to keep it up. Their general tone is different, I've found," said a 44-year-old man who had finished chemotherapy for lymphoma and was just finishing treatment. He was familiar with this situation, only too well, since he was both a patient and a Cancer Dad. He earned the second title only two years ago. He remains amazed that well-meaning people act oddly out of awkwardness.

CONSULTATION IN A BOX: IT'S ALL IN THE FAMILY

A 44-year-old man saw first-hand how people treat others after cancer when his son, who is now 22 years old, at the age of 12 was treated for childhood leukemia. Lucky to have a complete and enduring response from the first round of chemotherapy, he has been disease-free ever since. When his son finished 8 months with more days in the hospital than out and had not one hair left on his head, he was told by the pediatric oncologist that he could go back to class at school. Although he had missed the whole first part of the year, most of his current sixth-grade class was composed of his fifth-grade group, so apart from being "the cancer kid," he knew virtually all of his classmates. Having moved to middle school in the interim, he did not know Mrs. Fox, his homeroom teacher. The kindly Mrs. Fox, however, was not cancer smart, having not experienced cancer herself or through her family or friends. "I truly believe she thought my son, Jason, would split in half if he turned the wrong way." the father reported. She sent a message home saying that Jason's backpack was too heavy and too large for him. He was late a few times, due to car-pooling rather than his own doing, and his report card showed perfect attendance. Mrs. Fox was also his English teacher, well respected by the other parents since she was allergic to kids' cutting corners. She was a stickler for writing, good writing every day, and discouraged anyone from typing so they could develop reasonably readable penmanship in a world dominated by printed documents. Yet Mrs. Fox did not demand anything of Jason. All he had to do was show up (even late), and that was fine. Other parents described how tough she was, but Jason thought she was "nice" and "easy." Dad set up an appointment with Mrs. Fox, and at the meeting, she was pleasant but perplexed. "Jason is such a smart young

continued

CONSULTATION IN A BOX: IT'S ALL IN THE FAMILY

continued

man," she told him. When asked why she was going so easily on him while holding others to standards, she turned first very pale and then very red faced. In a flustered voice, she said, looking pained and quite sad, "I cannot imagine what he's been through. I just don't want him to die in my class. As long as he's breathing and alert . . . ." As her voice trailed off, listening to what she was saying, she looked even more distressed. She took a deep breath and, then with a visible tear, looked at Dad and said, "I guess I have been killing him with kindness." And then she apologized, pulled out her yellow pad, and said, "Let's make up for lost time. I owe it to you, Jason, and your family."

This poignant moment reverberated in the father's memory when he went back to work. Everyone came over to his cubicle and asked how he was. Dad explained how this made him feel. "I got tired of telling the same story over and over, and it seemed worse to me than living through it because of the repetition. Either they were being my Mrs. Fox, or they didn't feel they could count on me since I was out for a period of time. I decided to take an assertive approach. At a staff meeting, I asked that people not bring in lunch and that I would order in as a 'thank you' for covering my work during the time I was out. I thanked everyone for putting themselves out, said that to the best of the doctors' knowledge I was fine, and asserted that I was 'back to my fighting self' and would appreciate it if people would stop being so gentle. Worked like a dream, and I am glad to be back to myself, both in my own head and in others' view of me."

PEOPLE LOOK AT ME AS IF TODAY IS MY LAST

There are people who haven't seen you in a few months. They may be in your parking lot, on your commuter train, at work, school, or anywhere. You still don't look and feel like yourself. You're recognized, and there's that uncomfortable moment when someone says something clumsy. Prepare your script in advance. Everyone has his or her own words. "Yes," you say, "it's been a bad few months." Thank them for their concern. If the well-meaning acquaintance goes on, there is always, "It's a long story and I'm pooped just from telling it to so many people. But I'm OK/hanging in/going from day-to-day. Thanks again for asking."

■ *I can't believe my sexual desire has changed so much: Is this normal?*

You may be starting to feel something but are not sure. Maintain what you started at the beginning of treatment. Depending on which cancer you have and which treatment you received, there is a huge disparity at this point in time in how and when your sexual desire or function returns, and what, if anything, you need to do to nudge it along. It is not forgotten. Share your concerns with your spouse or partner. If you are dating, take it slowly and disclose your situation when you are ready. If your sexual function (desire or performance) does not approach what it was before he cancer, speak with one of the oncology team members. Make sure they have thought through the hormonal connections (see Hormones chapter). You may ask to be referred to a university-based program where both the physiological and psychological variables are evaluated serving as a basis for a treatment plan.

20 New Everyday Routines: Who Do I Call? Back to Work? Can the Personal Health Record Help?

■ *Does my primary care team talk to my oncology team?*

That depends. This is another one of those one-size-does-not-fit-all situations. Your primary care providers may be very comfortable and experienced dealing with the aftereffects of cancer. Or they may not. Ideally or at your request, your primary care provider has communicated with your oncologist. Which one? Well, at least the first one that confirmed the cancer diagnosis and the last one that was mainly responsible for your care. How do these providers communicate? That depends on the treatment setting. Information is shared in the hall at the hospital, through a phone call, e-mail, and/or sending copies of consultation and progress notes to each other. They will sometimes decide among themselves, and sometimes not. Less often, your insurance carrier may have decided who is in-charge at this point by allowing the primary care provider a certain number of follow-up visits. If that is the case, make a non-emergency appointment with the primary care provider and find out who should be your point provider for aftercare.

The "Personal Health Record" worksheet has a number of uses.

The LEARN System©

p. 277
Personal
Health
Record

CONSULTATION IN A BOX: GOOD COMMUNICATION PAYS OFF

A 60-year-old woman was treated for breast cancer with a lumpectomy, radiation therapy, chemotherapy and hormonal therapy. Three months after finishing her chemotherapy and one month after beginning hormonal treatment, she developed a cough. She did not know which doctor to call. She had no fever and was not coughing up any mucus or sputum. It was hard to tell how she actually felt since finishing her radiation therapy, because she was still tired. Each subspecialist thought something different: The surgeon didn't think that it was connected to the surgery, which was performed six months prior to the cough. The medical oncologist was thinking it could be pneumonia, though the woman was not feeling sick enough, or breast cancer metastasis to the lung. The radiation oncologist was thinking that it could be a yeast infection, though a little late, or radiation pneumonitis

continued

CONSULTATION IN A BOX: GOOD COMMUNICATION PAYS OFF

continued

(skin reaction in the lungs from the radiation), though the beam had been pointed away from her lungs. The primary care provider thought it was the woman's usual seasonal allergies, and asked the three oncologists if they were comfortable with conservative treatment for the moment: some over-the-counter cough medicine and antihistamine, repeating a scan in seven days if there was no improvement or the cough got worse. Luckily, the three oncology specialists participated in a weekly conference and could have a sidebar conversation. The medical oncologist who had seen the patient for her most recent checkup and wrote the prescription for the hormonal treatment called back the primary care provider to discuss the now consensus opinion. The primary care provider was thankful for the teamwork. The patient herself did get better after five days with some saline nose drops, a few doses of antihistamine, and decongestant—all over-the-counter. She agreed to go back to her allergist, since she had stopped her allergy shots six months previously at the time of the breast cancer surgery. The allergist repeated her skin tests and advised her to restart allergy shots so she would be less symptomatic by the next allergy season.

1. Exchanging of information between current providers
2. Documenting information for future providers
3. Chronicling of the things you need to know and do during and after treatment
4. Recording symptoms that need to be monitored and tests that need to be done in the future
5. Listing resources for the present and future

Call the provider who you think can be most helpful. If you can't figure it out or are too frightened to do so since you don't want to be wrong, call the last provider you have seen. As you think about your symptom keep "The Rules" in mind:

- Rule 1: If it comes and goes, it's not likely cancer.
- Rule 2: If it comes and stays, it needs to be checked.
- Rule 3: Follow Rules 1 and 2.
- Rule 4: Re-read Rules 1 and 2.

Personal health records (PHRs) are rather new on the health care scene. PHRs come in various forms, such as a paper document, an electronic document, or a medical record embedded into an electronic system that allows both provider and patient access. The advent of these documents brings up some fundamental questions about our health care information in general.

The information included can vary greatly. It can include personal information (individual, family, health care providers and contact information, insurers, history, pets), complaints (problem list), clinical encounters, diagnoses, procedures (surgeries, treatments), lab results, immunizations, allergies, medications, advance directives, nutrition and diet, exercise, personal comments, and information resources. Cancer-specific information should include the following:

- Immediate, expectable side effects of care
- Relapse/recurrence vigilance—who, what, how often
- Second primary cancers—who is monitoring
- Secondary cancers
- Screening for other cancers common to your age group—having one cancer predisposes you to others
- Imaging, tumor markers, CEA, CA-125, PSA, AFP
- Chemoprevention strategies
- Medications or supplements used preventively

A few progressive cancer centers that have successfully brought electronic medical records into their daily care have designed *patient portals* into their record systems. A patient portal is a way for patients to open their medical records from dedicated information kiosks in their centers or via the Internet, using security similar to what protects on-line banking or credit card accounts. Some major software development companies, interested in being a part of the electronic medical record revolution, are also developing systems for patients to securely access their records or maintain information online to be accessed by approved providers. These systems allow you to view a health summary, current medications, and test results as released by physicians; to review past and upcoming appointments as well as to request and cancel appointments; to receive important health reminders; to request prescription renewals; and even to notify your provider of changes to your mail or e-mail address.

A major initiative to bring PHRs directly to the public has been spearheaded by the American Society of Clinical Oncology (ASCO). In partnership with Journey Forward, a collaboration with the National Coalition for Cancer Survivorship, UCLA Cancer Survivorship Center, WellPoint and Genentech. Survivorship PHRs are also available through the ASCO patient website in the survivorship section (http://www. cancer.net) or Journey Forward (http://www.journeyforward.org). Updates and a

CONSULTATION IN A BOX: FINDING THE PAPER

AK, a 58-year-old man, had risen to be a supervisor in the light-bulb factory where he worked for 18 years. He was third in command after the owners, and the highest ranking employee who is not a blood relative of the owner. The owning family stuck by him despite his two rounds of treatment for lung cancer. Perhaps they were afraid that Mr. K would claim that the chemical exposures at work caused the cancer, but no one could tell him whether it was related or not. And besides, he felt a

continued

> **CONSULTATION IN A BOX: FINDING THE PAPER**
>
> *continued*
>
> special bond to the workers, as they did to him. As a result of a promotion upon return to work, he was no longer eligible for union medical benefits and he applied for new insurance. The insurance agent asked a lot of questions regarding his cancer treatment, including the exact dates of treatment but also *exactly* how much radiation therapy he had and at what angles, and the exact dosages of the chemotherapy he received. AK did not have these numbers and asked at the medical oncologist's office. "It was so long ago," the practice manager said, "that we have to send out to get an 'archived' chart, which will take a few days." He and his wife made a number of calls and visits to the office, only to find out that the chart could not be located. They even tried the family doctor, but he said that he had remembered many telephone calls to both the medical oncologist's and radiation oncologist's offices and had a copy of the chemotherapy clearance exam, but not the exact dosage of chemotherapy. In order to maintain his health insurance coverage without a gap, promotion was held up for almost a year until the office manger thought to get a copy of the inpatient hospital records from the hospital's storage area since he was admitted to the hospital with pneumonia after the last chemotherapy. If not for her good memory, Mr. K would never have gotten the promotion he deserved unless he had chosen to do without medical insurance.

page to share experiences with PHRs are available online at http://www.cancerknowanddo.com.

■ *How can I use the PHR?*

Look at the form or the printout. Some of the information (name, type of cancer) is easy. Other details—and here the details are very important—you may not know. An important purpose of doing even more work (yep, even more homework) is to collect the information while it is easily available.

■ *How do I know when to go back to work?*

You may want to go back before you are really ready. By following the LEARN System, you have already been self-monitoring and have a good idea measure of your capacities. Can you sustain all of your workday and the commute back and forth on your usual schedule? Your energy level needs to be able to match your desire if you are getting bored by being home. On your last check-up visit, had your blood counts returned to reasonably OK levels? Do your disability benefits allow you to go back part time or allow you to try to see if you are ready? That is often the best solution if it is feasible.

■ *I have heard the term the cancer ceiling. What is it?*

A variation of the *glass ceiling* where minority employees are kept from getting promotions or raises as discrimination, the *cancer ceiling* implies the imposition of some limitation to advancement in a corporation or one's field due to a cancer diagnosis. Such actual discrimination is hard to prove, but people do report that their reliability is in question after extended absences for cancer treatment, which can be the factor used to justify limiting professional advancement. The Americans with Disabilities Act, the Family Medical Leave Act, and the work of the Equal Employment Opportunities Commission all mandate certain federal protections. You may need legal assistance or advice about how to make an official report to your Human Resources Department if you work for a large business.

21 Back into the World

■ *When can I go back into crowds?*

Your ability to fight off infection is mostly attributed to your white cell count, part of your complete blood count. This protection may be compromised after treatment. With the use of bone-marrow-stimulating medications that help boost white cell counts during and right after chemotherapy, this vulnerable period has been greatly shortened. Your platelet count, also a component of the complete blood count, must be adequate for clotting should you fall or cut yourself. Otherwise, your general level of energy, unless your mobility is affected by neuropathy, will determine when you can be out and about. Old fashioned good hygiene, such as washing your hands or using water-free hand sanitizers, turning away from those who cough or sneeze in your path, and avoiding touching your hands to your face until washed, are all common sense ways of keeping infection to a minimum.

■ *Am I radioactive?*

Not unless you've been treated with some very specialized radiation therapy techniques. Anyone who has had radioactive iodine (I^{131}) for the treatment of thyroid cancer, and those who have had radioactive seed implants should get specific guidelines from their oncologist. Otherwise, you are not radioactive when receiving conventional radiation therapy.

BODY FUNCTIONS I NEED TO WORK ON/WITH

As your energy starts to return, with the activity you have been doing since your diagnosis, you will find an increase in your daily endurance. Celebrate it, and use it to your advantage by doing things you enjoy but have not gotten to during the initial treatment. One of the functions that is now likely to surface is sexual function.

You may have had the desire before this for sexual activity, but not the energy. Or it may be that the desire itself was gone earlier during treatment for many reasons: hormonal changes; being too scared; difficulties in being intimate either physically or emotionally with those you fear may survive you, are taking care of you, or whom you love very much.

■ *My hair skin and nails are not what they were either. Why?*

With all of the extra work that cancer treatment brings on, it may have been hard to justify spending time and attention on hair, skin, and nails from the beginning of treatment, but as you are emerging back into the world, you may have wished that you

MED SCHOOL IN A BOX: SEXUALITY AND CANCER

Sexuality after cancer has been a topic of burgeoning concern as the odds for survivorship have increased. After Helen Singer Kaplan, MD, developed the first medical school–based program for the diagnosis and treatment of sexual dysfunction, she trained Sarah Auchincloss, MD, a fellow at Memorial Sloan-Kettering across the street. Auchincloss was able to adapt Singer Kaplan's techniques for those who have received cancer treatment and was the first among many worldwide to heighten awareness about sexuality in cancer. Each type of cancer has physiological, psychological, social, and practical complications owing to the cancer or its treatment. Distilling such a complicated physical/emotional/practical human experience into outline form may be a bit simplistic, but it can be a useful starting point for more reading and discussion with your treatment team.

Colon Cancer: With a colostomy (temporary or permanent diversion of stool out through the abdomen), neuropathy from chemotherapy or surgery, and diarrhea from radiation of the pelvis can all physically interfere with sexuality.

Breast Cancer: Breasts may be an important part of your self-image and a source of pleasure during sexual activity. Many women who have implants or flap reconstruction report that the sense of feeling in that area has changed at first. It is not fully healed, and some sensation may return. Hormonal changes may be especially powerful on sexual function after chemotherapy, radiation therapy, or oophorectomy (removal of the ovaries). Younger, premenopausal women are likely more affected, but breast cancer patient is to some extent.

Gynecological Cancers: An obvious area of concern. Sexual desire may be totally absent. Sexual activity may hurt due to hormonal changes or surgery in the pelvic area than in breast cancer. There are a variety of lubricants on the market that my ease the friction and dryness. If you've had breast cancer, beware of prescription-only preparations that are likely to have hormones in their formula. Similarly, there are *natural* products that have many natural supplements whose claims need not be verified by clinical trials to the same extent that a prescription drug requires. Non-breast cancer patients should speak with their providers about estrogen that is mostly (but not completely) limited to the vaginal area, marketed in a cream or a ring that can be placed inside. Certain sexual positions are more likely to be comfortable. Alternatively, non-intercourse intimacy may be able to sustain you and your partner until you have healed and recovered.

Prostate Cancer: Reduction in testosterone levels can hurt desire and function. Weight changes may have been tempered by the LEARN System's

continued

MED SCHOOL IN A BOX: SEXUALITY AND CANCER

continued

early activity, affecting you less now than taking the "I'll get to this later" approach. The lack of testosterone really reduces desire, and painful ejaculation or urination can be equal deterrents even if you can have a complete or partial erection. Lubricants can help as well if you need to rely on manual manipulation to sustain a response.

Penile or Testicular Cancer: Penile cancer requires a huge adjustment, both physically and emotionally. The adjustment in both how a man thinks of himself and the changes in the mechanics of urination put sexual function as a lower priority. Having to find an alternate way to express sexuality likely will need specialized counseling. Testicular cancer brings other challenges, which are less disfiguring than penile cancer, but often involve multiple hormones through the pituitary and hypothalamus in the brain. Sexual response is changed, and recovery will involve proper hormonal replacement as well as counseling. Implants for inside the scrotum give the feeling of normal testicles. For those men who are in-between steady intimate relationships, how to tell and when to tell become critical. Since fertility, not only sexual desire and function, is affected, providers probably discussed the option of sperm or testicular banking during the initial work-up of your cancer.

had. If treatment caused your hair to fall out, little could have been done to avoid it. Ice packs cool the scalp so that less chemotherapy gets there, resulting in less hair falling out, leaving the scalp area unprotected against cancer growing there in the future. Your scalp may most likely itch or even hurt as your hair grows back. Some people say that the hair comes back in two stages, just the way newborns grow their hair. The first crop is fine and often falls out, making way for the thicker adult hair afterward. Hair generally grows about half an inch a month when your metabolism is at its peak. After treatment, it may be a little slower. Make sure your scalp is clean. Care for it the same way you would wash the skin on your face. Shampoo is generally ineffective on a scalp without hair. Save the gentle shampoo for when the hair returns. Make sure to dry your scalp well after washing, and moisturize it in any weather, using a product with sunscreen if you will spend any time out of doors, no matter the season. The skin on your head is very tender and is not used to sun exposure, so it is primed for sunburn. During and after treatment, just about any of the medications you have taken that have been stored in the skin can cause a *photosensitive reaction* when exposed to the sun. That is all the more reason to use sunscreen as even a little sun exposure can have a greater effect due to the photosensitivity.

■ *Which supplements should I be taking?*

> ## SUPPLEMENTS I SHOULD BE TAKING AFTER TREATMENT IS OVER
>
> 1. Multivitamin with a good coating on the pill
> 2. Calcium should come back into your routine (unless you have a high calcium level).
> 3. Vitamin D, dose based on blood level
> 4. Omega-3 fatty acids (fish oils), mostly EPA (eicosapentanoic acid)
> 5. Fiber

This is controversial because no good data exist and manufacturers want you to buy their products unqualified with testimonials that abound online and in print. Your basic nutrition should come from food with the usual heart-healthy/cancer-prevention message: whole grains, varied nonmeat proteins, and fruits and vegetables of many and deep colors. The deep-colored vegetables are the best sources of the important vitamins with fiber. If you are on solid food and cannot keep up with it, a quality multivitamin with a good coating to avoid dissolving in your esophagus and giving you distasteful heartburn is the best idea. Calcium and vitamin D should come back into your routine (unless you have a high calcium level). Once your cholesterol and triglyceride levels stabilize post-chemotherapy, there may be individualized adjustments to make. Fish oils (omega-3 fatty acids) are ever growing in popularity for both heart health and cancer. Studies to see if fish oils can relieve joint and muscle pain from estrogen- or testosterone-blocking treatments are underway. If you used fish oils to try to gain weight during your treatment, it may seem illogical to use them now for fear of gaining more weight, but that does not seem to be the case. Theoretically, it is thought that the omega-3s helped keep the bad effects of the *cytokines* at bay, and now having little or very low levels of circulating *cytokines*, it is believed the omega-3's do not affect the body in the same way.

Adequate fiber from food sources or even a fiber supplement is supposed to help push food (including impurities) through the digestive system. From a practical perspective, fluid and fiber keep bowels even and more on a schedule of convenience rather than urgency. Fiber is the main reason to have whole foods rather than to rely on *juicing* to replace and boost antioxidants in the fiber.

A Word on Detoxifying

The idea of *detoxifying* the body with a few days of fasting, with some electrolyte replacement in water or juice, seems attractive to cleanse the *cytokines* and the waste products from cell destruction from cancer treatment. The programs sound seductive and logical. Opponents believe that it is a risk with no benefit, since the body naturally detoxifies itself without a pricey product, and it can even be dangerous due to abrupt changes in electrolytes and fluids. For now, these regimens are *thumbs-down* after cancer.

■ *How can I help myself stay cancer free?*

ROLE OF ALCOHOL AND TOBACCO

Tobacco Products

Long-standing habits or even dependencies tend to come back now that the immediate crisis is over. This is a pivotal point in your care if you are dependent on these substances. No cancer whose recurrence or relapse rate is reduced using nicotine or other tobacco products. There is some reason to believe that a small to moderately small amount of alcohol in the daily diet for those without serious alcohol dependencies in the past *may* be helpful reducing recurrences of breast cancer and heart disease. No one is suggesting that if you are a nondrinker now is the time to start. Excessive alcohol or any nicotine/tobacco product use undoes what good treatment and hard work have done to help you.

Tobacco and nicotine products damage in a few ways. The actual nicotine itself changes the way our body digests many medications and food products. It actually causes us to extract *less* of the good resources from what we take or eat. The by-products in anything smoked actually irritate and inflame inside the mouth, lungs, and stomach. Chronic inflammation can encourage cancer re-growth. The usual cleaning mechanisms do not function properly with these by-products (such as tar) in the mouth, throat, or lungs.

Alcohol

Alcohol also affects the way we digest drugs and food as well as overworks the pancreas and liver. It is postulated that a minimal amount of alcohol may affect estrogen levels or some other intermediate chemical to be determined but, in general, causes lots of irritation in the mouth, throat, and esophagus. Alcohol has effects on *every* system in the body. Apart from the immediate *buzz* or relaxation that occurs within minutes and perhaps a small advantage in the hormonal profile that can minimally affect breast cancer risk or heart disease profile, alcohol does not do much good to any part of the body.

Resveratrol

Much has been written about the good antioxidant properties of resveratrol (3,5,4'-trihydroxy-trans-stilbene), which is a stilbenoid, a type of polyphenol, and a phytoalexin produced naturally by several plants. Some believe that this natural substance is helpful to metabolism and for heart health. Derived from grapes, it is bound in our thoughts and chemically to red wines, building an industry on this belief. The

HELP TO STOP SMOKING

1. Motivation—*key factor*
2. Learn which services are in your area.

   Your Primary Care Provider

   American Cancer Society

   County health department (or in some places, city or state health department)

   Local general hospital

   Your cancer center

   Faith-based programs (local church, synagogue)

   Health insurance plan
3. Know what the programs do.

   Individual and/or group counseling:

   Why do I smoke? What triggers a craving? Am I ready?

   What to do when a craving hits

   Buddy system
4. Nicotine replacement (gum, patch, spray)

   Anticraving medications: bupropion (Zyban® and others),

   varenicline (Chantix® and others)
5. Acupuncture
6. Pressure-point stimulation

resveratrol seems to be helpful, with little downside once divorced from the alcohol in grape products (skins, perhaps more than juice). Enjoy your resveratrol apart from the alcohol.

Cutting back, then stopping alcohol intake requires lots of determination and professional help. The scare of a cancer diagnosis can scare you into giving away your corkscrew and vowing "not to have another sip." Practically speaking, it is harder than that. Alcohol is all around us, in advertising and the fabric of many events. A large part of our travel and entertainment industry is centered around alcohol consumption, both a profit center and a way to promote good times. That cruise you may want to take after your treatment involves alcohol from the moment you walk on the ship until the last duty-free shop you will pass through at the airport.

The professional substance abuse community is split on approach. Some data point to full abstinence as the way to most guarantee no slippery slope into incremental

---

HOW I CAN STOP ALCOHOLIC DRINKS?

Reach out for guidance:

Your primary care provider

Your cancer center

Your health insurance carrier (often there is a special number to call listed on the card)

County-based substance abuse programs

Have a professional advise the best approach.

A formal *detox* (detoxification) inpatient or outpatient program

Maintenance program (such as Alcoholics Anonymous)

---

drinking. Other data reflect that one must live in the alcohol-soaked world as it exists, which means a realistic approach to modulation and moderation. But the goal is the same: eliminate or minimize alcohol. That is the most significant concept. How you go about it is more personal.

■ *What do I need to know about the human papilloma virus?*

The body's response to any viral exposure is affected by cancer and its treatment. Human papilloma virus (HPV) is implicated in the start of cervical cancer, and possibly many head and neck cancers. The vaccine (Gardasil®) that has been approved for use in young girls to avoid catching HPV during early sexual intercourse may actually be recommended for the wider population as knowledge is gained about its role in preventing other cancers. The sociology of HPV spread via unprotected oral sex or vaginal sex has taken it into the political realm and may affect public policy in the future. It is not easy to think that our children participate in sexual practices that can be risky. That realization is the first step to compel a national dialogue about preventing a sexually transmitted disease with a vaccine administered to our children. We did not face such a discussion with measles or smallpox. We did not face similar controversy where the public's health was clearly the greater good. We are not there yet with HPV.

EVERYONE HAS ADVICE FOR ME

The approach you have used thus far—thanking people for their interest and asking them to halt—may be wearing thin, but now you are more resilient to withstand the extra discussion and friendly advice. Try to balance your tolerance and their insistence.

VENTURING OUT

■ *I finally am ready to fly somewhere on a vacation or for work, but now I have many extra things to do. Any clues?*

We all want to travel safely. If you need to travel with more than three ounces of liquid supplements, declare them to the security agent before they are found. The Transportation Safety Administration (TSA) has relaxed the rules for baby formula and medical feedings. Best to carry a note, even a simple one scribbled on a prescription from your cancer center.

TRAVELS WITH MY CANCER

Carry a summary of records (such as a personal health record).

Make sure health insurance can be used for an emergency at your destination (foreign travel, travel outside of an HMO network region).

List all medicines and supplements, using generic and brand names as well dosages.

Find emergency services closest to where you are staying.

Take medicines in original bottles wherever possible in carry-on luggage (not in stowed luggage that can easily be lost).

Carry a note or card for any devices with metal parts that can set off security screening machines.

Have a provider note for Transportation Safety Administration (TSA) screeners for any liquids more than three ounces per bottle that together exceed a quart-size ziplock food-storage bag.

Take and *use* sunscreen.

Be careful about food and drink that may contain bacteria.

Use water-free hand sanitizers regularly.

Stay well hydrated.

Enjoy yourself!

For devices such as chemotherapy pumps, feeding pumps, opioid pumps, show them to the security agent and ask for a *hand check* as they will certainly sound an alarm when you go through security. A similar note on an Rx pad should satisfy the TSA.

For medications, carry a note as well as a list of exactly what you are taking with its generic as well as brand name. Outside of the United States, many brand names for the same substances are mostly different Although prescription drugs can sometimes seem like they are sold at *bargain prices* in some foreign cities, purity and quality control may not be what you've become used to, so it would be best to skip these travel bargains.

Have an emergency plan. Look ahead online and find out where the nearest emergency department is to your destination. Verify that your insurance covers reimbursement at your destination if outside of your own provider network. Carry your list of medications as well as the information on your treatment: chemotherapy agents, doses, dates as well as dates of radiation and portals. This is another practical use for a PHR. Make sure the emergency numbers for your treatment team are there as well, and if you do need to go to an emergency facility, be persistent in asking them to call your treating oncologist for discussion.

If you are traveling with any devices such as wheelchair, cane, or walker, ask the airline in advance for help so they are expecting you and the extra equipment.

Consider shipping your luggage in advance so there is less to carry onboard and less to do at the destination airport.

Cruises on large ships may also be ideal for your recovery period. You only unpack and pack once, and you can be active without overdoing. The food is plentiful, and shopping, cooking, and cleaning are taken care of for you. Large ships have sophisticated medical and nursing facilities to handle complicated medical problems until you can disembark in a port with specialized medical services or for transportation back to the closest center of excellence.

When traveling or even in your home port, be careful of the following: foods from street vendors, fruits or vegetables that can't be peeled, "native" ice cubes, and tap water in foreign countries. Obviously, the risk is different in different places. Snorkeling, scuba, skydiving, or long hikes may need to be reserved for the future when you have fully recovered your resistance, energy, and stamina.

QUESTIONS I WANT ANSWERED

When will I be myself? Will I have to keep paying special attention to all of this for the rest of my life?

■ *Where can I get more and reliable information?*

Refer to the list in the Resources. For specialized or up-to-date travel information, the TSA's website can help (http://www.tsa.gov); airline or cruise company websites, tourism bureaus, and hotel concierge desks at your destination all can help as well. Many teaching hospitals offer travel clinics for immunizations and preventive teaching. Your local health department (county, city, state) can also be a source of information. The Department of State as well as the Centers for Disease Control also house a significant amount of information on travel health and specific recommendations for potential epidemics.

The LEARN System©

p. 338
Trusted
Internet
Sites

Part V

Four to Six Months after Treatment

22 Living beyond Cancer—Four to Six Months

WHAT IS DIFFERENT NOW THAN BEFORE?

Another milestone in your posttreatment phase. By now you're less tired from treatment, but more weary of being a cancer survivor. While grateful to have reached this point, you just may wish that you could turn back the clock and have your record expunged. Not going to happen. But what you need to know and do has changed. You know a lot more than you did at the start and need to do much less. That alone is a relief. This course has had too many tiring assignments.

ADJUSTMENTS TO THE LEARN SYSTEM

Living

Making plans is still rough and unnerving. Will I have enough of a future to do so? You're still not sure, but you want to move on. Haven't finished the assignments from prior sections? Now is the time go back and complete them. Who wouldn't benefit from some reorganization of financial files? Personal documents need to be updated periodically. Now is a *good excuse* time to do so.

Education

There are still things to do, many of which would have been necessary anyway. Fewer people will think you will melt and you're not being treated you as if you are so fragile. If you've been open to friends and colleagues about your cancer, now is the time to reinforce that someone can survive cancer and move on, even with some of the physical and emotional scars that linger.

Activity

You are doing more each day and feel stronger with more stamina. It is less difficult. The neuropathy is interfering less than before, but the hormonal treatments still make you feel a little older than your chronological age and a bit dumb.

Rest

The resting comes more naturally as you are busier. You are still tired during the day, but less so.

Nutrition

Where are you in relation to your ideal body weight? Getting as close as possible to this ideal, as old as that sounds, is the best idea. Eating cancer-smart foods makes even more sense, though the message may already be tired. Wherever you live, there is likely a heart-healthy cooking seminar offered by the local hospital, YMCA, or cancer society. You may be in a bigger city with a cooking school. If not, well-made DVDs bring the experts to you. All the other survivors in your community need the same thing. Organize a cooking demonstration with the DVDs as your instructor. Donate the proceeds to the cancer-related program that helped you.

THINGS THAT MATTER NOW: PUTTING THE TREATMENT BEHIND

It's harder to do than you'd like to think. It is probably impossible to wipe it out of your personal history and pretend it did not happen. On the other hand, you're thinking less about the cancer and even trying to plan more for the future. Most people with good scans and exams at this time are trying to get back to their former state, but are a little older and a bit battered. It is possible that your treatment is extending beyond four months, and the treatment schedule does not allow you to advance to this point, yet. If that is so, read on to see where you may be headed and come back to re-read these sections a few months after your treatment is over.

■ *What do I need to know about* skeletal-related events *and* osteoporosis? *This is starting to sound like Halloween.*

Those television commercials discussing bone loss *do* apply to you. Chemotherapy and radiation therapy can thin bones to the point of their fracturing. This can happen on its own or at a spot where the cancer is growing (called a *pathologic fracture*). Bones need to stay strong and cancer free. A bone pain that does not go away needs follow-up, including an exam from your provider and some imaging. The medicines your friends are taking or from those television commercials (zolendronic acid or Zometa®; pamidronat or Aredia®; risedronate or Actonel®; alendronate or Fosamax®; or ibandronate or Boniva®) actually repair thin bones and can suppress growth of cancer in the bones as well. The intravenous forms are more often used after cancer treatment than the oral forms. The schedule varies with the agent chosen. Their use is controversial as there have been cases of *osteonecrosis,* a deterioration of the jaw bone when these medicines are used and dental work is needed that involves the bone. There is a current school of thought to use them for a shorter period of time, but the safety and risks as well as defining exactly how long that period of time is all being studied up in the air for now.

Other effective forms of prevention of skeletal-related events (SREs) or suppression of cancer progressing in the bone are yet to be found. What is considered preventive in osteoporosis (calcium vitamin D, weight-bearing exercise) has not definitively been found effective in preventing or delaying SREs. Bone density scans can help identify bone weakness in those who would naturally be prone to bone loss: over 65 years old, female, Asian ancestry, thin, history of previous fractures, use of tobacco products or alcohol, or previous use of corticosteroids. People with celiac disease, thyroid or para-thyroid problems, or vitamin D deficiency need to be monitored extra carefully. Effective chemotherapy or radiation therapy may be helpful, depending on the cancer or the location. Orthopedic stabilization remains a good option for patients who are otherwise in good health and whose cancer has achieved good control apart from the SRE.

Treatment for osteoporosis with weight-bearing exercise, calcium, and vitamin D with the judicious use of bisphosphonates is an area under a high level of scrutiny at this time. Minimal effective doses of bisphosphonates in both conditions is being reviewed. Other options for treatment can be *calcitonin* usually given by nasal spray.

■ *What is a* secondary cancer? *Is this something I need to worry about even more?*

POSSIBLE LONG-TERM EFFECTS OF CANCER TREATMENT

- Change in bone marrow's ability to produce red blood cells, white blood cells, or platelets (counts can be lower than usual)
- Neuropathy (pins and needles, hot and cold, numbness) in any *end organ* (fingers/hands, toes/feet, tip of nose, tip of tongue, ears, nipples, penis, or vagina)
- Small risk of *secondary* cancers (sarcoma, leukemia)
- Predisposition to other types of cancers
- Ongoing fatigue
- Reduced efficiency of liver and kidneys
- Fibrous muscles (tough and less flexible; after radiation therapy to that area)
- Cognitive difficulties
- Graft versus host disease (after bone marrow transplant)
- Kidney and liver less efficient

Less well tracked:

- Gastroparesis (slowed movement through the digestive tract leading to mild indigestion or constipation)
- Dry skin

This is confusing. Many people refer to *metastatic cancer,* one that has spread from one part of the body to another, as a *secondary cancer.* A secondary cancer more distinctly refers to getting one cancer as a result of having the first, treating it, and surviving it. These are rare but known circumstances. There is a bitter irony here: a hazard of having a response to initial cancer treatment is living with the risk of developing secondary cancers. Secondary cancers are generally leukemia or sarcomas. A portion of the patients with secondary cancers had treatment with older chemotherapy agents such as melphalan or higher doses of cyclophosphamide than used today. Monitoring for secondary cancers is an important component of follow-up care. What is checked (blood tests, imaging) and the frequency of testing needs to be somewhat individualized based on the kind of cancer previously treated, doses of chemotherapy or radiation therapy used, age, and other history. Such a plan should grow out of collaboration between the medical and radiation oncologists with the primary care provider.

CANCER SCREENING FOR ME

Know the current screening recommendations for anyone your age.

Women

- Mammograms
- Pap smears
- HPV tests
- Stool for fecal occult blood
- Sigmoidoscopy or colonoscopy
- Skin
- Mouth and throat

Men

- Prostate specific antigen (PSA)
- Stool for fecal occult blood
- Sigmoidoscopy or colonoscopy
- Skin
- Mouth and throat

Review optimal plan with your oncology or primary care provider about testing for recurrence, relapse, or secondary cancers.

■ *Which* regular *cancer screening tests do I need as a cancer survivor?*

This should be another point of discussion between your oncology sub-specialists and primary care provider. The use of screening tests for early detection of cancer for anyone is under serious evaluation as well. Both mammograms to detect breast cancer and prostate specific antigen (PSA) blood tests to find prostate cancer early are more and more debated but are still the standard of care (PSA for men older than 50, and mammograms for women starting at 40 years old.) Pap smears after being sexually active and a screen for colorectal cancer after the age of 50 years old, such as fecal occult blood (testing stool for hidden blood), flexible sigmoidoscopy, full colonoscopy, virtual colonoscopy, or double contrast CT scans are all used to find polyps or early stage cancer, depending on general health, age, and other medical conditions. You or your primary care provider can confirm the current screening guidelines at http://www.cancer.gov/cancertopics/pdq/screening/overview/healthprofessional.

The use of full body scans in the general non-cancer population remains controversial as a screening test for other cancers (but very useful to locate distant metastases) to avoid many unnecessary biopsies for shadows that may be benign. Scans are routinely used as follow-up once a cancer has been found and treated, a point less debated by public health experts. There has been some difference of opinion as to whether a man older than 70, for example, should get PSA tests or at what age women should stop mammograms as they survive other cancers.

■ *What are the long-term effects of chemotherapy that I need to know about and my primary care doctor needs to check for?*

Identifying which long-term side effects of chemotherapy are significant is more of a challenge than one would believe. Without a uniform electronic health record, side effects being treated as a result of standard chemotherapy do not get reported to any local or federal agency or pharmaceutical company unless they seem highly unusual to the treating staff. Information about reporting to the FDA is available at http://www.fda.gov/Safety/MedWatch/default.

The system in place does not collect information about less than life-threatening or unexpected side effects. There is no clearinghouse for information or way to reach into records to assemble such information. Privacy rights would need to be protected in order to do so. As a result of the limitations to farm medical information and absence of an electronic platform to do so, your treatment team members need to use their judgment and their personal knowledge of how much information you want to have as a caution about side effects. They need to know from you what you are experiencing. Your health history is also a big factor in judging what is *essential* for you rather than someone else.

For example, it is believed that someone with diabetes is more likely to get persistent neuropathy than someone who does not have another illness causing neuropathy. Someone with mild kidney insufficiency needs to have his or her kidney function monitored more often when taking cis-platinum. Preexisting heart problems (heart attack, angina, congestive heart failure, viral cardiomyopathy, and others) need to be taken in account, often with a formal consultation from your cardiologist before adriamycin, doxorubicin, or doxorubicin liposomal. If any of these situations was part of your history when staring chemotherapy, remind your primary care provider so that you can have proper follow-up during your survivorship period, especially if you are using a different primary care provider than while the cancer was treated.

Mild side effects rarely come to attention, even if they become long-standing, making it harder to know if something you are experiencing is from chemotherapy, the cancer, a separate problem, or advancing age. This is an unexpected revelation for most people. Most likely overlooking minor side effects occurs because the staff is vigilant about serious, life-threatening side effects (kidney failure, serious infection, high blood calcium levels) or watching for any sign of cancer spread (sudden incontinence or bowel activity, hemorrhage, quick-onset infections), so these less obvious and less significant occurrences seem trivial, until you've come to this point: grateful to have had a good treatment response, but contending with longer-term side effects.

Such side effects that are often associated with certain treatments are:

Persistent neuropathy: This includes numbness; burning; pins and needles feeling; hot and cold in hands, arms, feet, legs, or the tips of any *end organ* (breasts, nose, ears, penis); cramping or even color changes that come and go in the skin of end organs. Treatment remains the same as earlier in the period of survivorship, with physical therapy to strengthen the adjoining muscles and drug trials with antidepressants and anticonvulsants to minimize the misfirings of the nerve fibers, not because the trouble is related to either depression or seizures. Suffering is not inevitable. Treatment does not help everyone, but many. See specialists at your cancer center or get a proper referral to a specialist you can travel to and be covered by insurance reimbursement.

Persistent cognitive limitations: Two specific patterns have been identified, so far, this being such a new phenomenon. Long-term memories are preserved, but new information doesn't always get stored. So it is hard to do multiple tasks at once or keep track of seemingly basic things in everyday life. These effects can also be due to distraction from worry about the cancer or distress returning to work or school, but those are transient and less persistent.

Serious or major depression: A separate entity that gets unfortunately mixed up with the common everyday use of the term, this type of serious sadness and lack of motivation or enjoyment is out of context to the situation. Since most of the physical symptoms of major depression (change in sleep, appetite, energy) are part of cancer anyway, these are the things to bring to your provider's attention. If you ever had any episode of serious depression even if it wasn't treated, have alcohol or drug dependence, or have a close blood relative (child, parent, brother, or sister) with major depression, you are more likely than the average person to go through it. This is the type

---

SYMPTOMS THAT LIKELY MEAN I HAVE A DEPRESSION THAT NEEDS TREATMENT

- No enjoyment
- Little or no desire to do things that are necessary or fun
- Believing your situation is hopeless when there is a good chance of a treatment response for your cancer
- Can't stay asleep; awaken in middle of night and can't fall back asleep
- Serious thoughts or intention of killing yourself (more than feeling like a burden to others)

Other signs and symptoms of depression that can be due to cancer and its treatment and *may not* signal depression that needs treatment:

- Changes in appetite
- Change in energy level
- Change in ability to concentrate

of depression that responds to a combination of antidepressants and counseling the majority of the time. It is fixable. Do not hesitate to ask for help. These feelings are not the same as the usual and expected *distress* that is universal with cancer.

Distinguishing between what is major depression and what is expected *distress* requires lots of self-honesty and reflection. It is most obvious when you have the kind of cancer that responds well to treatment, yet your overwhelming feeling is hopelessness. If you have the type of cancer that has a small chance of response, pessimism is understandable but you can still get some satisfaction out of certain things in daily life. It is that feeling that nothing is pleasurable, even in a very limited way, which is worrisome and should signal formal evaluation.

MED SCHOOL IN A BOX: TREATMENT OF MAJOR DEPRESSION

Once your treatment team suspects a serious depression by your description of your mood, your inability to enjoy even the smallest nicety, or pessimism beyond what is expected, there are a few things to consider in getting some relief. Your providers can help or may refer you to trusted colleagues. Before referral, some specific considerations need to cross their minds:

- Is there any symptom of central nervous system involvement? Any weakness, headache, or other suspicious pattern?
- Is there any suspicion that the cancer is growing in a different place than has already been identified? General fatigue and moodiness can be common with growths in the pancreas, wall of stomach, or adrenal glands.
- Any symptoms of *hypothyroidism*? Tremor, constipation, lower energy, and lower voice can all be related to the cancer. Should a T4 and TSH test be done? Hypothyroidism can mimic depression.
- Any other unusual organ slowdown, particularly kidneys or liver?
- Is it really a feeling of *sadness,* or is that emotion a marker for other things: someone who asks a lot of questions (even good ones), someone who likes to "think the worst" to be relieved when the news is OK, but worries a lot along the way?

Use of antidepressants can be *extraordinarily* helpful. The "stigma problem" is still extraordinarily burdensome. Many people say to themselves, "Not only do I have cancer, but I am a wimp," implying that major depression is a failure of spirit or will. What do we know about depression in cancer? Quite a lot.

Major depression is associated with certain biochemical changes in the brain. The limbic system is home to emotional responses, including the crisis response, also known as *fight or flight.* Think of the neurons in

continued

MED SCHOOL IN A BOX:
TREATMENT OF MAJOR DEPRESSION

continued

the brain like the electrical system in your house. In your house, the wires have to physically touch each other (a *connection*) for current to go from one place to another. In the brain, these connections don't exist in the same way. There is a space (*synapse*) between the cells, and the transmission must jump this space. It does so millions of times for each movement or thought or sensation you have. This space is not empty. It is filled with fluids that contain chemical messengers, or *neurotransmitters,* that bring the message across the space very quickly, sort of like a ferryboat crosses a river. But very, very quickly. Imagine touching a hot stove. You know it is hot in less than a second and pull your hand back as a result of many connections and neurotransmitter ferries. The neurotransmitters dopamine, acetylcholine, and serotonin all must be in balance, and when depression becomes serious, they are not. They must also hit the dock and let the passengers out before pulling away. If the messenger pulls out of the chemical pier too quickly, the message is not effectively sent.

The logical person would say, "Well, why not put the neurotransmitters in a pill?" Great idea, if it were possible, but the neurotransmitters themselves are proteins that would get digested by the stomach and wouldn't get to the synapses. So medications have been designed to make the synaptic transmission more efficient. Discovery of effective drugs to alter this process has been tedious, because the positive effects still come with side effects on other neurotransmitters. Much progress has been made.

In the cancer treatment world, taking advantage of counseling and medications is the best route to treat a serious depression. A variety of medications is available, some affecting one neurotransmitter more than another. Just as when prescribing chemotherapy, the choice of agent and dosage is not random. The agent chosen should be the one that is likely best for you. A few of the antidepressants cause some sedation at the start, great if you are not sleeping well. So you can take them at night. The initial dose needs to be personalized (also within the parameters of your drug plan), and then the dose needs to be raised from one that is too small to one that is just right. Taking a full dose from the start may give you problematic side effects before good effects and keep you from continuing. Since these medications work so well, it is human nature to stop or forget the doses after a few weeks, but the best results require staying on them for a few months.

The best effect comes when coupled with some counseling. Clinicians sometimes think a particular type of counseling is best, but the studies show that what type matters less. What matters most is the human contact reinforces the medication effects, and together they make the most difference.

■ *I've heard of being* shell shocked *after being in battle, but does that apply after cancer? Is this a misunderstanding of the facts?*

No not at all. The more modern term for *shell shocked,* a common term after World War II, is *post-traumatic stress disorder* or *PTSD.* PTSD is a debilitating condition that can result after a person experiences a terrifying event or ordeal, such as a violent assault, a natural disaster, an accident, terrorism, military combat—or cancer! People with PTSD often relive the traumatic event in flashbacks, memories, or nightmares. Other symptoms include irritability, anger outbursts, intense guilt, and avoidance of thinking or talking about the traumatic ordeal. Persistent nightmares or flashbacks about treatment are disruptive to recovery and ruin quality of daily life. Treatment is essential and mirrors treatment for major depression: counseling and medications, most likely antidepressant medications. This is *not* because PTSD is hidden depression, but because some of the frightened and angry responses in the brain arise from the same location (the limbic system) and the same neurotransmitters involved in major depression.

SHELL SHOCKED: POST-TRAUMATIC STRESS DISORDER AND CANCER

Re-experiencing significant cancer-related events with hypervigilance, anger, and heightened arousal (always thinking about the incidents, reliving them over and over, and worried they will happen again).

Recurring memories of important experiences: receiving the diagnosis or taking the different diagnostic tests or treatments.

Repeated nightmares or flashbacks about the important cancer experiences, sometimes described as *reliving* them over and over.

■ *My doctor and nurse started to discuss* genetic testing *with me. They think my cancer can run in families, and they want to see if that is the case in my situation. Should I consider this?*

This is scary. "Not only do I have cancer, but to think I could give it to my kids!"

Since some cancers are the result of a genetic change from the material passed to you by your parents, it would be helpful to know if you or other family members are at risk for that or other types of cancer. There are 23 pairs of chromosomes that join together when an egg is fertilized by sperm, and those chromosomes carry many genes. A break in the sequence of proteins on the gene or change in its information can be inherited, and its presence may affect your treatment plan, in addition to direct family members. Each accredited cancer center has its own genetics counselor who can meet with you, review your family cancer history, and see if there are any known patterns that could show a genetic *predisposition* to getting a particular cancer. If there is not a suspicious pattern in your family, your insurance company probably would not approve the testing anyway. Best to ask. With the popularity of genealogical discovery on the web, such genetic testing adds another dimension to preventive care for a second malignancy or cancer in the family. Rarely is genetic testing important when you are dealing with the first few weeks after diagnosis. But as you feel less busy with treatment and ready to move on, it can be vital to you and your family. Fears that such information can be used against someone for employment or insurance purchase in the future have yet to be founded in fact. Stringent privacy and confidentiality laws are being updated to assure that such information is used constructively and not to deny care or a job.

GENETIC TESTING: WHO? ME?

Genetic testing may be recommended if you have two or more close relatives who had cancer, especially if they were diagnosed at a young age.

Inherited patterns of cancer are suspected or have been established in breast, colon, pancreatic, and ovarian cancers.

For other cancers, people in the same family who grew up in the same environment are likely to have the same chemical exposures or exposure to secondhand smoke.

Ask your providers if they believe that you should have genetic testing, and if they are not sure, ask to review your family history (*genogram* or *family pedigree*) with an experienced genetic counselor.

■ *My oncologist is sending me to my dentist. The cancer was not near the mouth. Is (s)he just making business for colleagues?*

Cancer affects the mouth as it affects various parts of the body even though the cancer is not located there. Both chemotherapy and radiation therapy affect the mouth. The mouth, like most of the digestive system, harbors good bacteria to aid in the process of digestion that can be affected by treatment. A low platelet count that can cause bleeding or oozing can occur in the mouth. Mouth sores are an uncomfortable side effect of most treatment. Your oncologist is probably sending you to the dentist for a thorough pretreatment exam and to fix what may give you trouble in the coming months. Dentists find it is hard or impossible to provide optimal care for you if you are going to have excessive bleeding or mucus, or if the healing will be delayed by chemotherapy's effects on the white blood cells.

After treatment, you will need a repeat exam and a good cleaning, since many of the medications used in treatment are drying, which can cause cavities or worsen infections. A dry mouth is very hard on the gums. Plaque and tarter that has accumulated during treatment can be skillfully scraped off. This is not a do-it-yourself project, even if you have good dexterity. Radiation to the mouth area can also affect the gums and teeth. These dental visits are part of good care. Dentists routinely check the mouth for unexpected growths or infections as part of healthy mouth care.

■ *So, I can understand seeing the dentist, but also the podiatrist? Isn't this an extreme suggestion?*

Well, no. What happens in the mouth also happens on the feet, particularly when the feet are in shoes that enclose them (making it a closed environment, like the mouth). Bleeding or infections can prevent you from walking, which is essential to "My Recovery Plan" in the *A,* or activity, category. Fungal infections on the hands are easy to spot. Many of us rarely look at the soles of our feet or in between our toes, places that fungus loves to live. Keeping your feet fungus free is one step (no pun intended) to being infection free. If you are diabetic or prediabetic, the associated neuropathy from treatment can cause rubs or abrasions that can easily bleed or get infected. Certain chemotherapies cause inflammation of the hands and feet. The targeted therapies also affect the skin on the feet. Feet are often a neglected part of skin cancer screening. This is an important component of good care at a time when healing is critical to recovery.

■ *What is* lymphedema, *and why is everyone so worried about it?*

Lymphedema is a technical term for when the arms, hands, legs, or feet (or even breasts) swell because they collect fluid. This can occur after surgery on any of these areas, or if the lymph channels draining the area are blocked. Lymphedema can be painful and holds back recovery because it limits activity and can be a source of infection or blood clots. Lymphedema can often be prevented in the same proactive way as many of the symptoms already discussed. Smaller, minimally invasive breast surgeries risk lymph node function in the arm on the side of the surgery less than larger procedures where with older procedures many lymph nodes were removed for examination (biopsy). A method to help minimize node removal in breast and melanoma surgery is the *sentinel node biopsy* in which a small amount of blue dye and radioactive tracer are injected into the end of the lymph node chain, so that an enlarged blue lymph node or one with a collection of the tracer is biopsied, but those without the blue dye or tracer are sampled. Many fewer nodes removed, leaving the nodes intact to do their drainage job in the healing process causing less potential swelling. Think of lymph nodes like the body's drainage system in a sink. Clean-flowing lymph is helpful in healing and removing fluid on a constant basis. Although lymphedema can occur way after surgery, that is rare.

Lymphedema specialists are often nurses or physical therapists with additional training and certification in lymphedema care.

One of the attractive *complementary-alternative* therapies involves lymphatic drainage and cleansing when lymphedema is not involved, as a way to rid the system of *toxins*. Sounds sensible but has not yet been shown to be beneficial. Approach such claims with a healthy amount of skepticism, and be sure to ask your oncology treatment team about such a treatment if you plan to try it out.

■ *Do I need my regular immunizations during cancer treatment? If cancer is largely immunologic, does it make sense to mix up the immune system even more than necessary?*

This is a common question, particularly when flu season arrives every autumn. The current recommendations favor immunization for most people undergoing treatment. A bad influenza can delay your chemotherapy or radiation therapy, and the reduction in your infection-fighting white blood cells may make the flu harder to shake. This is definitely a question for your treatment team and may change from year to year. The pneumonia vaccine (Pneumovax®) is also routinely offered to patients who will be immunosuppressed from treatment. If you are to be out and about where you can get cut with something rusty (practically anywhere), an up-to-date tetanus shot is in order. If you are offered a varicella vaccine (Varivax® or varicella-zoster vaccination for chicken pox), please be sure to defer until you speak with your cancer specialists. *Live attenuated* vaccine (processed live virus) can theoretically cause infection in those whose immune system is compromised from cancer and treatment.

INFORMATION FOR MY PRIMARY CARE PROVIDERS

■ *What should I be checking for? Since the busyness of treatment is over and I am recovering (mostly), am I at risk for other cancers now that I had the first?*

Pap smears, mammograms, stool tests for hidden (occult) blood, sigmoidoscopy or colonoscopy, skin checks, PSA blood tests, and digital rectal exams are necessary on schedule based upon age. A good check for neuropathy is essential using a clean flexible fiber, a small plastic pinwheel and some warm and cool water and a reflex hammer.

The American Cancer Society has up-to-date guidelines on its website (http://www.cancer.org/Healthy/FindCancerEarly/CancerScreeningGuidelines/american-cancer-society-guidelines-for-the-early-detection-of-cancer) as does the National Cancer Institute (http://www.cancer.gov/cancertopics/pdq/screening/overview/patient). Since these guidelines are regularly questioned and updated, the web is your best source of up-to-date information.

Questioning the need for some cancer screening in an older cancer survivor, especially for breast or prostate cancer in those over 70 years of age, is a current area of discussion and is an important individual decision among patients, their families, primary care providers, and oncology specialists. There is a growing sense that mammograms and prostate screenings may be less effective in this group, but there is no official set of guidelines yet.

■ *How often do I really need to see my cancer specialists?*

That depends upon who is doing most of follow-up care; unnecessary to duplicate, but be sure that it is a coordinated plan. There are not yet accepted guidelines; adherence to the schedule you are given is important, though. Using the PHRs provided at the end of this book to transmit information between providers will be essential unless they all work from a unified medical record in their offices that connects to the hospital, radiation therapy centers, laboratory processing blood and urine tests, and radiologist. Only very recently, likely due to the discussion sparked by the Institute of Medicine report, follow-up guidelines have been considered as part of accepted treatment guidelines. Such information can be specified by your treatment team on the worksheet pertaining to a particular kind of cancer.

The
LEARN
System©

p.277
Personal
Health
Record

CONSULTATION IN A BOX: OVERLAPPING CARE

AK is a 58-year-old woman who developed breast cancer while she was between jobs. She waited until she got coverage back at her new job about six months after she found the initial lesion, and during that time, it had grown to the point where she needed a full mastectomy, chemotherapy, radiation to the chest wall, and then reconstruction, followed by hormonal treatments. She actually did quite well through all the phases of her treatment, but developed high blood pressure and severe hot flashes despite her menopausal status, and required treatment for the hot flashes with acupuncture and fluoxetine. The fluoxetine caused hand tremors, which she felt a small price to pay as it completely controlled her hot flashes. As a result of a year's worth of treatment, her follow-up included seeing her primary care provider, her breast surgeon, a medical oncologist, a radiation oncologist, and a palliative care specialist (for the hot flashes and tremor). As a result, there was a lot of overlap in what the providers did. She spread out the visits to the medical, radiation, surgical, and reconstruction oncologists throughout the year as they each did a thorough breast exam on the remaining breast as well as the underarm area next to the reconstruction. She also separated the visits to the palliative care and primary care providers, who checked her blood pressure and agreed to order the same lab tests. She feels more confident that if she gets a recurrence, it will be found in its earliest stages since she gets so many professional breast exams. Since she has been following this routine for nine years, a superstitious streak encourages the routine that has served her so well.

Such communication is reflected in the "Personal Health Record" worksheet to help document what is necessary and foster communication between the providers.

Since your insurance plan may dictate who does what (based upon approvals requested by your primary care provider), sharing the "Personal Health Record" with the case manager at your insurance company, spreads the communication one step further.

QUESTIONS I WANT ANSWERED

The most common question people have but rarely ask is, *Will my cancer come back?* Or, *Is there a time that I can "breathe a sigh of relief"?* These are hard questions to answer. You will probably receive two types of responses from providers: the longer one that explains how it is impossible to know and the challenge of living with uncertainty, or the shorter but more limiting one that "you'll be fine." People differ in their preference for one type of answer or the other, and with the information shared on the "What Is Important to Me" worksheet, the style of response will fit in nicely.

The
LEARN
System©

p. 248
What Is
Important
to Me

23 Fertility

■ *I have not had children. I was too scared to ask about this before. Can I? When?*

It was the furthest thing from your mind when you heard about the cancer.

Sperm banking, egg cryopreservation—you may be astounded that these things are being offered to you. "How can I think about having children when I am secretly worried that I won't be around to bring them up?" is a common concern. The thought of childbearing may be right out of left field. Or it may be very much on your mind if you want to have children and suspect that your treatment can interfere with the potential to have a family in the future.

This is the time *for men as well as women* to have (yet another) serious discussion. *Discussing the options about fertility preservation can't be postponed.*

There are many options for consideration. They need to be thought out before chemotherapy or radiation therapy begins. In men, the treatments may very well affect your ability to have children, immediately if you can't have or sustain an erection. Both chemotherapy and radiation to the pelvis can also affect the genetic information in sperm. Your insurance is likely to cover all or part of the cost of collection and storage for a finite period of time. Though it may seem out of place, this is the time to make your deposit, even if you or your oncologist requests *gonadal shielding* during radiation therapy. A shield is a blanket with lead in between the layers that deflects radiation away from the part it is protecting. If your cancer or the initial surgery has interfered with your body's ability to make spermatic fluid or you can't ejaculate, banking a portion of your testicle is an option, though any use of the sperm without fluid is limited to this choice. Artificial insemination cannot be performed with dry sperm, and in vitro fertilization will need to be considered.

WOMEN HAVE FEWER OPTIONS

Gonadal shielding can also be done for women. If you are having radiation near the ovaries, then an *ovarian transposition* or *oophoropexy* can move them out of the treatment field. A discussion about embryo or egg *cryopreservation* (freezing) for later use is in order.

Fertile Hope is an organization with a mission to raise the awareness of patients with cancer about the ever-changing choices in preserving fertility. Their website is a wealth of good information (http://www.fertilehope.com).

There is no doubt that the technology to postpone pregnancy by artificial insemination or in vitro methods or the ever-changing egg preservation techniques are astounding. More frequent discussion about egg preservation is occurring, but less so than for sperm banking.

■ *But… the part of the discussion that rarely happens, but is on everyone's mind, must occur…*

What do most of us fear while having the *technical* discussion? That we may not survive to be a responsible parent or to witness our child's many milestones, from first tooth through college graduation or marriage and beyond. That is an unknown.

When you think about it, that is an unknown for all of us. At times, all parents may think that we could have an illness or accident that would keep us from effective parenting or experiencing the joys of child rearing. But being diagnosed with cancer, even a cancer with a good chance of five-year-plus survival and no recurrence or relapse, makes us think about our vulnerabilities and parental responsibilities. That is why it is so important to think the process through and decide about sperm or testicular banking or egg preservation.

The next part of the discussion, which also rarely happens when cancer is not part of the picture, can be even harder. What are the contingency plans if one parent for any reason gets sick, dies, or is unable to parent for any reason?, Can the other parent be the sole parent, financially and emotionally? Who else in the family can help in case of such a turn of events? Who can be there for the child at school plays or soccer games? Who has the financial acumen to provide for a child's expenses and wellbeing? Who can help with the myriad roles a parent takes on? Many families rise to the occasion, and good friends pitch in as family members. It is possible to make a solid contingency plan and many families do so even without the specter of cancer.

Decisions about sperm banking and egg preservation are a tough call. But this road has been traveled before. With a bit of time to think, *most people will decide to leave their options open,* either sperm banking (easy and less expensive), egg preservation (harder to find), or even testicular banking (available only at certain specialty centers around the country, but it is a growing program). A decision to use the donation can be—and probably should be—made later.

The usual fallback in these uncomfortable discussions involves the adoption option. Yet while viable, the survivorship fear is the same. Being alive and able to experience parenting is the same for a biological child or an adoptive one.

WHAT ABOUT THE COSTS?

A practical side to the answer also takes hold. Only a few insurance companies will cover the cost of sperm banking before cancer treatment. Some may not do so without special prior approval. This is another situation where working with the case manager or within the disease management program of your insurance company can make a difference. Fifteen states currently have mandated insurers to offer coverage. These laws vary widely by state, insurance carrier, and even within insurance carriers in the details of the individual policy. The costs include processing the donation and a finite period of time for storage. The donations are a once or twice event; the storage is ongoing. Find out also what co-pays are owed for storage. This is an area that can sometimes

CONSULTATION IN A BOX: THE GENETIC TRAIL

A 41-year-old woman was treated for breast cancer with lumpectomy, radiation therapy, and hormonal treatments. She would be scheduled to finish her hormonal treatments at age 46, outside of her zone of comfort to be pregnant. (With a constantly changing knowledge base, most breast cancer doctors can be comfortable with patients becoming pregnant after two years of cancer-free living after hormonal treatments have been completed. Hormonal treatments can block the pregnancy anyway by suppressing the hormones necessary to make it happen. Using hormonal supplements in later age pregnancy runs additional risks.)

As her mother had breast cancer at age 39 (and is a healthy long-term survivor) and her sister is also a breast cancer survivor (diagnosed at age 42), she was advised to get genetic counseling and was asked to take a BRCA1/2 test since there were two close relatives with breast cancer early in life. She was not at all surprised when the testing came back positive. Her thoughts about the pregnancy were clearly stated: "I am relieved, for the first time in many years, that I did not have a child when I was younger, and that my career took center stage. It is amazing for me to think this or say this since I beat myself up so hard for not having children when I could, especially after I found out about the breast cancer."

She went on to explain that her sister had adopted a son years ago, and adoption in her family does not require special explanation or thought. But her clear reaction was one of not "pre-loading" (her exact word) a child with breast cancer genes, and that with an adoption, "the child may have a fighting chance that the family legacy would not include breast cancer."

At age 46, she applied for adoption. The agency processing the application was doubly concerned, due to the age of the parents and the breast cancer history. A response is pending.

require a one-on-one negotiation with the business manager at the tissue bank. The benefit varies widely state by state for Medicaid programs or varies greatly between insurance carriers.

If you are not good at such haggling, or if you are just not up to it now, ask someone you know, a family member or friend, to intercede on your behalf (a signed privacy release may be necessary). It is also an area where grants may be available for your geographic region, your income level, or other factors.

An experienced oncology social worker can find what is out there. Some monies may be specifically earmarked for such purposes. Other foundations that help people with cancer in extraordinary circumstances may be interested in this specific situation as well. A bit of Internet searching may uncover programs. If no one in your area is fluent in these issues, call Cancer*Care* (800-813-HOPE) for direction.

What can make the experience even more cruel is a loophole in the definition of *infertility* that can exclude patients with cancer. Denials of coverage can occur because cancer treatment does not cause someone to be technically infertile. *Infertility* is defined as the absence of conception after at least one year of regular, unprotected intercourse to attempt pregnancy. Most newly-diagnosed cancer patients do not meet this definition—they are in a unique situation where they know they may become infertile from their treatments, but they do not meet such a definition when the benefit is being accessed by the insurance carrier.

The fertility question opens up much larger discussions. Sometimes these discussions never happen at all. It varies family by family. It is unfortunately forced by the tissue-banking question. And it comes at the least opportune time. Be prepared.

24 Giving Back/Giving Forward

■ *I have received a lot of help. I'd like to help someone else? How can I give forward?*

There are more than a few productive and satisfying ways to *give back* to those that have helped you and *give forward* to the next generation of cancer survivors. Here are some suggestions. Share your own suggestions for others on *LEARN To Live Through Cancer's* website at http://www.cancerknowanddo.com.

GIVING BACK AND GIVING FORWARD

Volunteerism:

Speak with newly diagnosed patients to answer questions about the personal effects of cancer you experienced

Arrange to speak to small groups at work or places of worship

Accompany other patients to chemotherapy or radiation treatments

Help other patients at home with chores

Fund-raising:

Your cancer center (if a not for profit or non-profit)

CancerCare, a *local* chapter of the American Cancer Society, or specialty organization

Make donations

Help with events (walks, runs, art shows, etc.), stuffing envelopes, phone calls, clerical work, and publicity to support other events

Share what works:

Recipes, ideas, tips, and suggestions can be posted on http://www.cancerknowando.com to give forward to the next generations of patients and caregivers.

VOLUNTEERISM

It's a great way to start. Find out what is available where you have received your treatment. The local American Cancer Society (ACS) office or, nationally, CancerCare may have ideas for you based upon your location and your skills. You may want to become a veteran patient, available to meet and speak (even by telephone) with newly diagnosed patients who will greatly benefit from hearing from someone who has "been there." Depending on your location and the type of cancer you have had, as well as the programs available locally, the above resources are the best places to start. Advocacy groups for individual or a group of cancers exist and can use help. The ACS, Cancer*Care,* or the National Coalition of Cancer Survivors (http://www.canceradvo-cacy.org) can point you in the right direction.

Speak informally with your minister or rabbi where you attend services, and see if there is anyone in your neighborhood in need of a friendly visit or practical help. Although that keeps the benefits of your services local, having an organized program can help you with some creative ideas and supervision. That may help you start your own services tailored to your own neighborhood. Yes, it does take a village, but all villages are not the same!

A number of local chapters of the ACS (http://www.cancer.org) are training volunteer patient navigators for local cancer centers. The program provides training and direction by experienced staff.

The ACS facilitates individual peer-to-peer speakers for local houses of worship, corporate health offices in sizeable companies, or even schools and universities as an adjunct to standard course work. You have experience that professionals don't have, and if programs are available in your area, this is a good way to pay it forward. Local television affiliates may want to interview you if there is an awareness month for the kind of cancer you have had. And if you have had an *unusual* cancer for your demographic or gender (e.g., breast cancer in men), or have had treatment involving a new technology, the local health reporter may want to hear your story to share it as a public service. Such interviews, however self-involved they may feel, have a widespread impact on the public, more than you imagine.

If you have been treated at a not-for-profit hospital, there is probably an active volunteer department and/or development department that should be more than happy to help you help others. You may be able to jump into one of their existing programs that combine your time and energy with their good contacts in the community.

The development department at your not-for-profit hospital is the place to start if you are interested in raising money for their programs or if you want to suggest programs. Getting help from experienced fund-raisers assures that your efforts are channeled into legitimate programs to avoid scams. Unfortunately, every few weeks the national news reports on someone who feigned illness in order to collect from unsuspecting donors. You do not want your efforts to be squandered with such associations. Contributions to a non-profit agency or hospital will come under their tax exempt status, so they are deductible expenses under IRS rules for those who contribute.

Due to the need to have tax exempt status to attract donors, fund-raising for cancer-related activities such as research or patient services is hard to manage on your own. Setting up a foundation or IRS code 501c3 organization so that donations can be tax deductible by contributors is complicated and needs professional oversight. There are marches, walks, runs, and other affinity programs throughout the country. Join one of them to see how things are done.

Giving back of time and/or money is a good way to move forward with the healing process for you and helps those who are just starting the process.

Due to federal protection of privacy and confidentiality under the Health Insurance Portability and Accountability Act, no one will be able to contact you without having one of your providers ask you first for consent. You, on the other hand, do not need their consent to ask. There can be a fine line between solicitation and privacy violation. Even more reasons to work with the professionals.

Just a small effort of an afternoon each month making friendly visits can mean so much to patients now in treatment and to the staff who see that you are giving their efforts forward. Meeting with a patient while he or she is in chemotherapy and discussing a book you are both reading, playing a few games of cards, or doing a crossword puzzle or playing Scrabble® together can mean so much. Giving back and giving forward also gives to yourself!

School health programs sometimes invite people from the community to discuss their personal experiences with students, taking age and sophistication into account. The school nurse or science coordinator/chairperson may be of help in setting you up to open the dialogue about cancer in your school. Your local ACS chapter may have materials for you to use. Speaking about the role that tobacco and alcohol may have played in the development of your cancer to young people whose habits are just forming may save many from future cancer treatment.

■ *Who am I helping: My community or myself?*

Simply, both. Not bad. A real two-for-one deal.

■ *I do not have the financial means to contribute. What else can I do?*

Share what has worked for you: tips, ideas, and recipes on http://www.cancerkknowanddo.com. Your experiences are a gift to current and future generations of patients and caregivers who are new visitors to the unusual land of cancer treatment. Pass along what works!

■ *Where can I get more and reliable information?*

Start with one of your cancer doctors. Many in private practices may have ties to a foundation or research group or may have veteran patients involved in their practices.

Part VI

Six Months and Beyond

25 Living Cancer Free

The recovery process is moving along. You are relieved to be feeling better and worried that you will learn that there is a recurrence or relapse. This is the odd, often unreal world that survivorship creates.

Adjustments to a healing body, mind, and spirit are occurring, so resulting adjustments to the LEARN System should also be continually occurring. In our technological world, the inevitable comparison to computer technology is made. So this phase is often called the *reboot,* when you reset the basic components that much more mirror your way of living before the cancer.

Fortunately, this is a crossroad point in your treatment. The hard questions you need to ask yourself have been those you have grappled with thus far in "My Recovery Plan" and the LEARN System. Deciding how long to follow its principles is the current task.

Does it "pay" to continue the higher level of adherence to a plan of good nutrition, extra activity, and assuring good rest and sleep at this point? If you have adopted the suggested improvements in diet, exercise, and rest, was it worth it? Do you think you feel better than if you would have waited for the "enlightenment?" There is no way to know. If your newly adopted habits are heart healthy, is that enough of a reason to continue? Your primary care provider and family probably resoundingly say, "Yes."

Take 30 minutes aside from the computer and telephone. Think back over the previous months and ask yourself the following:

- What would I have done differently? Knowing what I know now, would I have changed anything? Why is that important?
- If a relapse or recurrence is never to be, what have I learned that spilled over to the non-cancer parts of my life? Did I become more cynical, hardened, or jaded? Does the new appreciation for niceties continue, or do I now take people and situations for granted?
- What is my vision of the future? What will my life be like (we don't know for certain, that is true)? What are the possibilities? Thinking about the future is something you and your family may have suspended over the last few months, and if so, it is time to get back to your planning. Consider the changes in you that have likely affected your job (if you are working) or your employability (if you're not). Your work responsibilities may also have changed even if they weren't self-imposed. Many internal and external changes are very subtle and require some reflection and observation.
- Is a job or career change something to think about now? (Once federal protections for health insurance are in place in 2013, your answer may be different from now.) Having a major medical illness treated in the recent past (18 months in some localities) carries a *preexisting condition* rating to your insurability if you are going to cost out buying insurance on your own. That can get expensive. Such realities force some people to stay in a job that has outgrown them or that they have

outgrown. Having a pre-existing condition may unfortunately be an impediment to working in a small business. Ironically, if you are not working, your options may be greater today than in the past as many states opened up subsidized health insurance to non-working citizens when Medicaid was expanded to children and families. Specialized disease management programs are often part of these programs. Availability and eligibility vary by locale.

• Have I gone through any spiritual changes? It may actually be too soon to know as those adjustments often take longer than a few months. Do I treat others differently? Am I more impatient or more tolerant of others?

• Do I continue to *seize the day* and experience the moment?

LINGERING SIDE EFFECTS: ARE THEY MINE FOR THE REST OF MY LIFE?

Maybe. You will need to balance the relief of survival and the burdens of ongoing side effects—especially subtle ones that would normally be considered trivial but now loom large as you think of having a future. Long-term effects often include neuropathic pain and changes in taste or smell. Does it seem that food lingers longer in the stomach causing you to feel full? Has there been a permanent change in your bowel habits? Does it take longer for food to move through your system? Is there always a feeling of indigestion? Referred to as *gastroparesis,* these symptoms are sometimes reported after chemotherapy. If it seems that food is rushing through you and you've had radiation to the abdomen or pelvis, ask one of the cancer subspecialists for help, which may be medication to slow the speed down a bit, and then a referral to a gastroenterologist for a work-up.

Neuropathy may still be a problem, though less so than before. Taking care not to stumble and to be truly mindful of hot, cold, or irregular surfaces will save future injury. Wearing shoes or slippers all the time saves the scrape that may become infected, a stubbed toe that seems like it takes *forever* to heal, or a burn when you couldn't tell an object or the water was hot. Healing will be slower than before, so avoiding potentially problematic situations is key. But you also don't want to live in a bubble. It's a fine balance at times.

Any lingering problem that you bring up with your primary care provider may kick off a series of new doctor visits and testing. You need to ask yourself how subtle or prominent the symptom is to you and if it is worth these efforts. You need to ask your provider how important it is to look into. Sometimes it is, and sometimes it is not. The result of those two judgments will tell you how closely to pursue it.

■ *What should I be checking for?*

That depends upon what type of cancer you were treated for or what you were treated with. These lingering or late side effects *do not happen very often,* but when they are found, most people ask, "Why wasn't I warned?"

If you had:	**Check for:**
Radiation therapy:	any new lump that comes and stays in the field where you received treatment (sarcoma),

	muscle tightness (fibrosis) not getting better with heat or stretching
Radiation therapy to mouth:	tooth decay, jaw pain, osteoradionecrosis (thinning of the jaw bone at the site of radiation)
Radiation therapy to pelvis:	diarrhea, fistulas
Chemotherapy:	blood counts to monitor for leukemia
Breast cancer:	regular Pap smears with an occasional endometrial biopsy to rule out endometrial cancer, with slight increased risk from tamoxifen
Bisphosphonates with opening to jaw under teeth:	osteonecrosis of the jaw
Adriamycin or taxanes with radiation therapy:	radiation recall, red skin and pain in skin

Preparing for My First Anniversary

Plan for your first anniversary; mark the day to commemorate in some way. You can count it anyway you want from the day of a suspicious symptom, the day of official diagnosis, the day of surgery, or the day starting your first chemotherapy or radiation therapy. If you don't anticipate it, many people say they have a vague sense of something unusual happening that day but can't figure out what. Unusual feelings creep up on you if you don't plan ahead for them. It is an unusual type of anniversary or series of anniversaries. Some people don't celebrate them formally at the risk of tempting fate. Others mark the occasion.

Questions I Want Answered

Will you ever forget these past few months? Probably not. Will things ever be the same? Likely not. Will they have changed for the good or the bad? It depends on what you do with the experience. Use the anniversary as an impetus day to reach out as a veteran patient if you have not been able to in the last year. Use the day to make a donation to a cancer-related organization or volunteer for it. Call the people that helped you most to say thank you (or send a card or e-mail).

■ *Where can I get more and reliable information?*

One of the practical ways to put the anniversary concept to good use is to make it a signal to review the necessary screenings for your own situation, if there are published guidelines, or to follow the formula that you collaboratively developed with your providers. That funny feeling that comes on in a wave around the time of the anniversaries of significant cancer milestones can be put to good use.

26 Living with a Recurrence, Relapse, or Residual Cancer

No one wants to hear those words, especially after having done everything "the right way" for the past few months. It's even more upsetting if you have followed the cancer prevention and heart-healthy guidelines for many years. This was not supposed to happen.

QUESTIONS I'D LIKE TO ASK IF I HAVE MORE CANCER

- Why did the cancer come back?
- Can it be cured? Controlled? Put in remission?
- Will I recover and be myself?
- What will the treatment include?
- Can I continue to work?
- Should I re-consult the second opinion oncologist?
- Will I be more symptomatic with this round of treatment than the first?
- How should I alter my self-care this time?
- What will be affected by the cancer and by the treatments this time?
- Should there be any change in vitamins and supplements?
- Is this the time to look for a clinical trial?
- What is important to me now?
- What do I have to do to get better?
- When will I feel OK again?
- Will I be the same?
- Will the cancer come back again?
- How much time do I have?

Most people feel angry and cheated, and very, very disappointed. That being said, the words, even used all at once, do not adequately describe the feelings. As at the time of the original diagnosis, one often feels that getting cancer is a personal weakness in character, moral fortitude, or adherence. Many will also question their treatment choices. Did I go to the right doctors? The best hospital? Was it the best treatment? Did someone make a mistake? How can this have happened? Will I die from this?

Good questions with no easy answers. The first response is, "It depends." That is not comforting. Medicine relies on precision and critical thinking. Oncology is at the forefront of evidence-based medicine and proof-of-purchase using the placebo-controlled randomized clinical trial. Yes, but not everyone responds to any one regimen. There is nothing in cancer treatment, and very little in life, that is 100 percent.

First, a few definitions:

A *recurrence* refers to a solid tumor that has shown up after a period of time when it was not discoverable (it may have been there but was too small to detect, or it may be a brand-new growth with the same genetic information). A *second primary cancer* is the same type of cancer with a variation in its genetic fingerprint. A *relapse* is the same as a recurrence, but applies to leukemia, lymphoma or multiple myeloma. *Residual cancer* refers to the original cancer that is persistent, and has continued to grow in the same area of the body despite treatment. *Metastatic cancer* is the same cancer growing in a different part of the body.

So what are the variables?

1. Type of cancer. Even if it is a kind of cancer that is responsive to treatment, are there good options left? Due to the advances in the treatment of some cancers, particularly those that are hormone dependent (breast cancer, prostate cancer), spread to the bones is technically *late stage*. That is a deceptively unfortunate product of an old staging system in that it is often very controllable with ongoing maintenance treatment. Some second-, third-, or even fourth-line therapies are still effective.

2. How sensitive is it to second-line chemotherapy or radiation therapy (if radiation had not been part of the original treatment or has not been used to the maximum amount for that body part)? Third-, fourth-, and fifth-line drugs that have been FDA approved are often are active to treat with many cancers. Even if the response rates are less than you have heard at first, *someone* is in that group. It could be you.

3. Is your general health now good enough to withstand more treatment? Specifically, do you have an appetite, are you at the correct weight, and is your energy level up? Does your bone marrow have the resilience to replace new cells if it is to be suppressed by future chemotherapy?

4. Can you emotionally withstand more treatment now? Some people say it is easier the second time since they know what to expect and how to manage. Others say it is harder the second time as they sustained their hope through the first treatment with the idea that the cancer would be cured, and they won't be able to do so again with the same naïve confidence.

Next steps

1. Meet with your primary oncologists. That may be the surgeon, radiation oncologist, or medical oncologist. It may mean making three separate appointments. Find out what they are thinking and what your options are. Ask them to speak among themselves to come up with the best possible plan.

2. See if your case can be presented again at their Tumor Board for reconsideration by the larger group, so that they can cull ideas for you from their colleagues.

3. Ask about revisiting the oncologist who had provided a second opinion at the time of the original diagnosis. If you did not have the chance to have a second opinion then, now may be the time to do so.

4. Look online and see who the experts are and where they are in practice. There may very well be one in your area. If a general search engine does not reveal one, look at the National Cancer Institute (NCI) website for a list of clinical trials and enter information about your cancer, stage, and recurrence/relapse status (http://www.cancer.gov/clinicaltrials), not to find a trial but to see who is an investigator on your type of cancer, where he or she works, and if there is a co-investigator close to where you live. That oncologist will have more than the usual experience with your situation and may be the optimal second opinion.

5. If your health insurance needs prior approval, work with the disease management program or case manager (called by different names in different companies) not only to get authorization, but to be referred to a provider who is in network that has had treated a similar cancer that has not responded to first-line treatment. If the representative with whom you are speaking is not sure, ask him or her to speak with (or if you can speak with) a more senior nurse or the medical director. Try to have them work with you instead of adversarially. Appeal to them in a human-to-human way, focusing on wanting to find the best care, and play by the rules as any reasonable person would. They may be very willing to help or even see you as a high-cost customer who needs to overcome the obstacles their system has in place.

6. Ask about clinical trials. You will see from the NCI website that there are probably trials for you. Some may involve variations of FDA-approved treatments, or some use novel substances. Most likely, he list is likely technical. Ask for help from your own treatment team.

An online resource from the American Cancer Society (ACS) is the Clinical Trials Matching Service at http://www.cancer.org/treatment/treatmentsandsideeffects/clini caltrials/app/clinical-trials-matching-service (or you can get help over the telephone at 800-303-5691). Reading all of the information requires a certain amount of medspeak to sift through all of it and see what is practical for you. The NCI Cancer Information Service (1-800-4-CANCER) can also help you sort out the options.

■ *Despite everyone's best efforts, my health is declining. What should I do next?*

Do you still have the symptoms of cancer (pain, shortness of breath, anemia, repeat infections with multiple courses of antibiotics)? Or are you having trouble maintaining your energy, weight, and appetite while you seem to be getting weaker?

Schedule a *long* appointment with your main oncologist. Don't expect that the sub-specialists can all meet in-person with you at the same time, but if they work in the same place, it may be possible for them to consult. Or they may meet with one

The LEARN System©

p. 248
What Is Important to Me

MED SCHOOL IN A BOX: THE CONSPIRACY OF SILENCE

Although the words are strong, behind the concept is kindness stoked by fear. This idea has been applied to a phenomenon in medical care in which a hard choice has to be made, often through discussion, but each party is afraid to offend the other. In the context of cancer treatment, there are opposing forces at work. With some variations of this scenario, the basics apply to many situations. Here is what each party is thinking.

PROVIDER: I feel like a failure. I'm supposed to fix cancer, get people better. It hurts to bring this up because they will be angry with me and disappointed in me. We need a lot of time to have such a careful discussion. Having these discussions a few times a day takes a lot out of me with little time to recover. Then there are the phone calls, usually from relatives who are not here and do not know what is going on. So I will have to playback the conversations again for them. Maybe a few times. They will be angry too. They may threaten a lawsuit. It is easier to avoid this talk altogether and just move into the second-, third-, or fourth-line regimen and hope for the best. If I don't offer _____ treatment, I must be prepared to spend a lot of time and energy in controlling the symptoms.

PATIENT: I don't want to hear that I am doing badly, but I know it is so. I am really tired all of the time, and I have no appetite. I'm afraid to mention this to the doctor because (s)he will give up on me. I am really afraid of that happening, so when I am asked, "How do you feel?" my answer is, "Fine."

FAMILY: I just know that my _____ is too upset to hear bad news. (S)he so wants to get better, and if (s)he hears that there are few/no options of effective treatment left, (s)he will just give up and die. I can't bear to see that happen. (S)he has been so strong. (S)he just won't be able to take bad news without giving up.

Hence the *conspiracy of silence*. No one means harm. If anything, everyone is protecting everyone else—and him- or herself. It often works for a while, until the person gets really sick. If that happens, most often an inpatient hospitalization follows, and that hospitalization may fill the major part of the last few days or weeks of someone's life.

With the *conspiracy of silence*, the excessive burden of getting sicker and closer to dying is left to the patient himself or herself, unable to share it with close family and friends. He or she is grappling with the idea that death is closer and coping in isolation because the people who are close enough and skilled enough to help out—his/her providers and family members—are all being lovingly protective all around. Such is the case for many patients and families around the country. There are a few steps to take in this situation that can ease the burden for everyone. Reconnect with the social

continued

MED SCHOOL IN A BOX: THE CONSPIRACY OF SILENCE

continued

worker at your cancer center or the pastoral care chaplain. Make an appointment with your community spiritual leader to discuss the burden. If you cannot connect to those individuals in your area, be sure to call Cancer*Care* to discuss with one of the oncology social workers there by phone or e-mail. *It is unnecessary to go through this stage of care alone.*

Your insurance benefits can also help with a robust medical benefit embedded in Medicare, Medicaid, and most private health insurances. *Hospice is* one of the most generous and misunderstood managed care benefits around, yet nationally less than 43 percent of deaths occur while the patient is enrolled in a hospice program. Even fewer patients have access to palliative care in their hospitals or at home, although it is gaining momentum in larger urban academic hospitals as well as in smaller communities.

So how can one break the conspiracy of silence? By referring back to the "What Is Important to Me" worksheet, one of the first tasks in "My Recovery Plan", the proverbial ice has been broken. Please bring it with you to these longer appointments with your cancer subspecialists. Show it to them, and ask them how what is important to you meshes with their recommendations.

The burden should not be on you alone, and it is not.

The
LEARN
System©

p. 248
What Is
Important
to Me

another (and you) on a conference call. In any case, bring your relative or friend who knows you well, is a good listener and note taker, and can ask good questions.

Before this appointment, review the notes you made at the beginning of treatment on the "What Is Important to Me" worksheet. You should bring it with you or even show it to whomever is accompanying you to this appointment. Be prepared to ask some hard questions. This will be one of the most difficult visits you will make.

■ *I've heard of the living will. How is this document different?*

A living will is a document that allows you to specify, in advance, what *should* be done. When the living will is written, you really have to be clairvoyant, knowing what you're going to get and what will be available to treat that malady if and when you get it. Such foresight is a bit impossible. So a living will is really best suited for you to describe what you *don't want.* The "What Is Important to Me" worksheet is more specific in that it is completed after the cancer has been formally diagnosed and you are learning what treatment is planned. "What Is Important to Me" can be more specific to your own situation and is a summary of what should be done and how you want to be treated, not just what treatments you would consider.

■ *What are advance directives?*

An advance directive is a general term, which includes living wills as well as other types of documents in which you can name someone you trust to speak for you and make medical decisions in your place if you are unable to understand the details and speak up for yourself. It is a "power of Attorney" for medical decisions. It is more flexible than a living will in that you don't need to anticipate your illness and its potential treatment when the form is completed.

Although making your wishes known through these forms is a federal law, each state decides which format is acceptable, without uniformity across the United States.

The important element of course is the discussion of your goals and values. Using "My Recovery Plan," you have had those discussions, transforming the completion of the paperwork into the easiest part of the process.

■ *What happens next?*

During an office appointment with the main surgical or medical or radiation oncologist in combination or sequentially, you will hear what each thinks—or together they believe—what the next steps should be. Whatever their advice: to treat with anti-cancer therapy aggressively, to treat with anti-cancer therapy conservatively or not to focus on comfort and symptom relief, use "What Is Important to Me" to put the latest recommendations in context. For example:

"Thank you for considering what my options are. Let's see how that matches with what I/you/he/she thought at the time of diagnosis."

If the decision is made to proceed with symptomatic relief and comfort, the information from the form magically opens the door for honest discussion, and turns an awkward time into a purpose-driven one. Not by coincidence, the same techniques of self-care during cancer treatment in anticipation of good recovery are the same things you do now with a recurrence, relapse, or residual cancer. The activities may need to be adapted to being the primary modes of treatment, but the basics are the same.

BRING YOUR PRIMARY CARE PROVIDER BACK INTO THE CARE LOOP

If your primary care provider has been involved in the details of your care throughout your cancer treatment, or hasn't but your insurance no longer authorizes visits to the medical oncologist once off treatment, make a follow-up appointment with your primary care provider. Prepare the receptionist or assistant booking the appointment to leave a little extra time for an extended discussion. Perhaps the visit will be the first scheduled for the day, or the last, or on a day when the provider has shorter office hours but catches up on paperwork. This is not a seven-minute discussion. Depending upon the means of communication between the oncology sub-specialist and your primary care provider thus far, follow the same pattern and ask one to contact the other before your visit so they can be aligned with each other, not just through you.

ACTIVITIES OF DAILY LIVING (ADLs):

- feeding (eating and drinking)
- grooming: bathing, dressing
- transferring (between bed, chair, toilet)
- toileting
- managing finances
- housekeeping
- meal preparation
- taking medications (remembering, dispensing)
- using the telephone

■ *This is lousy. Everyone is in agreement. What are the next steps?*

That depends upon a number of personal decisions, but the main force driving those choices is likely, "What is my current level of functioning?" Specifically, go back to the "Activities of Daily Living" (ADLs) list. Can you do the following: walk (ambulate) or get around on your own or with an assistive device, go to the bathroom, get dressed, shower or bathe, eat, prepare food, do light household chores? Can you do these independently or do you need help? If you need help, is it assistance to complete these tasks or total help?

If you need assistance or total help, review the information you discovered about your health insurance. Do you have any coverage for home care? Has it been used up? Do you have any long-term care insurance? What are the thresholds that allow you to start collecting its benefits? Some policies state the number of ADLs you cannot do independently and even specify if *with assistance* or *unable* helps qualify to collect the benefits of the policy.

This review is very timely, even if you feel just fine and you can do all of the things listed without assistance. Extra work? Of course. Do you only participate in a fire drill if you're expecting a fire? No.

■ *My Medicare (or private insurance benefits) provides home care? Can that help?*

Home care benefits are designed to provide short-term help, often used after hospital discharge to keep the hospital stay as short as possible and prevent readmission within 30 days. To qualify for home care services, one must be homebound except for doctors' visits and have a *skilled nursing need.* That is a very specific set of needs and totally unlike what it seems. A *skilled nursing need* means care of a surgical drain or dressings or an intravenous line with fluids or medications running through. Only with a skilled need can other services be provided at home: social work, physical therapy, medical equipment (hospital bed, commode, shower/bath seat), and some home health aide time to help with the ADLs. This is a very short-term program. There are other alternatives, however, based on your insurance coverage.

The
LEARN
System©

p. 333
My Bucket
List

p. 248
What Is
Important
to Me

p. 335
My Personal
Affairs

SERVICES PROVIDED BY A CERTIFIED HOME HEALTH AGENCY (CHHA)

Skilled nursing needs (tasks only a nurse can do):

Dressing a wound

Maintaining an intravenous line or tube feedings

Monitoring rapidly changing needs such as:

cardiac or pulmonary function

nutritional status

physical, occupational, or speech therapy

LIFE IMITATES ART

It is supposed to be the other way around. But not always. Have you seen the 2007 movie *The Bucket List*? Morgan Freeman and Jack Nicholson identify and try to do the things they put on their *bucket list,* or the things they would do if their life expectancies were shorter than they had hoped. The comedic points cannot be described, but the principle can be. Have any of us whose life has not felt threatened made our bucket list? Or even thought about it or what's more, have we done any of those things? This may be the time to reconsider (see the "My Bucket List" worksheet).

It is not an easy list to make, forcing you to face your values head-on, and prioritize what gives you the most meaning or joy in your lives. Note that the things that give you meaning may *not* be the same things that give you joy. Most lists contain elements of both properties. Involve people you love in a discussion of what you choose, or have them help you. Start off by reviewing your "What Is Important to Me" worksheet. You are likely to find lots of overlap.

◼ *Is that what people mean when I hear "time to put your affairs in order?"*

Well it could be. Unfortunately, that dire directive is often used after fatigue and stamina are insufficient for anything but paperwork or quiet thought. You are probably ahead of that point since the "What Is Important to Me" worksheet has been an ongoing process. *Affairs* usually means legal and paperwork things, such as beneficiaries on accounts, making a last will and testament, and reviewing living wills and health care proxies (see the "My Personal Affairs" worksheet).

A bucket list is more comprehensive and can be more enjoyable.

◼ *I do need assistance with the ADLs. What are my options?*

The information you reviewed when you looked at your health insurance or long-term care benefits are coming in handy sooner than you would hope, in the context of your bucket list. Can you piece together the care that you need at home with personal care aides and visiting nurse services? A social worker at your cancer center, someone from the local chapter of the ACS or Cancer*Care* can help you figure this out.

■ *I am unable to put together enough help for now. It's even hard to get to doctors' appointments, but I am not bed bound. I'm too tired for any more treatment. What can I do?*

This situation calls for one of the most misunderstood concepts in health care: *hospice.*

Hospice is not a place to go (from the biblical reference). Hospice is not for the last hours or days of life. Hospice is an *added value* benefit. It does not take away services; it adds to them.

Hospice was proposed as part of the Medicare benefit in 1974, and after demonstrating effectiveness, was made permanent in 1986. Private insurance and Medicaid plans that include hospice benefits generally follow the Medicare guidelines, with small differences. Hospice programs are generally home care programs that bring services to you as you become unable to get to doctors' offices, pharmacies, and other outside offices. The benefit provides care for life-threatening illness (not just cancer), if

HOSPICE: THE MISUNDERSTOOD CARE SYSTEM

A benefit of Medicare (Part A) and many private insurance and Medicaid plans providing end-of-life care in a variety of settings: home, skilled nursing facility, hospital, or hospice residence. It is *not* limited to the last hours or days of life.

Hospice is not a *place*. It is care that is brought to the patient and family that focuses on symptom management and the relief of suffering. Most services are supplied in the patient's home.

The goal of hospice care is to maximize comfort and functional status through an active approach to symptom relief, psychosocial, and spiritual support.

There are an unlimited number of days, evaluated at 90 days, 180 days, and every 60 days thereafter with evidence of decline in functioning and worsening of disease.

No co-pays or deductibles (changing with some private insurance plans)
Services come to you:

Specialist-level physicians and nurses

Personal counseling by social workers and chaplains

Prescriptions to treat the life-limiting illness

Medical equipment needed due to limitations from life-limiting illness

Volunteer services

Home hospice aide services based on medical necessity

Physical, speech, nutritional therapies based on medical necessity

Respite or short inpatient stays to stabilize symptoms or for complex care there is steady decline in functioning (those ADLs again) and certain criteria are met. For Medicare recipients, it is part of the Part A benefit, and there are no co-pays or deductibles. (Unfortunately, co-pays are beginning to be applied by various insurance plans with some managed care contracts.) Surprisingly, for those with Medicare, the hospice benefit provides not only a few days or weeks of care, but actually for an unlimited period of time as long as there is decline in functioning. Absolutely the reverse of what people think. Even more backward is that for short-term home care, you must be homebound except for doctors' visits, and on hospice, you cannot only be mobile, but can travel around the country.

With cancer as the "hospice defining illness" there must be sign of spread outside the local area (or decline in blood counts in leukemia, for example). The benefit is designed to be used after chemotherapy and radiation therapy are completed when no further treatment is planned. The hospice benefit provides:

- specialist-level nurses coming to the home and coordinating care
- physician or nurse practitioner home visits
- counseling for the individual patient and family by social workers and chaplains
- volunteer services
- prescription drugs for the illness serious enough to enroll in hospice, called the "hospice defining illness"
- personal care aides for a few hours a week
- physical occupational and dietary services
- medical equipment for the hospice defining illness

Doctor visits, prescription drugs, or equipment for conditions unrelated to the cancer are reimbursed by regular medical insurance. Included in the benefit are also options to home care: respite inpatient admissions in your community or hospital stays if a serious need arises. Emergency room visits are often not necessary since the hospice team is available 24/7 for home-based intervention. If you need more care than is provided in the home, hospice is also licensed to visit in skilled nursing facilities to provide care in addition to what is routinely available. Many hospice programs support hospice residences in the area.

You and your doctors also have the chance to choose if they will still monitor your care and order whatever is necessary, or the hospice physician (hospice medical director) will do so, or a combination of the two. All of your doctors can continue to be involved in your care as long as their visits are coordinated through the registered nurse case manager who will visit you. There is simple paperwork for them to complete to get reimbursed by your insurance. The doctors and nurses who have been treating you have a longer-term familiarity with you, and the hospice medical director has the specialized expertise in pain and symptom management. Their working together is usually the optimal combination.

Amazingly, there are no or few co-pays and deductibles, and the services are brought to you. If you go to visit relatives, hospice programs cooperate with each other to give care at your destination. As soon as the hospice staff sets up the essentials of your care—medications, equipment delivery, review of your medical information to set a treatment plan—you can get to work on the really hard stuff that you have already started to do at the beginning of your treatment.

Whether you have hospice involved or are getting services via home care or a more informal network of family, friends, and privately hired caregivers or volunteers, there are a number of things to consider doing now.

You must review all of your important documents with someone who is familiar with your state laws. If you do not have a family attorney, there are many free or low-cost services available via the National Medical Legal Partnership (http://www.nmlp.org), LegalHealth (http://www.nylag.org). ACS (http://www.cancer.org), Cancer*Care* (http://www.cancercare.org), the local law schools, or the social workers at the hospice or home care program may likely have ideas about finding a lawyer if need be. Some are purely personal.

Here's the list of important documents to review:

- Last will and testament
- Health care proxy, living will, or other advance medical directive acceptable in your state
- Power of attorney (for bank, financial, pension, real estate transactions)
- List of bank accounts, pensions, insurance policies (with review of the beneficiaries or "in trust for…" designations)
- List of computer log-ons and passwords to access e-mail and electronic accounts
- Safe deposit box: location of box, key, and those authorized to access
- Registration and title for vehicles
- Special accommodations for dependent children or elderly
- Thoughts about memorial services, burial or cremation, including list of invitees
- Wording of obituary and where you'd like it submitted
- Letters and audio or video recordings you would like to leave for loved ones on upcoming milestones in their lives: school graduations, marriages, births, or other such momentous personal occasions
- "How I want you to remember me" thoughts. Written or recorded. This is something almost always neglected because the people who love you the most are afraid to bring it up to avoid scaring you that you are closer to death than you would believe (another *conspiracy of silence* thing).
- "What I know that you may not": genealogy, family history, stories, Grandma's cookie recipes, whatever is significant in your family's life
- "Permission slips": Regarding very personal and deep family issues: permission to move from the family house when the time is right, permission for a spouse to date or remarry (grist for many a made-for-television movie), permission to go back to school to finish a degree. There are many variations on this theme.
- "Thank you's" to family and friends who have helped with your care. In these times of e-mails, instant messaging, and social networking, a hand-written card really stands out because of the effort involved to write them. Why not thank those who have helped you when you needed it with a personal note. In addition

to expressing your gratitude, you may want to tell them about how their efforts allowed you to *give forward* to help others.

- "Thank you's" to staff members: Unless all of your treatment has been in a medical care system that is strictly for profit as it is in some states (yes, even some hospice programs are for profit), the treatment programs at not-for-profit organizations rely heavily on the generosity of grateful patients to meet the expenses that are not covered by shrinking reimbursements or to offer services beyond the usual scope of care. Although you may have said thank you to those staff members at each encounter, you can also recognize their efforts by directing something their way. If you have the ability to contribute, that's wonderful and it can have important positive consequences for your family and friends during their bereavement, as well as help patients who follow you in their care. If you cannot donate money, you can ask that memorial contributions be made to a certain program instead of flowers, or that everyone donate 20 hours of volunteer time. All not-for-profit health care organizations have staff members who know how to put such efforts to good use, and you should contact them while you can be in charge.

These activities are not fun, but they are useful to you as well as your family. Try not to make the "Affairs" tasks a full-time assignment. Do them a little at a time; engage family and friends or social workers or pastoral care staff to help you.

I'm done with my homework. I have finished everything that is on this list. What do I do now?

That depends upon your energy level and your own style. Some people at the end of life really value their privacy and time for the quiet that they did not have in their everyday lives. Others are just the opposite. Victoria Kennedy, the second wife of Senator Edward Kennedy, related that when the senator was at home in the last weeks of his life, what they wanted was to invite as many people over as possible for some good meals and good songs (perhaps a cultural stereotype, but that's what was portrayed in the media). Cost was not a consideration, and having a staff to help with the shopping, food preparation, and cleanup was not specified, though implied. The idea is good, even though the scale may be grander than you are able to manage. Some families besides famous ones actually have done things like this for years. A lavish meal is certainly lovely but not the main idea of this activity. Burdening caregivers with catering is often not helpful. Families have actually invited friends, neighbors, more distant family members, congregants from their houses of worship, and town or village leaders for potluck events where everyone brings something to relieve the caregivers of the strain of their daily cooking with leftovers, or two of whatever—one to use that day and one to keep. In many families, there is reason to believe that in addition to camaraderie and some food, there is good drink too, local and family customs respected.

27 The Next Word

Many of the suggestions in this book, including "My Recovery Plan" and using the LEARN System, involve a lot of busy work and tasks that prepare you and your family for either eventuality—long-term survivorship or end-of-life care. In both situations, using these techniques is the optimal accompaniment to high-tech, passive modern cancer treatments.

Patients and their families and friends see these recommendations as a guide in an extraordinarily variable journey. Things don't always go exactly as planned, even as prepared as anyone can be, when armed with the worksheets and best explanations from skilled and respectful caregivers.

If in your journey into the world of the modern cancer center, home care, and hospice services, there are things that you learned that are effective and helpful—share your new wisdom with others. It's easy and quick—just enter your ideas on Facebook at *Cancerknowanddo* or on the website at http://www.cancerknowanddo.com.

In this way, you can have the next word. Professionals have much experience and have seen their patients and families go through a lot, but the practical "I've been there" experience gets refined through your feedback.

Please pass along whatever you have learned in order to help the coming generations of people with cancer and their families so that after all these words, you, indeed, have the next word.

THE NEXT WORD IS MINE/OURS

What I have learned that will be valuable to the next generation of patients, families, caregivers, and providers:

Please pass this along to them so they can benefit from my experience, or enter it directly on the website at http://www.cancerknowanddo.com or find us on Facebook at *Learn to Live Through Cancer: What You Need to Know and Do.*

1._____

2._____

3._____

4._____

5._____

Resources & Worksheets

MY WEEKLY RECOVERY PLANNER
Using the LEARN System®

Copy this form regularly to set your course and chart your progress.
Check which stage of recovery you are in:

☐ post-operative

    ☐ chemotherapy ☐ radiation therapy

    ☐ combinations of above

☐ right after treatment

☐ more than three months after treatment

Living	Do:
	Done:
Education	Do:
	Done:
Activity	Do:
	Done:
Rest	Do:
	Done:
Nutrition	Do:
	Done:

WHAT IS IMPORTANT TO ME

I believe that life is precious and I want to continue living as well as I can for as long as I can.

At the time of my cancer diagnosis, I want to go through all of the necessary consultations and tests to determine, with the best medical expertise and judgment available:

- ■ The kind of cancer I have: _____
- ■ Where it is:
  - ❑ Locally advanced (where it started)
  - ❑ Lymph nodes
  - ❑ Other body systems; locations: _____
  _____

With treatment, it is my understanding that:

- ❑ I can be cancer-free for five years or more.
- ❑ I will likely need to be more treatment within the next five years.
- ❑ I will be on maintenance treatment for the rest of my life.

CHOOSE ONE (1) OF THE FOLLOWING:

❑ I am willing to do anything and everything necessary to control my cancer.

❑ I am interested in preserving my quality of life as well as surviving my cancer. With each proposed change in my treatment plan, please save a few minutes so we can discuss the benefit of the treatment and how I can expect to feel.

❑ I am more interested in preserving my quality of life if it is unlikely for me to survive my cancer for more than:

    ❑ 3 months   ❑ 6 months   ❑ 1 year   ❑ 2 years

❑ I am first and foremost interested in preserving my quality of life. If I do not get treatment or get abbreviated treatment, how will I feel?

_____

_____

CHOOSE ONE (1) OF THE FOLLOWING:

Whether my cancer responds to treatment or not, please be:

    ❑ as *optimistic* as possible in your advice

    ❑ as *pessimistic* as possible in your advice

    ❑ as *realistic* as possible in your advice

I think of myself as **strong** or **resilient**

    ❑ all of the time

    ❑ sometimes

    ❑ never

The worst thing in my life I have been through so far is:

_____

_____

_____

_____

_____

I got through it by doing the following:

_____

_____

_____

_____

_____

Here is other information you need to know about me and my family so that we can make the best possible decisions about my care:

_____

_____

_____

_____

_____

The answers to these questions are best supplemented by decisions regarding emergencies that may or may not happen in the course of cancer treatment. Each state has specific (and differing) laws regarding Health Care Power of Attorney, Living Will or Health Care Proxy forms and policies. One of the most useful forms to read, think about and complete is *Five Wishes*, produced by a private organization, *Aging With Dignity*. Find them at www.agingwithdignity.org or call 888-594-7743. *Five Wishes* adds to the depth of discussion.

DISTRESS THERMOMETER

Name:_____

Date: _____

Before you see your Nurse/Doctor, please complete this form. We would like to know how you are feeling and your concerns.

FIRST:
Please circle the number (0-10) that best describes *how much distress* you have been experiencing in the past week including today.

[name label]

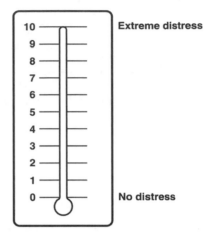

THEN: Please indicate WHICH of the following is a cause of distress. A staff member may call you to follow-up. At what telephone number would you like to be called?_____

Practical	**Physical**
☐ Housing	☐ Pain
☐ Insurance	☐ Nausea
☐ Work/school	☐ Fatigue [RN/MD: Hg:___ Hct:___]
☐ Transportation	☐ Sleep
☐ Child care	☐ Getting around
	☐ Bathing/dressing
Family	☐ Breathing
☐ Dealing with partner	☐ Mouth sores
☐ Dealing with children	☐ Eating
	☐ Indigestion
Emotional	☐ Constipation
☐ Worry	☐ Diarrhea
☐ Fears	☐ Changes in urination
☐ Sadness	☐ Fevers
☐ Depression	☐ Skin dry/itchy
☐ Nervousness	☐ Nose dry/congested
	☐ Tingling in hands/feet
Spiritual/Religious	☐ Feeling swollen
☐ Relating to God	☐ Sexual
☐ Loss of faith	☐ Legal

Other: _____

IMPORTANT BLOOD TESTS YOU NEED TO KNOW ABOUT

CBC (Complete Blood Count)

White Blood Cells (WBC)	fight infection; neutrophils are one type.
Hemoglobin (Hg)	carries oxygen to tissues in red blood cells that contain hemoglobin; low Hg can cause fatigue or breathlessness.
Platelets	control blood clotting

Basic Metabolic Panel (sometimes BNP)

Glucose	blood sugar
Calcium	muscle, heart, and thyroid function
Sodium (Na⁺)	*electrolyte* salt balance
Potassium (K⁺)	*electrolyte* salt balance
Chloride (Cl⁻)	*electrolyte* salt balance
Carbon dioxide (CO_2)	*electrolyte* salt balance
BUN (blood urea nitrogen)	kidney function
Creatinine	kidney function

Comprehensive Metabolic Panel (sometimes CMP)

All components of the *BNP*
   plus:

Total protein	general nutrition, liver function
Albumin	general nutrition, liver function
Alkaline phosphatase	liver function, muscle function
ALT (or SGOT)	liver function
ALP (or SGPT)	liver function
Bilirubin	liver function

Tumor Markers

CEA	colon cancer (carcinoembryonic antigen)
PSA	prostate cancer (prostate specific antigen)
CA-125	ovarian cancer
CA 15-3	breast cancer
AFP (alpha feto-protein)	liver, ovarian, brain cancers
Beta-2 microglobulin	chronic leukemia, non-Hodgkin's lymphoma, multiple myeloma
ER estrogen receptor	+ or – breast cancer
PR progesterone receptor	+ or – breast cancer

HER-2/neu

	Overexpressed (+) or underexpressed (–) breast cancer

MY RECOVERY PLAN COMMUNICATOR
BREAST CANCER

Name: _____

Date: _____

Today and in the last three (3) days:

Energy: ❑ Good   ❑ Fair   ❑ Poor
Weight _____   ❑ Gain   ❑ Loss   Appetite: ❑ Good ❑ Fair ❑ Poor
Hot Flashes   ❑ Yes: _____ per day   ❑ No

Chemo: Date last given: _____
White cell count _____ Hemoglobin _____ Platelet count _____
[ ] erythropoeitin   [ ] filgastrim
❑ Nausea or vomiting
❑ Pins and needles or numbness anywhere, place: _____

Radiation: Skin reaction   ❑ yes   ❑ no   [ ] Aquaphor® [ ] Aloe Vera

[ ] Biafene® [ ] Silvadene® [ ] Other: _____

Surgery: Postoperative healing   ❑ good   ❑ not healing

Medications: name and dose: _____

_____

_____

Complementary therapies: _____

Pain 0–10 (0 = no pain; 10 = worst pain): _____
Swelling of breast: ❑ yes
Lymphedema: ❑ yes
Cough: ❑ yes

MY RECOVERY PLAN COMMUNICATOR
PROSTATE CANCER

Name: _____

Date: _____

Today and in the last three (3) days:

Energy: ❑ Good   ❑ Fair   ❑ Poor
Weight _____   ❑ Gain   ❑ Loss   Appetite: ❑ Good ❑ Fair ❑ Poor
Urination: ❑ OK   ❑ Frequently   ❑ Need to go "right away"
❑ Can't urinate   ❑ Blood in urine   ❑ Pain
Hot Flashes   ❑ Yes: ____ per day   ❑ No

Chemo: White cell count _____ Hemoglobin _____ Platelet count _____
❑ Nausea or vomiting
❑ Pins and needles or numbness anywhere, place: _____

Radiation: Skin reaction   ❑ yes   ❑ no   Diarrhea   ❑ yes   ❑ no

Surgery: Postoperative healing   ❑ good   ❑ not healing

Medications: name and dose: _____

_____

_____

Complementary therapies: _____

Pain 0–10 (0 = no pain; 10 = worst pain):_____
Swelling of scrotum: ❑ yes
Lymphedema: ❑ yes
Cough: ❑ yes

MY RECOVERY PLAN COMMUNICATOR
LUNG OR ESOPHAGEAL CANCER

Name: _____

Date: _____

Today and in the last three (3) days:

Energy: ❑ Good ❑ Fair ❑ Poor

Weight _____ ❑ Gain ❑ Loss   Appetite: ❑ Good ❑ Fair ❑ Poor

Breathing: ❑ OK Short of breath: ❑ all of the time ❑ walking around

❑ Cough: ❑ No ❑ Yes: ❑ with mucus/phlegm ❑ with blood

❑ white "cheesy" spots in mucus ❑ dry

❑ Pain ❑ on breathing ❑ other part of body: name where: _____

❑ Difficulty swallowing

Skin reaction ❑ yes ❑ no [ ] Aquaphor® [ ] Aloe Vera [ ] Biafene®
[ ] Silvadene® [ ] Other: _____

❑ Pins and needles or numbness anywhere, place(s): _____

❑ Palpitations

Chemo: White cell count _____ Hemoglobin _____ Platelet count _____

❑ Nausea or vomiting

Radiation: Skin reaction ❑ yes ❑ no Diarrhea ❑ yes ❑ no

Surgery: Postoperative healing ❑ good ❑ not healing

Medications: name and dose: _____

_____

_____

Complementary therapies: _____

Pain 0–10 (0 = no pain; 10 = worst pain): _____

Swelling of neck: ❑ yes

Lymphedema: ❑ yes

Cough: ❑ yes

MY RECOVERY PLAN COMMUNICATOR
COLON, RECTAL, STOMACH, OR PANCREATIC CANCER

Name: _____

Date: _____

Today and in the last three (3) days:

Energy: ❏ Good   ❏ Fair   ❏ Poor

Weight _____   ❏ Gain   ❏ Loss   Appetite: ❏ Good ❏ Fair ❏ Poor

Breathing: ❏ OK   Short of breath: ❏ all of the time   ❏ walking around

Bowel movements: ❏ Well formed   ❏ Loose (diarrhea)   ❏ Soft
❏ Hard (constipated)

Skin reaction   ❏ yes   ❏ no [ ] Aquaphor® [ ] Aloe Vera [ ] Biafene®
[ ] Silvadene® [ ] Other: _____

❏ Pain ❏ No ❏ Yes: where: _____ when: ❏ sitting ❏ lying down on back

❏ Pins and needles, coldness or numbness anywhere, place: _____

Chemo: White cell count _____Hemoglobin _____ Platelet count _____
❏ Nausea or vomiting

Radiation: Skin reaction   ❏ yes   ❏ no

Surgery: Postoperative healing   ❏ good   ❏ not healing

Medications: name and dose: _____

_____

_____

Complementary therapies: _____

Pain 0–10 (0 = no pain; 10 = worst pain): _____
Swelling of abdomen or legs: ❏ yes
Lymphedema: ❏ yes
Cough: ❏ yes

MY RECOVERY PLAN COMMUNICATOR
OVARIAN, CERVICAL, OR UTERINE CANCER

Name: _____

Date: _____

Today and in the last three (3) days:

Energy: ❑ Good ❑ Fair ❑ Poor

Weight _____ ❑ Gain ❑ Loss   Appetite: ❑ Good ❑ Fair ❑ Poor

Vaginal bleeding: ❑ No ❑ Yes: number of pads used in 24 hours: _____

Skin reaction ❑ yes ❑ no [ ] Aquaphor® [ ] Aloe Vera [ ] Biafene®
[ ] Silvadene® [ ] Other: _____

Breathing: ❑ OK Short of breath: ❑ all of the time ❑ walking around

Bowel movements: ❑ Well formed ❑ Loose (diarrhea) ❑ Soft
❑ Hard (constipated)

Urination: ❑ OK ❑ Frequently ❑ Need to go "right away"
❑ Can't urinate ❑ Blood in urine ❑ Pain

Hot Flashes ❑ Yes: ____ per day ❑ No

❑ Pain ❑ No ❑ Yes: where: _____ when: ❑ sitting ❑ lying down on back

❑ Pins and needles, coldness or numbness anywhere, place: _____

Chemo: White cell count _____ Hemoglobin _____ Platelet count _____
❑ Nausea or vomiting

Radiation: Skin reaction ❑ yes ❑ no

Surgery: Postoperative healing ❑ good ❑ not healing

Medications: name and dose: _____

_____

_____

Complementary therapies:_____

Pain 0–10 (0 = no pain; 10 = worst pain):_____
Swelling of abdomen or legs: ❑ yes
Lymphedema: ❑ yes
Cough: ❑ yes

MY RECOVERY PLAN COMMUNICATOR
HEAD AND NECK CANCER

Name: _____

Date: _____

Today and in the last three (3) days:

Energy: ❑ Good ❑ Fair ❑ Poor

Weight _____ ❑ Gain ❑ Loss   Appetite: ❑ Good ❑ Fair ❑ Poor

Skin reaction ❑ yes ❑ no [ ] Aquaphor® [ ] Aloe Vera [ ] Biafene®
[ ] Silvadene® [ ] Other: _____

Breathing: ❑ OK   Short of breath: ❑ all of the time ❑ walking around

Swallowing: ❑ OK ❑ Painful ❑ Can't

Talking: ❑ OK ❑ Painful ❑ Can't

Mouth: ❑ Too dry ❑ Too much mucous ❑ Inflamed ❑ Can't chew
❑ Lockjaw

Taste: ❑ None ❑ Things don't taste like they are supposed to taste

Voice: ❑ Voice changes ❑ Hoarse

❑ Cough: ❑ No ❑ Yes: ❑ with mucus/phlegm ❑ with blood
❑ white "cheesy" spots in mucus ❑ dry

Bowel movements: ❑ Well formed ❑ Loose (diarrhea) ❑ Soft
❑ Hard (constipated)

❑ Pain ❑ No ❑ Yes: where: _____ when: ❑ sitting ❑ lying down on back

❑ Pins and needles, coldness or numbness anywhere, place: _____

Chemo: White cell count _____Hemoglobin _____ Platelet count _____
❑ Nausea or vomiting

Radiation: Skin reaction ❑ yes ❑ no

Surgery: Postoperative healing ❑ good ❑ not healing

Medications: name and dose: _____

_____

_____

Complementary therapies:_____

Pain 0–10 (0 = no pain; 10 = worst pain):_____

Swelling of face or neck: ❑ yes

Lymphedema: ❑ yes

Cough: ❑ yes

MY RECOVERY PLAN COMMUNICATOR
KIDNEY OF BLADDER CANCER

Name: _____

Date: _____

Today and in the last three (3) days:

Energy: ❑ Good   ❑ Fair   ❑ Poor

Weight _____   ❑ Gain   ❑ Loss   Appetite: ❑ Good ❑ Fair ❑ Poor

Urination: ❑ OK   ❑ Frequently   ❑ Need to go "right away"
❑ Blood in urine   ❑ Pain

Bowel movements: ❑ Well formed   ❑ Loose (diarrhea)   ❑ Soft
❑ Hard (constipated)

Breathing: ❑ OK   Short of breath: ❑ all of the time   ❑ walking around

Swelling: ❑ legs   ❑ hands

Skin reaction   ❑ yes   ❑ no [ ] Aquaphor® [ ] Aloe Vera [ ] Biafene®
[ ] Silvadene® [ ] Other: _____

Chemo: White cell count _____Hemoglobin _____ Platelet count _____
❑ Nausea or vomiting
❑ Pins and needles or numbness anywhere, place: _____

Radiation: Skin reaction   ❑ yes   ❑ no   Diarrhea   ❑ yes   ❑ no

Surgery: Postoperative healing   ❑ good   ❑ not healing

Medications: name and dose: _____

_____

_____

Complementary therapies: _____

Pain 0–10 (0 =no pain; 10 = worst pain): _____
Swelling of abdomen or legs: ❑ yes
Lymphedema: ❑ yes
Cough: ❑ yes

MY RECOVERY PLAN COMMUNICATOR
BRAIN OR SPINAL CORD CANCER

Name: _____

Date: _____

Today and in the last three (3) days:

Energy: ❑ Good   ❑ Fair   ❑ Poor
Weight _____   ❑ Gain   ❑ Loss   Appetite: ❑ Good   ❑ Fair   ❑ Poor
Urination: ❑ OK   ❑ Frequently   ❑ Need to go "right away"
❑ Blood in urine   ❑ Pain
Bowel movements: ❑ Well formed   ❑ Loose (diarrhea)   ❑ Soft
❑ Hard (constipated)

❑ Changes in ability to move: part of body: _____
❑ Involuntary movements   ❑ seizure activity
❑ Changes in sensations: part of body: _____
❑ Changes in speech
❑ Change in ability to retain information

Chemo: White cell count _____Hemoglobin _____ Platelet count _____
❑ Nausea or vomiting
❑ Pins and needles or numbness anywhere, place: _____

Radiation: Skin reaction   ❑ yes   ❑ no   Diarrhea   ❑ yes   ❑ no

Surgery: Postoperative healing   ❑ good   ❑ not healing

Medications: name and dose: _____

_____

_____

Complementary therapies:_____

Pain 0–10 (0 = no pain; 10 = worst pain):_____
Swelling of head or neck: ❑ yes
Lymphedema: ❑ yes

IMPORTANT REVELATIONS TO MY TREATMENT TEAM

Please complete as many of the items that pertain to you and your family. Some of this information may be personal or embarrassing. Being candid will ease your treatment so that your needs can be best anticipated.

PART 1

Personal information:

I am the kind of person who likes *a lot/little* information.

Family history of important conditions that will affect my treatment:

Cancer (type, age) (For more detailed family history, see Family History Form)

Serious depression (even if never treated)

Significant drinking or drug (substance abuse problems)

Conditions important to consider during cancer treatment (see worksheet):

Motion sickness (trains, planes, car, bus)

Comfort level in closed spaces

Nausea/vomiting during pregnancy

Reactions to pain medicines if used in past

Reactions to steroid medicines if used in past

History of serious depression (even if never treated)

Authentic estimate of use of tobacco products

Authentic estimate of use of alcoholic beverages

IMPORTANT REVELATIONS TO MY TREATMENT TEAM

Use this checklist to prepare for your Initial Consultation. Its purpose is to have you think in advance about the information you may be asked.

PART 2

List of all the medicines I take: prescriptions; over-the-counter medications; vitamin, mineral, or nutritional supplements

_____

_____

Past illnesses and treatments

_____

_____

List all surgeries: type, date. Reactions to coming out of anesthesia (no one does it well).

_____

_____

Allergies (serious reactions with hives, rash, wheezing, or couldn't breathe)

_____

_____

Side effects I commonly get from medications (not the same as allergies)

_____

_____

❑ I am the kind of person who needs (a lot/little) information to make decisions.

❑ I want to be included in the decision-making process or I want to be given the resulting decision. If not myself, I trust _____ to speak for me.

❑ In my family, I suspect or am sure that these people had cancer and what kind. (See "Family History Form")

❑ I become frightened in closed spaces.

❑ I get train, car, bus, or plane sick regularly.

❑ When I was pregnant, I had bad nausea and/or vomiting during the early part of the pregnancy.

❑ I have regularly used strong "narcotic" opioid pain medicine for periods of time at significant doses when younger. I got "high" when I used them for pain relief. (yes/no; yes/no).

❑ I regularly used marijuana as a teenager or young adult. It did/did not make me "high."

❑ *Social drinking* to me means:_____.

❑ I do/do not get drunk regularly where I pass out or get mean.

❑ A close blood relative of mine (not someone who married into the family) has serious drinking or drug problems.

❑ I remember when my mother went through menopause and it was easy/hard.

❑ I have had periods of depression where I took to bed and couldn't function, whether they were treated or not.

❑ I have close blood relatives who had similar experiences.

❑ In my lifetime, the worst thing I have been through was: _____ and this is what I did to get through:_____

FAMILY HISTORY FORM

Patient Name: _____ D.O.B._____ Today's Date: _____

<u>Directions</u>: Please list **all** of your <u>biological</u> (blood) relatives **below including those who have not had cancer**. **If someone is deceased, please put an asterisk (*) in the age column next to the age at death.** Use an additional page if you need extra space. You may not know each piece of information we are asking for. If you are unsure of something, give your best guess and put a question mark (?) next to it. It may be helpful to contact family members who may know additional information, but if this is not possible, we will do our best with the information you can give us.

Relationship to You	Name or initials	Current age or age at death (mark* if deceased)	Date of birth (approximate if unsure)	Cancer type (s) If person has not had cancer, leave blank.	Age at cancer diagnosis
Your Children	List your children below. In the first column, circle son or daughter for each child.				
Son / Daughter					
Son / Daughter					
Son / Daughter					
Son / Daughter					
Son / Daughter					
Son / Daughter					
Your Brothers and Sisters	List each of your brothers and sisters below. If half-sibling, specify which parent you share.				
Brother / Sister					
Brother / Sister					
Brother / Sister					
Brother / Sister					
Brother / Sister					
Brother / Sister					
Nieces/Nephews	List any of your nephews or nieces **IF** they have had cancer				
Niece / Nephew					
Niece / Nephew					
Niece / Nephew					
Niece / Nephew					

* Reprinted with permission: Norris Cotton Cancer Center, New Hampshire.

Patient Name: _____ D.O.B._____ Today's Date: _____

MOTHER'S SIDE OF THE FAMILY

Relationship to You	Name or initials	Current age or age at death (mark* if deceased)	Date of birth (approximate if unsure)	Cancer type (s) If person has not had cancer, leave blank.	Age at cancer diagnosis
Mother					
Mother's mother					
Mother's father					
Mother's Brothers/Sisters:	List each of you mother's brothers and sisters (your aunts and uncles) below, even if they did not have cancer. Circle aunt or uncle in the first column for each person.				
Aunt / Uncle					
Aunt / Uncle					
Aunt / Uncle					
Aunt / Uncle					
Aunt / Uncle					
Aunt / Uncle					
Aunt / Uncle					
Aunt / Uncle					
Aunt / Uncle					
Cousins	List any cousins on your mother's side who have had cancer. Specify who is his/her parent in the first column, i.e. Alice's daughter.				
Distant Relatives	List more distant relatives (i.e. great-aunts/uncles or great-grandparents) who had cancer. Specify how you are related in the first column, i.e. my mother's father's sister (great-aunt)				

* Reprinted with permission: Norris Cotton Cancer Center, New Hampshire.

Continued

Patient Name: _____ D.O.B._____ Today's Date: _____

FATHER'S SIDE OF THE FAMILY

Relationship to You	Name or initials	Current age or age at death (mark* if deceased)	Date of birth (approximate if unsure)	Cancer type (s) If person has not had cancer, leave blank.	Age at cancer diagnosis
Father					
Father's mother					
Father's father					
Father's Brothers/Sisters	List each of you father's brothers and sisters (your aunts and uncles) below, even if they did not have cancer. Circle aunt or uncle in the first column for each person.				
Aunt / Uncle					
Aunt / Uncle					
Aunt / Uncle					
Aunt / Uncle					
Aunt / Uncle					
Aunt / Uncle					
Aunt / Uncle					
Aunt / Uncle					
Cousins	List any cousins on your father's side who have had cancer. Specify who is his/her parent in the first column, i.e. Alice's daughter.				
Distant Relatives	List more distant relatives (i.e. great-aunts/uncles or great-grandparents) who had cancer. Specify how you are related in the first column, i.e. my father's mother's sister (great-aunt)				

* Reprinted with permission: Norris Cotton Cancer Center, New Hampshire.

QUESTIONS I WANT ANSWERED

How will I feel?

Will I recover and be myself?

What will the treatment include?

Can I continue to work?

How can I arrange for a second opinion? (No offense, please, but this is serious and I need to know.)

Who can help with my kids? Will I need help at home?

What do I need to do during my treatment? Eating, exercise?

What will be affected by the cancer and by the treatments?

What about vitamins and supplements?

What are *clinical trials*?

What is important to me now?

What do I have to do to get better?

When will I feel OK again? Will I be the same?

Will the cancer come back?

Is it familial?

What do my family and friends need to know?

Will I be able to forget all of what is happening?

How long will I need follow-up care? What will it be?

Will I be OK?

What if nothing works?

What will happen if I get sicker?

Will you stick by me if treatment does not work?

How...and when will I die?

WHAT I AM SUPPOSED TO BE EATING OR DRINKING WHEN I CAN'T EAT ANYTHING

Right after chemotherapy or during radiation therapy (involving the mouth, neck, and esophagus or if mouth sores develop from any treatment):

I FEEL TOO SICK OR NAUSEOUS. WHAT IF READING THIS MAKES ME NOT FEEL WELL?

Pass the worksheet to someone else to read who can help.

Ask your oncologist or oncology nurse if your regimen is highly emetogenic, moderately emetogenic or minimally emetogenic. The higher the chance of nausea and/or vomiting (emetogenesis), the longer it will take to move through the phases (1, 2, etc.). Some combinations will not cause much nausea the first few days due to the anti-nausea medication cocktail that accompanies it, others can show a surge 5–10 days afterward. Understand the usual pattern connected with your chemotherapy drugs and anti-nausea drugs so you can move through the Phases as quickly as possible.

Phase 1

You really need to make sure that fluids are moving in (and out). At a bare minimum. If it's early in the day (equivalent to breakfast time), try some juice of your choice, diluted with water. Half juice and half water. This will keep you from getting dehydrated (in any climate). A sports drink (Gatorade® and others) is fine. Put it in a sports cup with a straw, and sip a little bit at a time, so that the cup is emptied within a few hours or sooner. Optional addition to juice/water: 1/2 teaspoon of Morton's Lite Salt® or similar (or any potassium-based salt substitute) will replace some of the potassium your body loses, unless your oncologist or nurse tells you it is not necessary for you, based on the blood tests taken before chemotherapy (700 mg of potassium in 1/2 teaspoon is about 18 mEq of potassium).

Important Note: If your chemotherapy contained cis-platin or cyclophosphamide, this fluid is more than essential. Without it, the chemotherapy stays too long in your kidneys and bladder and is damaging.

For later in the day, clear broth of your choice (chicken, beef, vegetable) is ideal if that's the most complex food you can tolerate. If you have not added the Lite Salt to juice earlier in the day, add it to one of the cups of broth. Make it moderately warm. Or even cold if you are in a very hot climate. Sip a little at a time.

If you can tolerate, add some type of fiber, such as brown rice, whole wheat pasta (cooked way too much for general use so it is soft).

Thick or thin? Although our first impulse is to reach for some water (how much more basic can we get?) as the first thing to swallow, it may be among the hardest choices due to the thin consistency. For any and all foods, thin foods can be made thicker with a commercially made product (Thick-it® or similar). Made of malto-dextrin and corn starch, such additives can be thought of as a "bridge" to regular consistency foods rather than an additive to use for a long time. Depending upon the food, unflavored gelatin may be a more healthful alternative. Gelatin is usually added right before eating as a thickener to hot foods or else the proteins are denatured by the heat and the food returns to its original consistency. It has a small amount of protein and no carbohydrate. To use gelatin effectively, sprinkle it into warm (not boiling water) so that it rests on the surface for 10–15 minutes, then mix the gelatin with the food to be thickened just before it is served or in the very last minutes of cooking.

I FEEL A BIT HUNGRY. WHAT'S NEXT?

Phase 2

You've been able to tolerate the diluted juice and soup. Let's ramp up one small notch. Try a smoothie shake (see recipe or a commercially sold drink, such as Ensure Plus®, Boost®, or Nutren 1.5® and others. Compare labels to maximize proteins and minimize sugars to taste. Those with diabetes have other options, such as Glucerna® and others). Use the sports bottle, sip a bit at a time. Can be diluted, but more to drink. Use them as you can but continuously.

Smoothie Shake *(courtesy of Bridget Bennett, MS, RD)*

Basic Ingredients:

- 1 cup any liquid (whole milk, soy milk, rice milk, almond milk, etc.; use more than 1 cup if needed to blend.)
- 2 tablespoons protein powder (any type: soy, whey, egg)
- 1 tablespoon canola, olive or other oil
- 1 banana or other fresh or frozen fruit

For added protein, calories, and fiber, the following items can also be added:

- 1/2 cup plain or flavored organic yogurt, soy yogurt or soft tofu
- 1 tablespoon peanut butter, almond butter, cashew butter
- 1 tablespoon ground flaxseeds (optional)

Instructions:

- Blend all of the ingredients together to your desired consistency.
- Add additional liquid or ice to the blender if needed to thin out consistency for better blending. You may need more or less liquid to make the mixture blend.
- Add flavors or extracts if desired.
- Be creative.
- Store any excess in the refrigerator & give a quick re-blend before drinking.

Variation: See *Bridget's Basic Recipe* to create on your own.

MAN (WOMAN) DOES NOT LIVE BY SMOOTHIES ALONE. I NEED MORE!

Phase 3

Move up to something a little more substantial. Smooth warm cereals work well and provide protein, complex carbohydrates and fiber.

Early in the day: *Oatmeal, Cream of Wheat,* or *Cream of Rice* flavored with a small amount of butter, honey, and/or fresh fruit.

If you are getting radiation to the mouth, neck or chest, choose the smoothest type (oatmeal that is constantly stirred when made so it is creamier).

Later in the day: *Polenta* can be made the same way or with more savory flavoring as lunch or dinner. Can use olive oil instead of butter.

Options besides cornmeal (polenta): *buckwheat groats, couscous, pastina* (very small pasta pieces). *Quinoa* is actually not a grain but the seed of a leafy plant related to spinach. It has more protein than other carbohydrate grains, and cooks up into a smooth cereal-like consistency that adopts the flavors of the foods that are combined with it.

PRINCIPLES OF FLAVORING AFTER CHEMOTHERAPY OR DURING RADIATION THERAPY (OF THE MOUTH, NECK, OR CHEST)

Think of the taste buds having four primary flavors that work together to form the thousands of flavors we experience (similar to colors where all colors are mixtures of the primary colors: red, blue and yellow): bitter, acid, sweet, salty, and umami. All of the taste buds will not go into suspended animation at once, so familiar foods may taste odd (bitter dessert instead of sweet, vinegar sweet instead of bitter, etc.).

To compensate, make the flavor that is missing more intense to see if it breaks through the taste buds that are still functioning, even if not at capacity OR concentrate on foods that expectedly taste like the flavors you *can* taste.

For later in the day eating, can add the same broths used previously (may think about fish stock, based upon food preferences in addition to vegetable, chicken or beef). Some people like to graduate to tomato bases, even starting with tomato juices (or a vegetable fortified one, like V-8® and others). Adding some mild cheese can also vary the taste with additional protein. Plain cheeses (low-fat cottage cheese or ricotta cheese) are the easiest to tolerate, then can graduate to aged, sharper cheeses (cheddar, parmesan or Romano types). Using a stock made from mushrooms (Portobello, for example) adds even a different flavor dimension.

Can even move into whole wheat pasta (whole wheat better than regular, but regular will do) that is cooked on the softer side—unless you're up to al dente—and made slippery with mild sauces, or even butter-flavored olive oils with herbs, tomato sauces, or cheese sauces (from bland to spicy based upon food preferences and tasting abilities).

269

I'M TOO TIRED TO CHEW AND EAT REGULAR FOOD. IDEAS?

Phase 4

Use the vegetable, chicken, beef or fish stocks to make thicker soups. Think about what are really favorites—this is not hospital food. Even favorites become boring day after day, and if the goal is proper nutrition, then boring is counterproductive. Vary the recipes between the basic stocks and add whatever you like. Well-cooked lean meats, chicken, turkey or soft poached fish matched with the stock flavor of your choice. Add vegetables of as many different colors as you can. Cook well. At first, be prepared to put the resulting soup in a blender or food processor if it seems like too much work to chew and swallow, or the consistency is irritating to the mouth or esophagus. Judge what size pieces are tolerable, and may reach the point where well-cooked soft contents are fine on their own without processing.

Soft foods that are *slicked* with an oil or liquid. Think about poached egg whites (OK; whole eggs of course; unless your cholesterol levels were dangerously high before the cancer) with butter or butter-flavored oils. Some naturally slippery foods may be quite a treat (even something like a steamed oyster or clam; raw is not a good idea due to the risk of infection) slathered in a sauce or butter/oil.

For a treat, add puddings in the flavors you like, ice cream (or sorbets, unless high blood sugars or hypoglycemic reactions make such a load of simple sugars a bad idea). To be the most careful, many brands of commercially prepared ice cream come in *no sugar added* formulations. (Can use them on their own or add to smoothie drinks.)

Vary phases 1, 2, 3, and 4 during treatment, based upon tolerance. Of course, be prepared to jump back to phase 1 foods with each chemotherapy cycle, then advance as tolerated.

MORE THAN CHIPS AND CANDY…GOOD SNACKS?

Snacks (courtesy of Bridget Bennett, MS, RD):

Each of these has about 1 serving of carb and 1–2 oz. protein, for a nice balance.

¼ cups nuts and dried fruit or a piece of fresh fruit, take with lots of water or herbal tea

1 tablespoon natural peanut butter spread on 2–3 Ryvita crackers (high fiber)

1 low-fat string cheese with any piece of fresh fruit

1/3 cup low-fat cottage cheese with 1 cup fruit salad

1 low-fat yogurt, add some nuts to it

1 Balance bar or Luna Bar (has protein, vitamins/minerals, and carbs) if you're craving sweet

Small cup of bean or chicken soup if you're craving savory

Tips for Adding Calories

- Eat snacks between meals and at bedtime—choose peanut butter, hummus or bean dip, dried fruit and nuts if tolerated, custards, string cheese, drinkable yogurt, smoothies, and so forth.
- Add olive oil or butter to warm prepared dishes such as eggs, sweet potatoes, soups, pasta, and so forth.
- Drink high-calorie beverages such as smoothies, shakes, nectars, juice, whole milk, and nutritional supplements, which have more calories than water, coffee, or tea.
- Add avocado or mayonnaise to dishes and use other sauces liberally to moisten foods.
- Make your own shakes with whole or soy milk, fruit, peanut butter, frozen yogurt, ice cream, protein powder, honey, and so forth.
- Substitute milk for water when making soups, pudding, and warm cereals such as oatmeal or grits.

Tips for Adding Protein

- High protein foods include meat, poultry, fish, eggs, beans, cheese, tofu, and other soy products as well as most dairy products. Whole grains, such as quinoa, bulgur, and barley, also contain protein. Nuts, nut butters, and seeds contain protein as well as healthy fats.
- Add protein powder (whey, egg, or soy based) or dry milk powder to foods and drinks such as soups, smoothies, milkshakes, casseroles, sauces, cooked cereals, eggs, and mashed potatoes.
- Blend chopped hard-cooked eggs into soups or casseroles. DON'T EAT RAW EGGS.
- Mash cooked beans and use as a dip or spread.
- Add canned or cooked beans to salads or rice or use as a side dish.
- Add grated cheese to top warm dishes such as eggs, soups, casseroles, and vegetables.
- Add tofu to soups or salads or blend into liquids (soft tofu).
- Use 4 percent cottage cheese as a side dish or with fruit.
- Sprinkle flaxseed meal or wheat germ to vegetables, cereal, ice cream, or yogurt. A word of caution: Uncooked vegetables and unwashed fruits can harbor bacteria. Best to peel or wash fruits and vegetables well, including those labeled, "prewashed".

Bridget Bennett, MS, RD, is an Oncology Nutritionist working with patients with cancer and their families for many years. She serves as the senior Oncology Nutritionist at the Continuum Cancer Centers of New York.

Bridget is reluctant to admit that her movie career skyrocketed with her appearance as the dietician in Super Size Me, *a film about the fast-food industry.*

Bridget's Basic Recipe

Use the following recipe for the base, meaning a *very plain* liquid, to which you may add foods.

Basic Recipe	Calories	Protein	Carbohydrate	Fat
Whole milk 1 cup	150	8 g	12 g	8 g
Canola oil, olive oil, etc. 1 tablespoon	120	0	0	14 (unsat.)
Protein powder (whey, soy, egg) 1 scoop: varied, see label	100	20 g	1 g	1 g
Total =	370	28 g	13 g	23 g

To this base an endless variety of additions can be added and blended in as desired, based on a person's taste, tolerance, and nutritional needs.

Nutritional Breakdown

The basic recipe will have about 300–400 calories and 20–30 grams of protein per 1 cup or so, but these values will increase with any additions you make to your own personal smoothie!

"THE IDEAL COUPLE"

An ideal pairing of rustic whole wheat bread and omega-3 fatty acid fish oils* together can supply good complex carbohydrates and the omega-3s. It's like eating in a fine restaurant where the butter brought with the bread has been switched to flavored olive oil. The added calories plus fiber and oil lubrication against constipation makes this snack an *ideal couple.*

Make sure the *rustic* whole what bread actually contains whole wheat flour, not just various seeds added to make it appear healthy.

Add a small amount of the herb of your choice (rosemary is a favorite), and you'll almost think you're in Tuscany (maybe).

* There are a variety of omega-3 oils on the market, some are already flavored (lemon flavored oil goes great with the rosemary). On the Internet, use your favorite search engine for "omega 3 oils" or "omega 3 oils lemon" to see what is available and where you can purchase it. You can certainly mix omega-3 oils with some olive oil for taste, but keep the majority as omega-3.

I'VE RECOVERED ENOUGH TO GET BACK TO REGULAR FOODS. I MADE THE PROMISE TO EAT MORE HEALTHFULLY. WHERE CAN I GET INSPIRATION? (IS PHASE 5 THE LAST PHASE?)

Dana's Recipes

Dana Jacobi, a well-respected chef, has been working with the special needs of the cancer community for many years. She writes a column for the American Institute for Cancer Research (AICR) and is the author of a number of creative, practical, and beautiful books: Cook & Freeze: 150 Delicious Dishes to Serve Now and Later, Dana's Market Basket, *and* The 12 Best Foods Cookbook: Over 200 Recipes Featuring the 12 Healthiest Foods.

Dana's columns are available through the AICR at www.aicr.org, along with sound nutritional information. Dana's additional work can be viewed at www.dana-jacobi.com and by blogging at www.danasmarketbasket.com.

The following suggestions may even be considered phase 5, since their flavors and textures are more complex. These recipes provide examples of good foods that can be prepared nutritiously at the end of treatment and further into survivorship to counteract our reliance on processed foods with enriched flour and sugar products. The corn pudding requires more time in the kitchen. Many more appear in Dana's books, and serve as examples of how we can alter our diet without sacrificing taste.

Cocoa Nutty Smoothie

Chocoholics love this rich smoothie. It offers a perfect balance of cocoa flavor, peanut butter, and sweetness from a frozen banana. Serves 1.

1 cup chocolate milk (almond, hemp, or coconut can be substituted for dairy milk)

1 small banana, sliced and frozen

2 tablespoons natural smooth peanut butter

2 tablespoons unsweetened cocoa powder

2 ice cubes

1. Combine the milk, banana, peanut butter, and cocoa in a blender. Blend until creamy. With the blender running, add the ice cubes and blend until smooth. Pour into a tall glass and serve.

California Date Shake

Southern Californians have long enjoyed this thick, creamy milk shake. The secret to making this fiber-rich smooth drink is using moist Medjool dates and blending them with hot water before adding the other ingredients. A touch of coffee adds an interesting note, if you wish. Serves 2.

1/2 cup chopped, pitted Medjool dates (4–6 dates)
1 cup vanilla ice cream or frozen yogurt
1 cup milk
1/2 teaspoon ground cinnamon
4 ice cubes

1. Place the dates and 1/2 cup boiling water in a blender, and whirl to purée.
2. Add the frozen yogurt, milk, cinnamon, and ice cubes. Whirl until the ice is blended. Divide between two tall glasses and drink immediately.

Baked Oatmeal

This is a great way to enjoy oatmeal. Dried fruits and an apple make this a more complete breakfast. Serves 4.

1-3/4 cups milk
1 tablespoon unsalted butter
1/8 teaspoon salt
1 cup old-fashioned rolled oats
1/4 cup dried apricots
1/4 cup raisins
3 tablespoon lightly packed brown sugar, divided
1/2 Golden Delicious apple, peeled
3 tablespoons chopped walnuts

1. Preheat the oven to 350°F.
2. In a 2-quart microwaveable, ovenproof casserole, heat the milk and butter until the milk steams. Mix in the salt and oats and set aside.
3. Chop the apricots. Mix the apricots, raisins, and 1 tablespoon of the sugar into the oats. Shred the apple into the oats and mix to combine.
4. Bake the oats, uncovered, for 15 minutes. Stir, then top with the remaining sugar and the nuts. Bake 15 minutes longer, or until the oats are chewy. Divide the oatmeal among four bowls. Serve immediately, accompanied by a pitcher of cold milk.

Baked Corn Pudding

This colorful casserole is equally good as a meatless main course or as a side dish with pork chops or roast chicken or pork chops. Serves 6–8.

1/2 cup stone-ground yellow corn meal

1/2 cup all-purpose flour

1 teaspoon baking powder

2 tablespoon sugar

1 small onion, chopped

1/2 cup chopped scallions, green and white parts

4 tablespoons unsalted butter, melted

1 can (15¼ oz.) corn, drained

1 can (14¾ oz.) creamed corn

1 large egg, beaten

1 cup shredded cheddar cheese, divided

1/2 teaspoon salt

1/8 teaspoon freshly ground pepper

1 (4 oz.) can green chiles, drained

1. Preheat the oven to 350°F. Coat an 8-inch square baking dish with cooking spray and set aside.
2. In a bowl, combine the corn meal, flour, baking powder, and sugar, and set aside.
3. Place onions and scallions in strainer and plunge them into a medium pot of boiling water for 30 seconds. Cool the vegetables under cold running water, drain very well, and set aside.
4. In large mixing bowl, combine the corn, creamed corn, egg, and butter. Add the dry ingredients and mix just to combine. Mix in the onions, scallions and 1/2 cup of the cheese. Spread the pudding in prepared baking dish. Sprinkle the remaining 1/2 cup cheese over top of pudding.
5. Bake the casserole for 40 minutes, until the pudding is puffed and golden on top and a knife inserted into the center comes out clean. Cool the pudding on a wire rack for 15 minutes before serving.

Three Bean Salad with Mustard Dressing

Using mayonnaise and yogurt to make a creamy dressing gives this popular salad a different twist. Serves 4.

1 cup canned chickpeas, rinsed and drained

1 cup canned Great Northern beans, rinsed and drained

1 cup canned kidney, rinsed and drained

1/2 cup finely chopped red onion

2 tablespoons yogurt

1 tablespoon mayonnaise

1 tablespoon Dijon-style mustard

1 teaspoon white vinegar

2 dashes hot pepper sauce

1/2 teaspoon salt

1/4 teaspoon ground black pepper

2 teaspoons extra virgin olive oil

1/2 cup chopped fresh dill or flat-leaf parsley

1. In a mixing bowl, combine the drained beans with the onion.
2. For the dressing, whisk together the yogurt, mayonnaise, mustard, vinegar, hot sauce, salt and pepper. Continuing to whisk, drizzle in the oil. Add the dressing to the beans and mix to combine. If serving immediately, mix in the dill or parsley. Or, cover the dressed beans and refrigerate for up to 8 hours, and add the herbs just before serving.

Share Your Ideas!

These recipes are here for your convenience and immediate use but should also serve as a springboard for creativity.

To *Give Forward* to future generations of patients and their caregivers, share your successes on   www.cancerknowanddo.com.

YOUR PERSONAL HEALTH RECORD

The text describes in more detail how a personal health record (PHR) can help you focus your care after treatment has completed.

Many PHRs now exist using a similar template. This version for a variety of cancers stresses what *you* need to do after treatment, more than a catalog of treatment you have received.

Treatments change over time, so it is possible that the chemotherapy or type of radiation therapy listed does not match yours. Please personalize these forms on the following pages so that they remain current and meaningful to you.

The American Society of Clinical Oncology's patient resource site (http://www.cancer.net) has a selection of specialized forms using the same format. Journey Forward (http://www.journeyforward.org) has similar documents available through its website. LiveStrong—The Lance Armstrong Foundation (http://www.livestrong.org) has funded seminal programs in this area. New formats will continually be improved and available.

To Use Your Personal Health Record

Each PHR has two pages. Page 1 is tailored to many specific cancers. If your type is not listed, use the "General template". Page 2 applies to each type of cancer listed. Please be sure to copy **both pages** for each PHR.

PHR forms

PERSONAL HEALTH RECORD

Last Name: First Name:
DOB: Age: Gender: Date:
Day Phone: Evening Phone:
Address: City: State: Zip:
Email:
My Insurance: Policy #:

Spouse/Relative/Caretaker: Phone:
Health Care Proxy: Phone:

MEDICAL INFORMATION

Type of Cancer: Date of diagnosis:
Staging   T: N: M:

My Health Care Team   **Phone:**   **Email:**
Medical Oncologist:
Radiation Oncologist:
Surgeon:
Fellow:
Nurse Practitioner:
Integrative Oncology Nurse:
Speech/Swallowing Therapist:
Pain/Symptom Management:
Dentist/Orthodontist:
Nutritionist:
Physical Therapist:
Social Worker:

Treatments received:
Surgical Procedures:

Chemotherapy: ☐   (mg)   ☐   (mg)   ☐   (mg)
☐   (mg)   ☐   (mg)   ☐ other
Freq: Total Dose:

Radiation Therapy:
Area treated:
☐ External Beam Radiation Therapy
(EBRT)   Last Date: Dose:
☐ Brachytherapy   Last Date: Procedure: Dose:

FOLLOW-UP APPOINTMENTS:

Follow-ups: *Remember to follow up with your providers on a regular schedule*

☐ Surgical: ☐ Radiation Oncology: ☐ Medical Oncology:
☐ Cancer Supportive Services: ☐ Pain/Symptom Management: ☐ Nutrition:

☐ Speech/Swallowing Therapy: ☐ Physical Therapy: ☐ Social Work:

☐ Dental:

IMPORTANT FOLLOW-UP CARE:

Physical Therapy: *Practice the exercises you have been given by our staff to manage the following*   **Contact:** _____

☐ Secretions   ☐ Pain   ☐ Fatigue   ☐ Neck Mobility

Nutritional Management: *See your nutritionist within 1 month post treatment to develop a plan for optimal nutrition and to manage symptoms* **Contact:** _____

Height: Current Weight: Ideal Body Weight: Weight History:
PEG placed: PEG removed: Formula:
                       Recommendations:
Eating orally? ☐ Yes ☐ No   - Weaning from a PEG is a <u>process</u> and it <u>can't be done immediately</u>
                       - Food progression is <u>gradual</u>
Texture tolerance:
Follow up with the Nutritionist to address ongoing concerns related to nutrition, weight status and eating including any of the following symptoms:
☐ Chewing   ☐ Sore throat
☐ Dry/sensitive mouth   ☐ Mouth sores
☐ Changes in taste

Treatment-Related Medications:	*Remember to take your medicines as scheduled*

Exams: *Do the appropriate exams as scheduled*
Blood tests: Thyroid function:

Scans:
X-ray: PET/CT: CT: Other:
Self exams:

Integrative Oncology: *Follow up as needed*   Contact: _____

☐ Acupuncture
Breath/relaxation techniques: ☐ Guided imagery   ☐ Progressive relaxation   ☐ Autogenics
Energy therapy: ☐ Reiki   ☐ Therapeutic Touch   ☐ Acupressure

Speech and Swallowing: *Practice what you have been taught by our staff*   Contact: _____

- Follow up with your speech and swallowing therapist after completing treatment
- If you had surgery, get a baseline swallowing test after your surgeon clears you for eating orally
Speech Evaluation: ☐ Yes ☐ No
Results:
Swallowing Evaluation: ☐ Yes ☐ No
Results:
Acceptable diet choices:
☐ Thin Liquids   ☐ Thick liquids   ☐ Purees
☐ Soft Solids   ☐ Unrestricted diet

Dental Care: *See your dentist for routine checkups*   Contact: _____
- Teeth/gums care: thoroughly brush your teeth; floss carefully and avoid gum irritation
- Fluoride regimen: apply fluoride in a prescribed manner
- Other oral care:

Breathing: *Practice what you have been taught by our staff*
☐ Stoma care

Other:

ADJUSTING TO SURVIVORSHIP

*Contact your social worker if you are experiencing distress
in any of the following areas*   Contact: _____

☐ Body-image   ☐ Eating/sleeping patterns   ☐ Disinterest in activities that you enjoy
☐ Pervasive concerns and worry   ☐ Relationships with your family   ☐ Relationship with partner
                              and friends
☐ Changes in mood   ☐ Sadness   ☐ Fears
☐ Nervousness

WELLNESS

Avoid: Maintain:
☐ Nicotine and Tobacco Products   ☐ Healthy nutrition
☐ Alcohol use   ☐ Physical activity
☐ Drug use   ☐ Screening for other cancers
☐ Overexposure to the sun

Screening for other cancers:
☐ Colonoscopy   ☐ Mammogram   ☐ PSA/Digital Rectal exam   ☐ PAP/HPV tests   ☐ Skin exam

ADDITIONAL INFORMATION

Organizations/Programs:	Contact Info:	Website:
Alcoholics Anonymous (AA)	Many local groups exist	http://www.alcoholics-anonymous.org
Narcotics Anonymous (NA)	Many local groups exist	http://www.na.org

Cancer Support Groups:	Contact Info:	Website:
American Cancer Society	1-800-ACS-2345	http://www.cancer.org
Cancer*Care*	1-800-813-HOPE	http://www.cancercare.org
People Living With Cancer		http://www.cancer.net
National Cancer Institute (NCI)	1-800-4-CANCER	http://www.cancer.gov
NCI Office of Cancer Survivorship	1-301-402-2964	http://dccps.nci.nih.gov/ocs
Gilda's Club	1-888-GILDA-4-U	http://www.gildasclubnyc.org
LIVESTRONG	1-866-235-7205	http://www.livestrong.org

PERSONAL HEALTH RECORD
BRAIN OR SPINAL CORD CANCER

Last Name: First Name:
DOB: Age: Gender: Date:
Day Phone: Evening Phone:
Address: City: State: Zip:
Email:
My Insurance: Policy #:

Spouse/Relative/Caretaker: Phone:
Health Care Agent: Phone:

MEDICAL INFORMATION

Cell type: Topography (location)   Date of diagnosis:
WHO Classification

My Health Care Team   **Phone:**   **Email:**
Medical Oncologist:
Radiation Oncologist:
Surgeon:
Fellow:
Nurse Practitioner:
Integrative Oncology Nurse:
Speech/Swallowing Therapist:
Pain/Symptom Management:
Dentist/Orthodontist:
Nutritionist:
Physical Therapist:
Social Worker:

Treatments received:
Surgical Procedures:

Chemotherapy: ☐ temozolomide (mg)   ☐ CCNU (mg)   ☐ procarbazine (mg)
☐ vincristine (mg)   ☐ bevacizumab (mg)   ☐ other
Freq: Total Doses:

Radiation Therapy:
Area treated:
☐ External Beam Radiation Therapy   Last Date: Dose:
(EBRT)
☐ Stereotactic Radiosurgery   Date: Procedure: Dose:

FOLLOW-UP APPOINTMENTS:
Follow-ups: *Remember to follow up with your providers on a regular schedule*

☐ Surgical: ☐ Radiation Oncology: ☐ Medical Oncology:
☐ Cancer Supportive Services:
                               ☐ Pain/Symptom Management: ☐ Nutrition:
☐ Speech/Swallowing Therapy:
                               ☐ Physical Therapy: ☐ Social Work:
☐ Dental:

IMPORTANT FOLLOW-UP CARE:

Physical Therapy: *Practice the exercises you have been given by our
staff to manage the following*   Contact: _____

☐ Movement or   ☐ Pain   ☐ Fatigue   ☐ Cognitive impairment
Strength

Nutritional Management: *See your nutritionist within 1 month post
treatment to develop a plan for optimal nutrition and to manage symptoms*   Contact: _____

Height: Current Weight: Ideal Body Weight: Weight History:
PEG placed: PEG removed: Formula:
                     Recommendations:
Eating orally? ☐ Yes ☐ No   - Weaning from a PEG is a <u>process</u> and it <u>can't be done immediately</u>
                             - Food progression is <u>gradual</u>
Texture tolerance:
*Follow up with the Nutritionist to address ongoing concerns related to nutrition, weight status and eating including any of the
following symptoms:*
☐ Chewing   ☐ Sore throat
☐ Dry/sensitive mouth   ☐ Mouth sores
☐ Changes in taste

280

Treatment-Related Medications: *Remember to take your medicines as scheduled*

Exams: *Do the appropriate exams as scheduled*
Blood tests: Thyroid function:

Scans:
X-ray: PET/CT: CT: Other:
Self exams:

Integrative Oncology: *Follow up as needed*   Contact: _____

☐ Acupuncture
Breath/relaxation techniques: ☐ Guided imagery   ☐ Progressive relaxation   ☐ Autogenics
Energy therapy: ☐ Reiki   ☐ Therapeutic Touch   ☐ Acupressure

Speech and Swallowing: *Practice what you have been taught by our staff*
                                                        Contact: _____

- Follow up with your speech and swallowing therapist after completing treatment
- If you had surgery, get a baseline swallowing test after your surgeon clears you for eating orally
Speech Evaluation: ☐ Yes ☐ No
Results:
Swallowing Evaluation: ☐ Yes ☐ No
Results:
Acceptable diet choices:
☐ Thin Liquids   ☐ Thick liquids   ☐ Purees
☐ Soft Solids   ☐ Unrestricted diet

Dental Care: *See your dentist for routine checkups*   Contact: _____
  - Teeth/gums care: thoroughly brush your teeth; floss carefully and avoid gum irritation
  - Fluoride regimen: apply fluoride in a prescribed manner
  - Other oral care:

Breathing: *Practice what you have been taught by our staff*
☐ Stoma care

Other:

ADJUSTING TO SURVIVORSHIP

*Contact your social worker if you are experiencing distress
in any of the following areas*   Contact: _____

☐ Body-image   ☐ Eating/sleeping patterns   ☐ Disinterest in activities that you enjoy
                             ☐ Relationships with your family
☐ Pervasive concerns and worry and friends   ☐ Relationship with partner
☐ Changes in mood   ☐ Sadness   ☐ Fears
☐ Nervousness

WELLNESS

Avoid: **Maintain:**
☐ Nicotine and Tobacco Products   ☐ Healthy nutrition
☐ Alcohol use   ☐ Physical activity
☐ Drug use   ☐ Screening for other cancers
☐ Overexposure to the sun

Screening for other cancers:
☐ Colonoscopy   ☐ Mammogram   ☐ PSA/Digital Rectal exam   ☐ PAP/HPV tests   ☐ Skin exam

ADDITIONAL INFORMATION

Organizations/Programs:	**Contact Info:**	**Website:**
Alcoholics Anonymous (AA)	Many local groups exist	http://www.alcoholics-anonymous.org
Narcotics Anonymous (NA)	Many local groups exist	http://www.na.org

Cancer Support Groups:	**Contact Info:**	**Website:**
American Cancer Society	1-800-ACS-2345	http://www.cancer.org
CancerCare	1-800-813-HOPE	http://www.cancercare.org
People Living With Cancer		http://www.cancer.net
National Cancer Institute (NCI)	1-800-4-CANCER	http://www.cancer.gov
NCI Office of Cancer Survivorship	1-301-402-2964	http://dccps.nci.nih.gov/ocs
Gilda's Club	1-888-GILDA-4-U	http://www.gildasclubnyc.org
LIVESTRONG	1-866-235-7205	http://www.livestrong.org

PERSONAL HEALTH RECORD
BREAST CANCER

Last Name: First Name:
DOB: Age: Gender: Date:
Day Phone: Evening Phone:
Address: City: State: Zip:
Email:
My Insurance: Policy #:

Spouse/Relative/Caretaker: Phone:
Health Care Agent: Phone:

MEDICAL INFORMATION

Type of Breast Cancer: Date of diagnosis:
Staging   T: N: M:

My Health Care Team   **Phone:**   **Email:**
Medical Oncologist:
Radiation Oncologist:
Surgeon:
Fellow:
Gynecologist
Nurse/Nurse Practitioner:
Integrative Oncology Nurse:
Lymphedema Specialist:
Pain/Symptom Management:
Social Worker:
Nutritionist:
Physical Therapist:
Patient Navigator:

Treatments received:
Surgical Procedures:

Chemotherapy: ☐ adriamycin   (mg) ☐ cyclophosphamide   (mg)   ☐ pactitaxel   (mg)
☐ 5-FU   (mg)   ☐ Herceptin   (mg)   ☐ other
Freq: Total Dose:
Hormonal Treatments: ☐ Arimidex ☐ tamoxifen ☐ Femara (letrozole)
Radiation Therapy:
Area treated:
☐ External Beam Radiation Therapy
(EBRT)   Last Date: Dose:
☐ Brachytherapy   Last Date: Procedure: Dose:

FOLLOW-UP APPOINTMENTS:
Follow-ups: *Remember to follow up with your providers on a regular schedule*

☐ Surgical: ☐ Radiation Oncology: ☐ Medical Oncology:
☐ Cancer Supportive Services:
                             ☐ Pain/Symptom Management: ☐ Nutrition:
☐ Gynecological   ☐ Physical Therapy: ☐ Social Work:

IMPORTANT FOLLOW-UP CARE:
Hot Flashes: number per day   interferes with comfort or functioning
Cognitive Impairment ("chemobrain")
Physical Therapy: *Practice the exercises you have been given by our*
staff to manage the following   **Contact:** _____
☐ Swelling of Arm   ☐ Pain   ☐ Weight Gain   ☐ Fatigue   ☐ Range of Motion

Nutritional Management: *See your nutritionist within 1 month post*
treatment to develop a plan for optimal nutrition and to manage symptoms **Contact:** _____

Height: Current Weight: Ideal Body Weight: Weight History:
Weight gain or loss:

Follow up with the Nutritionist to address ongoing concerns related to nutrition, weight status and eating including any of the
following symptoms:
☐ Relying on comfort foods   ☐ Changes in taste
☐ Dry/sensitive mouth   ☐ Mouth sores
☐ Changes in taste

Treatment-Related Medications: *Remember to take your medicines as scheduled*

Exams: *Do the appropriate exams as scheduled*
Blood tests: Thyroid function:

Scans:
X-ray: PET/CT: CT: Other:
Self exams:

Integrative Oncology: *Follow up as needed*   Contact: _____

☐ Acupuncture
Breath/relaxation techniques: ☐ Guided imagery   ☐ Progressive relaxation   ☐ Autogenics
Energy therapy: ☐ Reiki   ☐ Therapeutic Touch   ☐ Acupressure

---

Speech and Swallowing: *Practice what you have been taught by our staff*   Contact: _____

- Follow up with your speech and swallowing therapist after completing treatment
- If you had surgery, get a baseline swallowing test after your surgeon clears you for eating orally
Speech Evaluation: ☐ Yes ☐ No
Results:
Swallowing Evaluation: ☐ Yes ☐ No
Results:
Acceptable diet choices:
☐ Thin Liquids   ☐ Thick liquids   ☐ Purees
☐ Soft Solids   ☐ Unrestricted diet

Dental Care: *See your dentist for routine checkups*   Contact: _____
- Teeth/gums care: thoroughly brush your teeth; floss carefully and avoid gum irritation
- Fluoride regimen: apply fluoride if advised
- Other oral care:

Breathing: *Practice what you have been taught by our staff*
☐

Other:

ADJUSTING TO SURVIVORSHIP

*Contact your social worker if you are experiencing distress
in any of the following areas*   Contact: _____

☐ Body-image   ☐ Eating/sleeping patterns   ☐ Disinterest in activities that you enjoy
☐ Pervasive concerns and worry   ☐ Relationships with your family   ☐ Relationship with partner
                                   and friends
☐ Changes in mood   ☐ Sadness   ☐ Fears
☐ Nervousness

WELLNESS

Avoid: **Maintain:**
☐ Nicotine and Tobacco Products   ☐ Healthy nutrition
☐ Alcohol use   ☐ Physical activity
☐ Drug use   ☐ Screening for other cancers
☐ Overexposure to the sun

Screening for other cancers:
☐ Colonoscopy   ☐ Mammogram   ☐ PSA/Digital Rectal exam   ☐ PAP/HPV tests   ☐ Skin exam

ADDITIONAL INFORMATION

Organizations/Programs:	Contact Info:	Website:
Alcoholics Anonymous (AA)	Many local groups exist	http://www.alcoholics-anonymous.org
Narcotics Anonymous (NA)	Many local groups exist	http://www.na.org

Cancer Support Groups:	Contact Info:	Website:
American Cancer Society	1-800-ACS-2345	http://www.cancer.org
Cancer*Care*	1-800-813-HOPE	http://www.cancercare.org
People Living With Cancer		http://www.cancer.net
National Cancer Institute (NCI)	1-800-4-CANCER	http://www.cancer.gov
NCI Office of Cancer Survivorship	1-301-402-2964	http://dccps.nci.nih.gov/ocs
Gilda's Club	1-888-GILDA-4-U	http://www.gildasclubnyc.org
LIVESTRONG	1-866-235-7205	http://www.livestrong.org

PERSONAL HEALTH RECORD
COLORECTAL OR GASTRIC CANCER

Last Name: First Name:
DOB: Age: Gender: Date:
Day Phone: Evening Phone:
Address: City: State: Zip:
Email:
My Insurance: Policy #:

Spouse/Relative/Caretaker: Phone:
Health Care Agent: Phone:

MEDICAL INFORMATION

Type of cancer: Date of diagnosis:
Staging   T: N: M:

My Health Care Team   **Phone:**   **Email:**
Medical Oncologist:
Radiation Oncologist:
GI Surgeon:
Fellow:
Gastroenterologist:
Nurse/Nurse Practitioner:
Integrative Oncology Nurse:
Pain/Symptom Management:
Social Worker:
Nutritionist:
Physical Therapist:
Patient Navigator:
Enterostomal Therapist:
Treatments received:
Surgical Procedures:

Chemotherapy: ☐ 5-FU   (mg)   ☐ oxaliplatin   (mg)   ☐ Avastin   (mg)
☐ capecitabine
(mg)   ☐ leucovorin   (mg)   ☐ other
Freq: Total Dose:
Hormonal Treatments: ☐ ☐ ☐
Radiation Therapy:
Area treated:
☐ External Beam Radiation Therapy
(EBRT)   Last Date: Dose:
☐ Brachytherapy Last Date: Procedure: Dose:

FOLLOW-UP APPOINTMENTS:
Follow-ups: *Remember to follow up with your providers on a regular schedule*

☐ Surgical: ☐ Radiation Oncology: ☐ Medical Oncology:
☐ Cancer Supportive Services:
                             ☐ Pain/Symptom Management: ☐ Nutrition:
☐ Gastroenterologist   ☐ Physical Therapy: ☐ Social Work:

IMPORTANT FOLLOW-UP CARE:
Shortness of Breath   Blood when: number per day
Taper and avoid nicotine products   Avoid alcoholic beverages
Physical Therapy: *Practice the exercises you have been given by our
staff to manage the following*   **Contact:** _____
☐ Trouble urinating   ☐ Pain when urinating   ☐ Pain in pelvis   ☐ Fatigue

Nutritional Management: *See your nutritionist within 1 month post
treatment to develop a plan for optimal nutrition and to manage symptoms* **Contact:** _____

Height: Current Weight: Ideal Body Weight: Weight History:
Weight gain or loss:

*Follow up with the Nutritionist to address ongoing concerns related to nutrition, weight status and eating including any of the
following symptoms:*
☐ Relying on comfort foods   ☐ Breathing exercise; rehabilitation
☐ Dry/sensitive mouth   ☐ Mouth sores
☐ Changes in taste

Treatment-Related Medications: *Remember to take your medicines as scheduled*

Exams: *Do the appropriate exams as scheduled*
Blood tests: Thyroid function:

Scans:
X-ray: PET/CT: CT: Other:
Self exams:

Integrative Oncology: *Follow up as needed*   Contact: _____

☐ Acupuncture
Breath/relaxation techniques: ☐ Guided imagery   ☐ Progressive relaxation   ☐ Autogenics
Energy therapy: ☐ Reiki   ☐ Therapeutic Touch   ☐ Acupressure

Speech and Swallowing: *Practice what you have been taught by our staff*   Contact: _____

- Follow up with your speech and swallowing therapist after completing treatment
- If you had surgery, get a baseline swallowing test after your surgeon clears you for eating orally
Speech Evaluation: ☐ Yes ☐ No
Results:
Swallowing Evaluation: ☐ Yes ☐ No
Results:
Acceptable diet choices:
☐ Thin Liquids   ☐ Thick liquids   ☐ Purees
☐ Soft Solids   ☐ Unrestricted diet

Dental Care: *See your dentist for routine checkups*   Contact: _____
- Teeth/gums care: thoroughly brush your teeth; floss carefully and avoid gum irritation
- Fluoride regimen: apply fluoride if advised
- Other oral care:

Breathing: *Practice what you have been taught by our staff*
☐ Stoma care

Other:

ADJUSTING TO SURVIVORSHIP

*Contact your social worker if you are experiencing distress
in any of the following areas*   Contact: _____

☐ Body-image   ☐ Eating/sleeping patterns   ☐ Disinterest in activities that you enjoy
☐ Pervasive concerns and worry   ☐ Relationships with your family   ☐ Relationship with partner
                            and friends
☐ Changes in mood   ☐ Sadness   ☐ Fears
☐ Nervousness

WELLNESS

Avoid: **Maintain:**
☐ Nicotine and Tobacco Products   ☐ Healthy nutrition
☐ Alcohol use   ☐ Physical activity
☐ Drug use   ☐ Screening for other cancers
☐ Overexposure to the sun

Screening for other cancers:
☐ Colonoscopy   ☐ Mammogram   ☐ PSA/Digital Rectal exam   ☐ PAP/HPV tests   ☐ Skin exam

ADDITIONAL INFORMATION

Organizations/Programs:	Contact Info:	Website:
Alcoholics Anonymous (AA)	Many local groups exist	http://www.alcoholics-anonymous.org
Narcotics Anonymous (NA)	Many local groups exist	http://www.na.org

Cancer Support Groups:	Contact Info:	Website:
American Cancer Society	1-800-ACS-2345	http://www.cancer.org
CancerCare	1-800-813-HOPE	http://www.cancercare.org
People Living With Cancer		http://www.cancer.net
National Cancer Institute (NCI)	1-800-4-CANCER	http://www.cancer.gov
NCI Office of Cancer Survivorship	1-301-402-2964	http://dccps.nci.nih.gov/ocs
Gilda's Club	1-888-GILDA-4-U	http://www.gildasclubnyc.org
LIVESTRONG	1-866-235-7205	http://www.livestrong.org

PERSONAL HEALTH RECORD
GYNECOLOGIC CANCER

Last Name: First Name:
DOB: Age: Gender: Date:
Day Phone: Evening Phone:
Address: City: State: Zip:
Email:
My Insurance: Policy #:

Spouse/Relative/Caretaker: Phone:
Health Care Agent: Phone:

MEDICAL INFORMATION

Type of cancer: Date of diagnosis:
Staging   T: N: M:

My Health Care Team   **Phone:**   **Email:**
Medical Oncologist:
Radiation Oncologist:
GI Surgeon:
Fellow:
Gynecologist:
Nurse/Nurse Practitioner:
Integrative Oncology Nurse:
Pain/Symptom Management:
Social Worker:
Nutritionist:
Physical Therapist:
Patient Navigator:
Enterostomal Therapist:
Treatments received:
Surgical Procedures:

Chemotherapy: ☐ carboplatinum   ☐ paclitaxel   (mg)   ☐ PEG-adriamycin
                     (mg)   (mg)
☐   (mg)   ☐   (mg)   ☐ other
Freq: Total Dose:
Hormonal Treatments: ☐ ☐ ☐
Radiation Therapy:
Area treated:
☐ External Beam Radiation Therapy   Last Date: Dose:
(EBRT)
☐ Brachytherapy   Last Date: Procedure: Dose:

FOLLOW-UP APPOINTMENTS:
Follow-ups: *Remember to follow up with your providers on a regular schedule*

☐ Surgical: ☐ Radiation Oncology: ☐ Medical Oncology:
☐ Cancer Supportive Services:
                               ☐ Pain/Symptom Management: ☐ Nutrition:
☐ Gastroenterologist   ☐ Physical Therapy: ☐ Social Work:

IMPORTANT FOLLOW-UP CARE:
Shortness of Breath   Blood when: number per day
Taper and avoid nicotine products   Avoid alcoholic beverages
Physical Therapy: *Practice the exercises you have been given by our*   **Contact:** _____
staff to manage the following
☐ Trouble urinating   ☐ Pain when urinating   ☐ Pain in pelvis   ☐ Fatigue

Nutritional Management: *See your nutritionist within 1 month post*
treatment to develop a plan for optimal nutrition and to manage symptoms   **Contact:** _____

Height: Current Weight: Ideal Body Weight: Weight History:
Weight gain or loss:

Follow up with the Nutritionist to address ongoing concerns related to nutrition, weight status and eating including any of the
following symptoms:
☐ Relying on comfort foods   ☐ Breathing exercise; rehabilitation
☐ Dry/sensitive mouth   ☐ Mouth sores
☐ Changes in taste

Treatment-Related Medications: *Remember to take your medicines as scheduled*

Exams: *Do the appropriate exams as scheduled*
Blood tests: Thyroid function:

Scans:
X-ray: PET/CT: CT: Other:
Self exams:

Integrative Oncology: *Follow up as needed*   **Contact:** _____

- ☐ Acupuncture
- Breath/relaxation techniques: ☐ Guided imagery ☐ Progressive relaxation ☐ Autogenics
- Energy therapy: ☐ Reiki ☐ Therapeutic Touch ☐ Acupressure

Speech and Swallowing: *Practice what you have been taught by our staff*   **Contact:** _____

- Follow up with your speech and swallowing therapist after completing treatment
- If you had surgery, get a baseline swallowing test after your surgeon clears you for eating orally
Speech Evaluation: ☐ Yes ☐ No
Results:
Swallowing Evaluation: ☐ Yes ☐ No
Results:
Acceptable diet choices:
- ☐ Thin Liquids   ☐ Thick liquids   ☐ Purees
- ☐ Soft Solids   ☐ Unrestricted diet

Dental Care: *See your dentist for routine checkups*   **Contact:** _____
- Teeth/gums care: thoroughly brush your teeth; floss carefully and avoid gum irritation
- Fluoride regimen: apply fluoride if advised
- Other oral care:

Breathing: *Practice what you have been taught by our staff*
☐ Stoma care

Other:

ADJUSTING TO SURVIVORSHIP

Contact your social worker if you are experiencing distress
in any of the following areas   **Contact:** _____

- ☐ Body-image   ☐ Eating/sleeping patterns   ☐ Disinterest in activities that you enjoy
- ☐ Pervasive concerns and worry   ☐ Relationships with your family and friends   ☐ Relationship with partner
- ☐ Changes in mood   ☐ Sadness   ☐ Fears
- ☐ Nervousness

WELLNESS

Avoid:
- ☐ Nicotine and Tobacco Products
- ☐ Alcohol use
- ☐ Drug use
- ☐ Overexposure to the sun

Maintain:
- ☐ Healthy nutrition
- ☐ Physical activity
- ☐ Screening for other cancers

Screening for other cancers:
☐ Colonoscopy   ☐ Mammogram   ☐ PSA/Digital Rectal exam   ☐ PAP/HPV tests   ☐ Skin exam

ADDITIONAL INFORMATION

Organizations/Programs:	Contact Info:	Website:
Alcoholics Anonymous (AA)	Many local groups exist	http://www.alcoholics-anonymous.org
Narcotics Anonymous (NA)	Many local groups exist	http://www.na.org

Cancer Support Groups:	Contact Info:	Website:
American Cancer Society	1-800-ACS-2345	http://www.cancer.org
CancerCare	1-800-813-HOPE	http://www.cancercare.org
People Living With Cancer		http://www.cancer.net
National Cancer Institute (NCI)	1-800-4-CANCER	http://www.cancer.gov
NCI Office of Cancer Survivorship	1-301-402-2964	http://dccps.nci.nih.gov/ocs
Gilda's Club	1-888-GILDA-4-U	http://www.gildasclubnyc.org
LIVESTRONG	1-866-235-7205	http://www.livestrong.org

PERSONAL HEALTH RECORD
HEAD AND NECK CANCERS

Last Name: First Name:
DOB: Age: Gender: Date:
Day Phone: Evening Phone:
Address: City: State: Zip:
Email:
My Insurance: Policy #:

Spouse/Relative/Caretaker: Phone:
Health Care Agent: Phone:

MEDICAL INFORMATION

Type of Cancer: Date of diagnosis:
Staging   T: N: M:

My Health Care Team   **Phone:**   **Email:**
Medical Oncologist:
Radiation Oncologist:
Surgeon:
Fellow:
Nurse Practitioner:
Integrative Oncology Nurse:
Speech/Swallowing Therapist:
Pain/Symptom Management:
Dentist/Orthodontist:
Nutritionist:
Physical Therapist:
Social Worker:

Treatments received:
Surgical Procedures:

Chemotherapy: ☐ cisplatin   (mg)   ☐ carboplatin   (mg)   ☐ pactitaxel   (mg)
☐ 5-FU   (mg)   ☐ cetuximab   (mg)   ☐ other
Freq: Total Dose:

Radiation Therapy:
Area treated:
☐ External Beam Radiation Therapy
(EBRT)   Last Date: Dose:
☐ Brachytherapy   Last Date: Procedure: Dose:

FOLLOW-UP APPOINTMENTS:

Follow-ups: *Remember to follow up with your providers on a regular schedule*

☐ Surgical: ☐ Radiation Oncology: ☐ Medical Oncology:
☐ Cancer Supportive Services: ☐ Pain/Symptom Management: ☐ Nutrition:
☐ Speech/Swallowing Therapy: ☐ Physical Therapy: ☐ Social Work:
☐ Dental:

IMPORTANT FOLLOW-UP CARE:

Physical Therapy: *Practice the exercises you have been given by our
staff to manage the following*   **Contact:** _____

☐ Secretions   ☐ Pain   ☐ Fatigue   ☐ Neck Mobility

Nutritional Management: *See your nutritionist within 1 month post
treatment to develop a plan for optimal nutrition and to manage symptoms* **Contact:** _____

Height: Current Weight: Ideal Body Weight: Weight History:
PEG placed: PEG removed: Formula:
Eating orally? ☐ Yes ☐ No
Texture tolerance:
*Follow up with the Nutritionist to address ongoing concerns related to nutrition, weight status and eating including any of the
following symptoms:*
☐ Chewing   ☐ Sore throat
☐ Dry/sensitive mouth   ☐ Mouth sores
☐ Changes in taste

Treatment-Related Medications: *Remember to take your medicines as scheduled*

Exams: *Do the appropriate exams as scheduled*
Blood tests: Thyroid function:

Scans:
X-ray: PET/CT: CT: Other:
Self exams:

Integrative Oncology: Contact:

☐ Acupuncture
Breath/relaxation techniques: ☐ Guided imagery ☐ Progressive relaxation ☐ Autogenics
Energy therapy: ☐ Reiki ☐ Therapeutic Touch ☐ Acupressure

Speech and Swallowing: *Practice what you have been taught by our staff* Contact:

- *Follow up with your speech and swallowing therapist after completing treatment*
- *If you had surgery, get a baseline swallowing test after your surgeon clears you for eating orally*
Speech Evaluation: ☐ Yes ☐ No
Results:
Swallowing Evaluation: ☐ Yes ☐ No
Results:
Acceptable diet choices:
☐ Thin Liquids ☐ Thick liquids ☐ Purees
☐ Soft Solids ☐ Unrestricted diet

Recommendations:
- Weaning from a PEG is a <u>process</u> and it <u>can't be done immediately</u>
- Food progression is <u>gradual</u>

Dental Care: *See your dentist for routine checkups* Contact:
  • Teeth/gums care: thoroughly brush your teeth; floss carefully and avoid gum irritation
  • Fluoride regimen: apply fluoride in a prescribed manner
  • Other oral care:

Breathing: *Practice what you have been taught by our staff*
☐ Stoma care

Other:

ADJUSTING TO SURVIVORSHIP

*Contact your social worker if you are experiencing distress
in any of the following areas* Contact:

☐ Body-image ☐ Eating/sleeping patterns ☐ Disinterest in activities that you enjoy
☐ Relationships with your family
☐ Pervasive concerns and worry and friends ☐ Relationship with partner

☐ Changes in mood ☐ Sadness ☐ Fears
☐ Nervousness

WELLNESS

Avoid: Maintain:
☐ Nicotine and Tobacco Products ☐ Healthy nutrition
☐ Alcohol use ☐ Physical activity
☐ Drug use ☐ Screening for other cancers
☐ Overexposure to the sun

Screening for other cancers:
☐ Colonoscopy ☐ Mammogram ☐ PSA/Digital Rectal exam ☐ PAP/HPV tests ☐ Skin exam

ADDITIONAL INFORMATION

Organizations/Programs:	Contact Info:	Website:
Alcoholics Anonymous (AA)	Many local groups exist	http://www.alcoholics-anonymous.org
Narcotics Anonymous (NA)	Many local groups exist	http://www.na.org

Cancer Support Groups:	Contact Info:	Website:
American Cancer Society	1-800-ACS-2345	http://www.cancer.org
Cancer*Care*	1-800-813-HOPE	http://www.cancercare.org
People Living With Cancer		http://www.cancer.net
National Cancer Institute (NCI)	1-800-4-CANCER	http://www.cancer.gov
NCI Office of Cancer Survivorship	1-301-402-2964	http://dccps.nci.nih.gov/ocs
Gilda's Club	1-888-GILDA-4-U	http://www.gildasclubnyc.org
LIVESTRONG	1-866-235-7205	http://www.livestrong.org

PERSONAL HEALTH RECORD
HEPATOBILIARY CANCER

Last Name: First Name:
DOB: Age: Gender: Date:
Day Phone: Evening Phone:
Address: City: State: Zip:
Email:
My Insurance: Policy #:

Spouse/Relative/Caretaker: Phone:
Health Care Agent: Phone:

MEDICAL INFORMATION

Type of cancer: Date of diagnosis:

Staging   T: N: M:

Grade: Fibrosis Score

My Health Care Team   **Phone:**   **Email:**
Medical Oncologist:
Radiation Oncologist:
GI Surgeon:
Fellow:
Gastroenterologist:
Nurse/Nurse Practitioner:
Integrative Oncology Nurse:
Pain/Symptom Management:
Social Worker:
Nutritionist:
Physical Therapist:
Patient Navigator:
Enterostomal Therapist:
Treatments received:
Surgical Procedures:

Chemotherapy: ☐ sorafenib   (mg)   ☐ 5-FU   (mg)   ☐ mitomycin   (mg)
☐ intrahepatic FUDR   ☐ Yttrium90 microspheres   ☐ other
Freq: Total Dose:

Radiation Therapy:
Area treated:
☐ External Beam Radiation Therapy   Last Date: Dose:
(EBRT)
☐ Brachytherapy   Last Date: Procedure: Dose:

FOLLOW-UP APPOINTMENTS:
Follow-ups: *Remember to follow up with your providers on a regular schedule*

☐ Surgical: ☐ Radiation Oncology: ☐ Medical Oncology:
☐ Cancer Supportive Services: ☐ Pain/Symptom Management: ☐ Nutrition:
☐ Gastroenterologist   ☐ Physical Therapy: ☐ Social Work:

IMPORTANT FOLLOW-UP CARE:
Shortness of Breath   Swelling feet or abdomen   Blood tests: AFP every 3 months x 2 years, then every 6 months
Imaging: every 3-6 months x 2 years, then every year
Taper and avoid nicotine products   Avoid alcoholic beverages
Physical Therapy: *Practice the exercises you have been given by our*   **Contact:** _____
staff to manage the following
☐ range of motion   ☐ fatigue/general deconditioning   ☐ shortness of breath

Nutritional Management: *See your nutritionist within 1 month post*
treatment to develop a plan for optimal nutrition and to manage symptoms   **Contact:** _____

Height: Current Weight: Ideal Body Weight: Weight History:
Weight gain or loss:

Follow up with the Nutritionist to address ongoing concerns related to nutrition, weight status and eating including any of the following symptoms:
☐ Relying on comfort foods   ☐ Breathing exercise; rehabilitation
☐ Dry/sensitive mouth   ☐ Mouth sores
☐ Changes in taste

Treatment-Related Medications: *Remember to take your medicines as scheduled*

Exams: *Do the appropriate exams as scheduled*
Blood tests: Thyroid function:

Scans:
X-ray: PET/CT: CT: Other:
Self exams:

Integrative Oncology: *Follow up as needed*   Contact: _____

☐ Acupuncture
Breath/relaxation techniques: ☐ Guided imagery   ☐ Progressive relaxation   ☐ Autogenics
Energy therapy: ☐ Reiki   ☐ Therapeutic Touch   ☐ Acupressure

---

Speech and Swallowing: *Practice what you have been taught by our staff*   Contact: _____

- Follow up with your speech and swallowing therapist after completing treatment
- If you had surgery, get a baseline swallowing test after your surgeon clears you for eating orally
Speech Evaluation: ☐ Yes ☐ No
Results:
Swallowing Evaluation: ☐ Yes ☐ No
Results:
Acceptable diet choices:
☐ Thin Liquids   ☐ Thick liquids   ☐ Purees
☐ Soft Solids   ☐ Unrestricted diet

Dental Care: *See your dentist for routine checkups*   Contact: _____
   ▪   Teeth/gums care: thoroughly brush your teeth; floss carefully and avoid gum irritation
   ▪   Fluoride regimen: apply fluoride if advised
   ▪   Other oral care:

Breathing: *Practice what you have been taught by our staff*
☐ Stoma care

Other:

---

*Contact your social worker if you are experiencing distress
in any of the following areas*   Contact: _____

☐ Body-image   ☐ Eating/sleeping patterns   ☐ Disinterest in activities that you enjoy
                               ☐ Relationships with your family
☐ Pervasive concerns and worry   and friends   ☐ Relationship with partner
☐ Changes in mood   ☐ Sadness   ☐ Fears
☐ Nervousness

WELLNESS

Avoid: **Maintain:**
☐ Nicotine and Tobacco Products   ☐ Healthy nutrition
☐ Alcohol use   ☐ Physical activity
☐ Drug use   ☐ Screening for other cancers
☐ Overexposure to the sun

Screening for other cancers:
☐ Colonoscopy   ☐ Mammogram   ☐ PSA/Digital Rectal exam   ☐ PAP/HPV tests   ☐ Skin exam

---

ADDITIONAL INFORMATION

Organizations/Programs:	Contact Info:	Website:
Alcoholics Anonymous (AA)	Many local groups exist	http://www.alcoholics-anonymous.org
Narcotics Anonymous (NA)	Many local groups exist	http://www.na.org

Cancer Support Groups:	Contact Info:	Website:
American Cancer Society	1-800-ACS-2345	http://www.cancer.org
CancerCare	1-800-813-HOPE	http://www.cancercare.org
People Living With Cancer		http://www.cancer.net
National Cancer Institute (NCI)	1-800-4-CANCER	http://www.cancer.gov
NCI Office of Cancer Survivorship	1-301-402-2964	http://dccps.nci.nih.gov/ocs
Gilda's Club	1-888-GILDA-4-U	http://www.gildasclubnyc.org
LIVESTRONG	1-866-235-7205	http://www.livestrong.org

PERSONAL HEALTH RECORD
KIDNEY OR BLADDER CANCER

Last Name: First Name:

DOB: Age: Gender: Date:

Day Phone: Evening Phone:

Address: City: State: Zip:

Email:

My Insurance: Policy #:

Spouse/Relative/Caretaker: Phone:

Health Care Agent: Phone:

MEDICAL INFORMATION

Type of Cancer: Date of diagnosis:

Staging   T: N: M:

My Health Care Team   **Phone:**   **Email:**

Medical Oncologist:

Radiation Oncologist:

Surgeon:

Fellow:

Nurse Practitioner:

Integrative Oncology Nurse:

Speech/Swallowing Therapist:

Pain/Symptom Management:

Dentist/Orthodontist:

Nutritionist:

Physical Therapist:

Social Worker:

Treatments received:

Surgical Procedures:

Chemotherapy: ☐ cisplatin   (mg)   ☐ gemcitabine   (mg)   ☐ methotrexate   (mg)

☐ paclitaxel   (mg)   ☐ doxorubicin   (mg)   ☐ other

Freq: Total Dose:

☐ sunitinib   (mg) ☐ temsirolimus   (mg) ☐ bevacizumab   (mg) ☐ pazopanib   (mg)

BCG into bladder:

Radiation Therapy:

Area treated:

☐ External Beam Radiation Therapy (EBRT)   Last Date: Dose:

☐   Last Date: Procedure: Dose:

FOLLOW-UP APPOINTMENTS:

Follow-ups: *Remember to follow up with your providers on a regular schedule*

☐ Urine cytology or cystoscopy :   Chest, abdomen & pelvis imaging every 6 mo

Surgical: ☐ Radiation Oncology: ☐ Medical Oncology:

☐ Cancer Supportive Services: ☐ Pain/Symptom Management: ☐ Nutrition:

☐ Speech/Swallowing Therapy: ☐ Physical Therapy: ☐ Social Work:

☐ Dental:

IMPORTANT FOLLOW-UP CARE:

Blood work and imaging above

Physical Therapy: *Practice the exercises you have been given by our staff to manage the following*   **Contact:** _____

☐ Secretions   ☐ Pain   ☐ Fatigue   ☐ Neck Mobility

Nutritional Management: *See your nutritionist within 1 month post treatment to develop a plan for optimal nutrition and to manage symptoms*   **Contact:** _____

Height: Current Weight: Ideal Body Weight: Weight History:

PEG placed: PEG removed: Formula:

                         Recommendations:

Eating orally? ☐ Yes ☐ No   - Weaning from a PEG is a process and it can't be done immediately

                        - Food progression is gradual

Texture tolerance:

Follow up with the Nutritionist to address ongoing concerns related to nutrition, weight status and eating including any of the following symptoms:

☐ Chewing   ☐ Sore throat

☐ Dry/sensitive mouth   ☐ Mouth sores

☐ Changes in taste

Treatment-Related Medications: *Remember to take your medicines as scheduled*

Exams: *Do the appropriate exams as scheduled*
Blood tests: Thyroid function:

Scans:
X-ray: PET/CT: CT: Other:
Self exams:

Integrative Oncology: *Follow up as needed*   **Contact:** _____

☐ Acupuncture
Breath/relaxation techniques: ☐ Guided imagery   ☐ Progressive relaxation   ☐ Autogenics
Energy therapy: ☐ Reiki   ☐ Therapeutic Touch   ☐ Acupressure

Speech and Swallowing: *Practice what you have been taught by our staff*   **Contact:** _____

- Follow up with your speech and swallowing therapist after completing treatment
- If you had surgery, get a baseline swallowing test after your surgeon clears you for eating orally
Speech Evaluation: ☐ Yes ☐ No
Results:
Swallowing Evaluation: ☐ Yes ☐ No
Results:
Acceptable diet choices:
☐ Thin Liquids   ☐ Thick liquids   ☐ Purees
☐ Soft Solids   ☐ Unrestricted diet

Dental Care: *See your dentist for routine checkups*   **Contact:** _____
   • Teeth/gums care: thoroughly brush your teeth; floss carefully and avoid gum irritation
   • Fluoride regimen: apply fluoride if advised
   • Other oral care:

Breathing: *Practice what you have been taught by our staff*
☐ Stoma care

Other:

ADJUSTING TO SURVIVORSHIP

Contact your social worker if you are experiencing distress   **Contact:** _____
in any of the following areas
☐ Body-image   ☐ Eating/sleeping patterns   ☐ Disinterest in activities that you enjoy
                              ☐ Relationships with your family
☐ Pervasive concerns and worry   and friends   ☐ Relationship with partner

☐ Changes in mood   ☐ Sadness   ☐ Fears
☐ Nervousness

WELLNESS

Avoid: **Maintain:**
☐ Nicotine and Tobacco Products   ☐ Healthy nutrition
☐ Alcohol use   ☐ Physical activity
☐ Drug use   ☐ Screening for other cancers
☐ Overexposure to the sun

Screening for other cancers:
☐ Colonoscopy   ☐ Mammogram   ☐ PSA/Digital Rectal exam   ☐ PAP/HPV tests   ☐ Skin exam

ADDITIONAL INFORMATION

Organizations/Programs:	Contact Info:	Website:
Alcoholics Anonymous (AA)	Many local groups exist	http://www.alcoholics-anonymous.org
Narcotics Anonymous (NA)	Many local groups exist	http://www.na.org

Cancer Support Groups:	Contact Info:	Website:
American Cancer Society	1-800-ACS-2345	http://www.cancer.org
CancerCare	1-800-813-HOPE	http://www.cancercare.org
People Living With Cancer		http://www.cancer.net
National Cancer Institute (NCI)	1-800-4-CANCER	http://www.cancer.gov
NCI Office of Cancer Survivorship	1-301-402-2964	http://dccps.nci.nih.gov/ocs
Gilda's Club	1-888-GILDA-4-U	http://www.gildasclubnyc.org
LIVESTRONG	1-866-235-7205	http://www.livestrong.org

PERSONAL HEALTH RECORD
LEUKEMIA

Last Name: First Name:
DOB: Age: Gender: Date:
Day Phone: Evening Phone:
Address: City: State: Zip:
Email:
My Insurance: Policy #:

Spouse/Relative/Caretaker: Phone:
Health Care Agent: Phone:

MEDICAL INFORMATION

Type of Leukemia: Subtype: Stage: Date of diagnosis:

My Health Care Team   **Phone:**   **Email:**
Medical Oncologist:
Radiation Oncologist:
Surgeon:
Fellow:
Nurse Practitioner:
Integrative Oncology Nurse:
Hematologist:
Pain/Symptom Management:
Dentist/Orthodontist:
Nutritionist:
Physical Therapist:
Social Worker:

Treatments received:
Surgical Procedures:
Chemotherapy: ☐ doxorubicin   bleomycin   mg   vincistine   mg   dacarbazine   mg   rituximab   mg
                   prednisone   mg   cyclophosphamide   mg ☐   (mg) ☐ l   (mg)
☐ fludarabine   (mg) ☐ chlorambucil   (mg)
☐ Allopurinol   (mg) ☐ cetuximab   (mg)   ☐ rasburicase   (mg)
                         ☐ other
Freq: Total Doses:
Radiation Therapy:
Area treated:
☐ External Beam Radiation Therapy
(EBRT)   Last Date: Dose:

FOLLOW-UP APPOINTMENTS:

Follow-ups: *Remember to follow up with your providers on a regular schedule*

☐ Surgical: ☐ Radiation Oncology: ☐ Medical Oncology:
☐ Cancer Supportive Services: ☐ Pain/Symptom Management: ☐ Nutrition:

☐ Speech/Swallowing Therapy:
                             ☐ Physical Therapy: ☐ Social Work:
☐ Dental:

IMPORTANT FOLLOW-UP CARE:

Physical Therapy: *Practice the exercises you have been given by our
staff to manage the following*   **Contact:** _____

☐ Fatigue/general   ☐ Shortness of breath ☐ Pain ☐ Fatigue

Nutritional Management: *See your nutritionist within 1 month post
treatment to develop a plan for optimal nutrition and to manage symptoms* **Contact:** _____

Height: Current Weight: Ideal Body Weight: Weight History:
PEG placed: PEG removed: Formula:
                         Recommendations:
Eating orally? ☐ Yes ☐ No   - Weaning from a PEG is a process and it can't be done immediately
                             - Food progression is gradual
Texture tolerance:
*Follow up with the Nutritionist to address ongoing concerns related to nutrition, weight status and eating including any of the
following symptoms:*
☐ Chewing   ☐ Sore throat
☐ Dry/sensitive mouth   ☐ Mouth sores
☐ Changes in taste

Treatment-Related Medications: *Remember to take your medicines as scheduled*

Exams: *Do the appropriate exams as scheduled*
Blood tests: Thyroid function:

Scans:
X-ray: PET/CT: CT: Other:
Self exams:

Integrative Oncology: *Follow up as needed*   Contact: _____

☐ Acupuncture
Breath/relaxation techniques: ☐ Guided imagery   ☐ Progressive relaxation   ☐ Autogenics
Energy therapy: ☐ Reiki   ☐ Therapeutic Touch   ☐ Acupressure

---

Speech and Swallowing: *Practice what you have been taught by our staff*   Contact: _____

- Follow up with your speech and swallowing therapist after completing treatment
- If you had surgery, get a baseline swallowing test after your surgeon clears you for eating orally
Speech Evaluation: ☐ Yes ☐ No
Results:
Swallowing Evaluation: ☐ Yes ☐ No
Results:
Acceptable diet choices:
☐ Thin Liquids   ☐ Thick liquids   ☐ Purees
☐ Soft Solids   ☐ Unrestricted diet

Dental Care: *See your dentist for routine checkups*   Contact: _____
- Teeth/gums care: thoroughly brush your teeth; floss carefully and avoid gum irritation
- Fluoride regimen: apply fluoride if advised
- Other oral care:

Breathing: *Practice what you have been taught by our staff*
☐

Other:

ADJUSTING TO SURVIVORSHIP

*Contact your social worker if you are experiencing distress
in any of the following areas*   Contact: _____

☐ Body-image   ☐ Eating/sleeping patterns   ☐ Disinterest in activities that you enjoy
☐ Pervasive concerns and worry   ☐ Relationships with your family   ☐ Relationship with partner
                             and friends
☐ Changes in mood   ☐ Sadness   ☐ Fears
☐ Nervousness

WELLNESS

Avoid: **Maintain:**
☐ Nicotine and Tobacco Products   ☐ Healthy nutrition
☐ Alcohol use   ☐ Physical activity
☐ Drug use   ☐ Screening for other cancers
☐ Overexposure to the sun

Screening for other cancers:
☐ Colonoscopy   ☐ Mammogram   ☐ PSA/Digital Rectal exam   ☐ PAP/HPV tests   ☐ Skin exam

ADDITIONAL INFORMATION

Organizations/Programs:	Contact Info:	Website:
Alcoholics Anonymous (AA)	Many local groups exist	http://www.alcoholics-anonymous.org
Narcotics Anonymous (NA)	Many local groups exist	http://www.na.org

Cancer Support Groups:	Contact Info:	Website:
American Cancer Society	1-800-ACS-2345	http://www.cancer.org
Cancer*Care*	1-800-813-HOPE	http://www.cancercare.org
People Living With Cancer		http://www.cancer.net
National Cancer Institute (NCI)	1-800-4-CANCER	http://www.cancer.gov
NCI Office of Cancer Survivorship	1-301-402-2964	http://dccps.nci.nih.gov/ocs
Gilda's Club	1-888-GILDA-4-U	http://www.gildasclubnyc.org
LIVESTRONG	1-866-235-7205	http://www.livestrong.org

PERSONAL HEALTH RECORD
LUNG CANCER

Last Name: First Name:
DOB: Age: Gender: Date:
Day Phone: Evening Phone:
Address: City: State: Zip:
Email:
My Insurance: Policy #:

Spouse/Relative/Caretaker: Phone:
Health Care Agent: Phone:

MEDICAL INFORMATION

Type of cancer: Date of diagnosis:
Staging   T: N: M:

My Health Care Team   **Phone:**   **Email:**
Medical Oncologist:
Radiation Oncologist:
Thoracic Surgeon:
Fellow:
Pulmonologist:
Nurse/Nurse Practitioner:
Integrative Oncology Nurse:
Pain/Symptom Management:
Social Worker:
Nutritionist:
Physical Therapist:
Patient Navigator:

Treatments received:
Surgical Procedures:

Chemotherapy: ☐ carboplatin   (mg)   ☐ paclitaxel   (mg)   ☐ Avastin   (mg)
☐ Alimpta   (mg)   ☐ cisplatin   (mg)   ☐ other
Freq: Total Dose:
Hormonal Treatments: ☐
Radiation Therapy:
Area treated:
☐ External Beam Radiation Therapy   Last Date: Dose:
(EBRT)
☐ Brachytherapy   Last Date: Procedure: Dose:

FOLLOW-UP APPOINTMENTS:
Follow-ups: *Remember to follow up with your providers on a regular schedule*

☐ Surgical: ☐ Radiation Oncology: ☐ Medical Oncology:
☐ Cancer Supportive Services: ☐ Pain/Symptom Management: ☐ Nutrition:
☐ Pulmonologist   ☐ Physical Therapy: ☐ Social Work:

IMPORTANT FOLLOW-UP CARE:
Shortness of Breath   Blood whens: number per day
Taper and avoid nicotine products   Avoid alcoholic beverages
Physical Therapy: *Practice the exercises you have been given by our*
staff to manage the following   **Contact:** _____
☐ Trouble urinating   ☐ Pain when urinating   ☐ Pain in pelvis   ☐ Fatigue

Nutritional Management: *See your nutritionist within 1 month post*
treatment to develop a plan for optimal nutrition and to manage symptoms   **Contact:** _____

Height: Current Weight: Ideal Body Weight: Weight History:
Weight gain or loss:

Follow up with the Nutritionist to address ongoing concerns related to nutrition, weight status and eating including any of the
following symptoms:
☐ Relying on comfort foods   ☐ Breathing exercise; pulmonary rehabilitation
☐ Dry/sensitive mouth   ☐ Mouth sores
☐ Changes in taste

Treatment-Related Medications: *Remember to take your medicines as scheduled*

Exams: *Do the appropriate exams as scheduled*
Blood tests: Thyroid function:

Scans:
X-ray: PET/CT: CT: Other:
Self exams:

Integrative Oncology: *Follow up as needed*   **Contact:** _____

☐ Acupuncture
Breath/relaxation techniques: ☐ Guided imagery   ☐ Progressive relaxation   ☐ Autogenics
Energy therapy: ☐ Reiki   ☐ Therapeutic Touch   ☐ Acupressure

---

Speech and Swallowing: *Practice what you have been taught by our staff*
                                              Contact: _____

- Follow up with your speech and swallowing therapist after completing treatment
- If you had surgery, get a baseline swallowing test after your surgeon clears you for eating orally
Speech Evaluation: ☐ Yes ☐ No
Results:
Swallowing Evaluation: ☐ Yes ☐ No
Results:
Acceptable diet choices:
☐ Thin Liquids   ☐ Thick liquids   ☐ Purees
☐ Soft Solids   ☐ Unrestricted diet

Dental Care: *See your dentist for routine checkups*   **Contact:** _____
- Teeth/gums care: thoroughly brush your teeth; floss carefully and avoid gum irritation
- Fluoride regimen: apply fluoride if advised
- Other oral care:

Breathing: *Practice what you have been taught by our staff*
☐ Stoma care

Other:

ADJUSTING TO SURVIVORSHIP

Contact your social worker if you are experiencing distress
in any of the following areas   **Contact:** _____

☐ Body-image   ☐ Eating/sleeping patterns   ☐ Disinterest in activities that you enjoy
☐ Pervasive concerns and worry   ☐ Relationships with your family   ☐ Relationship with partner
                                and friends
☐ Changes in mood   ☐ Sadness   ☐ Fears
☐ Nervousness

WELLNESS

Avoid: **Maintain:**
☐ Nicotine and Tobacco Products   ☐ Healthy nutrition
☐ Alcohol use   ☐ Physical activity
☐ Drug use   ☐ Screening for other cancers
☐ Overexposure to the sun

Screening for other cancers:
☐ Colonoscopy   ☐ Mammogram   ☐ PSA/Digital Rectal exam   ☐ PAP/HPV tests   ☐ Skin exam

---

ADDITIONAL INFORMATION

Organizations/Programs:	Contact Info:	Website:
Alcoholics Anonymous (AA)	Many local groups exist	http://www.alcoholics-anonymous.org
Narcotics Anonymous (NA)	Many local groups exist	http://www.na.org

Cancer Support Groups:	Contact Info:	Website:
American Cancer Society	1-800-ACS-2345	http://www.cancer.org
CancerCare	1-800-813-HOPE	http://www.cancercare.org
People Living With Cancer		http://www.cancer.net
National Cancer Institute (NCI)	1-800-4-CANCER	http://www.cancer.gov
NCI Office of Cancer Survivorship	1-301-402-2964	http://dccps.nci.nih.gov/ocs
Gilda's Club	1-888-GILDA-4-U	http://www.gildasclubnyc.org
LIVESTRONG	1-866-235-7205	http://www.livestrong.org

PERSONAL HEALTH RECORD
LYMPHOMAS

Last Name: First Name:
DOB: Age: Gender: Date:
Day Phone: Evening Phone:
Address: City: State: Zip:
Email:
My Insurance: Policy #:

Spouse/Relative/Caretaker: Phone:
Health Care Agent: Phone:

MEDICAL INFORMATION

Type of Lymphoma: Date of diagnosis:
Staging   Stage: Lymphovascular   Residual

My Health Care Team   **Phone:**   **Email:**
Medical Oncologist:
Radiation Oncologist:
Surgeon:
Fellow:
Nurse Practitioner:
Integrative Oncology Nurse:
Hematologist:
Pain/Symptom Management:
Dentist:
Nutritionist:
Physical Therapist:
Social Worker:

Treatments received:
Surgical Procedures:
Chemotherapy: ☐ doxorubicin ☐ bleomycin   mg   ☐ vincistine   mg   ☐ dacarbazine   mg
            ☐ rituximab   mg   ☐ prednisone   mg ☐ cyclophosphamide   mg   ☐   (mg) ☐   (mg)
            ☐ ara C   (mg)   ☐ fludarabine   (mg)   ☐ chlorambucil   (mg)
                                                        ☐ other
Freq: Total Dose:

Radiation Therapy:
Area treated:
☐ External Beam Radiation Therapy
(EBRT)   Last Date: Dose:

FOLLOW-UP APPOINTMENTS:
Follow-ups: *Remember to follow up with your providers on a regular schedule*

☐ Surgical: ☐ Radiation Oncology: ☐ Medical Oncology:
☐ Cancer Supportive Services:
                               ☐ Pain/Symptom Management: ☐ Nutrition:
☐ Speech/Swallowing Therapy:
                               ☐ Physical Therapy: ☐ Social Work:
☐ Dental:

IMPORTANT FOLLOW-UP CARE:

Physical Therapy: *Practice the exercises you have been given by our*   **Contact:** _____
staff to manage the following

☐ Shortness of breath   ☐ Pain   ☐ Fatigue   ☐

Nutritional Management: *See your nutritionist within 1 month post*
treatment to develop a plan for optimal nutrition and to manage symptoms   **Contact:** _____

Height: Current Weight: Ideal Body Weight: Weight History:
PEG placed: PEG removed: Formula:
                     Recommendations:
Eating orally? ☐ Yes ☐ No   - Weaning from a PEG is a <u>process</u> and it <u>can't be done immediately</u>
                             - Food progression is <u>gradual</u>
Texture tolerance:
Follow up with the Nutritionist to address ongoing concerns related to nutrition, weight status and eating including any of the
following symptoms:
☐ Chewing   ☐ Sore throat
☐ Dry/sensitive mouth   ☐ Mouth sores
☐ Changes in taste

298

Treatment-Related Medications: *Remember to take your medicines as scheduled*

Exams: *Do the appropriate exams as scheduled*
Blood tests: Thyroid function:

Scans:
X-ray: PET/CT: CT: Other:
Self exams:

Integrative Oncology: *Follow up as needed*   Contact: _____

☐ Acupuncture
Breath/relaxation techniques: ☐ Guided imagery   ☐ Progressive relaxation   ☐ Autogenics
Energy therapy: ☐ Reiki   ☐ Therapeutic Touch   ☐ Acupressure

---

Speech and Swallowing: *Practice what you have been taught by our staff*   Contact: _____

- Follow up with your speech and swallowing therapist after completing treatment
- If you had surgery, get a baseline swallowing test after your surgeon clears you for eating orally
Speech Evaluation: ☐ Yes ☐ No
Results:
Swallowing Evaluation: ☐ Yes ☐ No
Results:
Acceptable diet choices:
☐ Thin Liquids   ☐ Thick liquids   ☐ Purees
☐ Soft Solids   ☐ Unrestricted diet

Dental Care: *See your dentist for routine checkups*   Contact: _____
  • Teeth/gums care: thoroughly brush your teeth; floss carefully and avoid gum irritation
  • Fluoride regimen: apply fluoride if prescribed
  • Other oral care:

Breathing: *Practice what you have been taught by our staff*
☐

Other:

---

*Contact your social worker if you are experiencing distress
in any of the following areas*   Contact: _____

☐ Body-image   ☐ Eating/sleeping patterns   ☐ Disinterest in activities that you enjoy
☐ Pervasive concerns and worry ☐ Relationships with your family   ☐ Relationship with partner
                                 and friends
☐ Changes in mood   ☐ Sadness   ☐ Fears
☐ Nervousness

WELLNESS

Avoid: **Maintain:**
☐ Nicotine and Tobacco Products   ☐ Healthy nutrition
☐ Alcohol use   ☐ Physical activity
☐ Drug use   ☐ Screening for other cancers
☐ Overexposure to the sun

Screening for other cancers:
☐ Colonoscopy   ☐ Mammogram   ☐ PSA/Digital Rectal exam   ☐ PAP/HPV tests   ☐ Skin exam

---

ADDITIONAL INFORMATION

Organizations/Programs:	Contact Info:	Website:
Alcoholics Anonymous (AA)	Many local groups exist	http://www.alcoholics-anonymous.org
Narcotics Anonymous (NA)	Many local groups exist	http://www.na.org

Cancer Support Groups:	Contact Info:	Website:
American Cancer Society	1-800-ACS-2345	http://www.cancer.org
Cancer Care	1-800-813-HOPE	http://www.cancercare.org
People Living With Cancer		http://www.cancer.net
National Cancer Institute (NCI)	1-800-4-CANCER	http://www.cancer.gov
NCI Office of Cancer Survivorship	1-301-402-2964	http://dccps.nci.nih.gov/ocs
Gilda's Club	1-888-GILDA-4-U	http://www.gildasclubnyc.org
LIVESTRONG	1-866-235-7205	http://www.livestrong.org

PERSONAL HEALTH RECORD
MYELOMA

Last Name: First Name:
DOB: Age: Gender: Date:
Day Phone: Evening Phone:
Address: City: State: Zip:
Email:
My Insurance: Policy #:

Spouse/Relative/Caretaker: Phone:
Health Care Agent: Phone:

MEDICAL INFORMATION

Plasmacytoma: Asymptomatic: Symptomatic: Date of diagnosis:

My Health Care Team   **Phone:**   **Email:**
Medical Oncologist:
Radiation Oncologist:
Surgeon:
Fellow:
Nurse Practitioner:
Integrative Oncology Nurse:
Hematologist:
Pain/Symptom Management:
Dentist:
Nutritionist:
Physical Therapist:
Social Worker:

Treatments received:
Surgical Procedures:
Chemotherapy: ☐ (mg) ☐ I (mg)
     ☐ bortezomib (mg)   ☐ lenalidomide (mg)   ☐ dexamethasone (mg)
     ☐ melphalan (mg)   ☐ thalidomide (mg)   ☐ vincristine (mg)   ☐ other
Freq: Total Doses:

Radiation Therapy:
Area treated:
☐ External Beam Radiation Therapy   Last Date: Dose:
(EBRT)

FOLLOW-UP APPOINTMENTS:
Follow-ups: *Remember to follow up with your providers on a regular schedule*

☐ Surgical: ☐ Radiation Oncology: ☐ Medical Oncology:
☐ Cancer Supportive Services: ☐ Pain/Symptom Management: ☐ Nutrition:

☐ Speech/Swallowing Therapy: ☐ Physical Therapy: ☐ Social Work:

☐ Dental:

IMPORTANT FOLLOW-UP CARE:

Physical Therapy: *Practice the exercises you have been given by our staff to manage the following:*   **Contact:** _____
☐ general deconditioning/fatigue   ☐ balance
☐ SPEP every   weeks   ☐ CBC for anemia   ☐ Lytes for renal func every   ☐ Bone density & ?
                            every   weeks   weeks   bisphosphonates
      avoid NSAIDs   avoid IV contrast

Nutritional Management: *See your nutritionist within 1 month post treatment to develop a plan for optimal nutrition and to manage symptoms*   **Contact:** _____

Height: Current Weight: Ideal Body Weight: Weight History:
PEG placed: PEG removed: Formula:
                    Recommendations:
Eating orally? ☐ Yes ☐ No   - Weaning from a PEG is a <u>process</u> and it <u>can't be done immediately</u>
                    - Food progression is <u>gradual</u>
Texture tolerance:
Follow up with the Nutritionist to address ongoing concerns related to nutrition, weight status and eating including any of the following symptoms:
☐ Chewing   ☐ Sore throat
☐ Dry/sensitive mouth   ☐ Mouth sores
☐ Changes in taste

Treatment-Related Medications: *Remember to take your medicines as scheduled*

Exams: *Do the appropriate exams as scheduled*
Blood tests: Thyroid function:

Scans:
X-ray: PET/CT: CT: Other:
Self exams:

Integrative Oncology: *Follow up as needed*   **Contact:** _____

☐ Acupuncture
Breath/relaxation techniques: ☐ Guided imagery   ☐ Progressive relaxation   ☐ Autogenics
Energy therapy: ☐ Reiki   ☐ Therapeutic Touch   ☐ Acupressure

Speech and Swallowing: *Practice what you have been taught by our staff*
                                                                   Contact: _____

- *Follow up with your speech and swallowing therapist after completing treatment*
- *If you had surgery, get a baseline swallowing test after your surgeon clears you for eating orally*
Speech Evaluation: ☐ Yes ☐ No
Results:
Swallowing Evaluation: ☐ Yes ☐ No
Results:
Acceptable diet choices:
☐ Thin Liquids   ☐ Thick liquids   ☐ Purees
☐ Soft Solids   ☐ Unrestricted diet

Dental Care: *See your dentist for routine checkups*   **Contact:** _____
  - Teeth/gums care: thoroughly brush your teeth; floss carefully and avoid gum irritation
  - Fluoride regimen: apply fluoride if advised
  - Other oral care:

Breathing: *Practice what you have been taught by our staff*
☐

Other:

ADJUSTING TO SURVIVORSHIP

*Contact your social worker if you are experiencing distress
in any of the following areas*   **Contact:** _____

☐ Body-image   ☐ Eating/sleeping patterns   ☐ Disinterest in activities that you enjoy
                             ☐ Relationships with your family
☐ Pervasive concerns and worry   and friends   ☐ Relationship with partner
☐ Changes in mood   ☐ Sadness   ☐ Fears
☐ Nervousness

WELLNESS

Avoid: **Maintain:**
☐ Nicotine and Tobacco Products   ☐ Healthy nutrition
☐ Alcohol use   ☐ Physical activity
☐ Drug use   ☐ Screening for other cancers
☐ Overexposure to the sun

Screening for other cancers:
☐ Colonoscopy   ☐ Mammogram   ☐ PSA/Digital Rectal exam   ☐ PAP/HPV tests   ☐ Skin exam

ADDITIONAL INFORMATION

Organizations/Programs:	Contact Info:	Website:
Alcoholics Anonymous (AA)	Many local groups exist	http://www.alcoholics-anonymous.org
Narcotics Anonymous (NA)	Many local groups exist	http://www.na.org

Cancer Support Groups:	Contact Info:	Website:
American Cancer Society	1-800-ACS-2345	http://www.cancer.org
CancerCare	1-800-813-HOPE	http://www.cancercare.org
People Living With Cancer		http://www.cancer.net
National Cancer Institute (NCI)	1-800-4-CANCER	http://www.cancer.gov
NCI Office of Cancer Survivorship	1-301-402-2964	http://dccps.nci.nih.gov/ocs
Gilda's Club	1-888-GILDA-4-U	http://www.gildasclubnyc.org
LIVESTRONG	1-866-235-7205	http://www.livestrong.org

PERSONAL HEALTH RECORD
PANCREATIC CANCER

Last Name: First Name:
DOB: Age: Gender: Date:
Day Phone: Evening Phone:
Address: City: State: Zip:
Email:
My Insurance: Policy #:

Spouse/Relative/Caretaker: Phone:
Health Care Agent: Phone:

MEDICAL INFORMATION

Type of cancer: Date of diagnosis:
Staging   T: N: M:

My Health Care Team   **Phone:**   **Email:**
Medical Oncologist:
Radiation Oncologist:
GI Surgeon:
Fellow:
Gastroenterologist:
Nurse/Nurse Practitioner:
Integrative Oncology Nurse:
Pain/Symptom Management:
Social Worker:
Nutritionist:
Physical Therapist:
Patient Navigator:

Treatments received:
Surgical Procedures:
☐ nerve block
Chemotherapy: ☐ 5-FU   (mg)   ☐ oxaliplatin   (mg)   ☐ gemcitabine   (mg)
☐ capecitabine
(mg)   ☐ leucovorin   (mg)   ☐ other
Freq: Total Dose:
☐ pancreatic enzymes
Radiation Therapy:
Area treated:
☐ External Beam Radiation Therapy
(EBRT)   Last Date: Dose:
☐ Brachytherapy   Last Date: Procedure: Dose:

FOLLOW-UP APPOINTMENTS:
Follow-ups: *Remember to follow up with your providers on a regular schedule*

☐ Surgical: ☐ Radiation Oncology: ☐ Medical Oncology:
☐ Cancer Supportive Services:
                               ☐ Pain/Symptom Management: ☐ Nutrition:
☐ Gastroenterologist   ☐ Physical Therapy: ☐ Social Work:

IMPORTANT FOLLOW-UP CARE:
Shortness of Breath   Blood cough up: in stool
Taper and avoid nicotine products   Avoid alcoholic beverages
Physical Therapy: *Practice the exercises you have been given by our*   **Contact:** _____
staff to manage the following
☐ Trouble urinating   ☐ Pain when urinating   ☐ Pain in pelvis   ☐ Fatigue

Nutritional Management: *See your nutritionist within 1 month post*
treatment to develop a plan for optimal nutrition and to manage symptoms   **Contact:** _____

Height: Current Weight: Ideal Body Weight: Weight History:
Weight gain or loss:
Supplements

*Follow up with the Nutritionist to address ongoing concerns related to nutrition, weight status and eating including any of the
following symptoms:*
☐ Relying on comfort foods   ☐ Breathing exercise; rehabilitation
☐ Dry/sensitive mouth   ☐ Mouth sores
☐ Changes in taste

Treatment-Related Medications: *Remember to take your medicines as scheduled*

Exams: *Do the appropriate exams as scheduled*
Blood tests: Thyroid function:

Scans:
X-ray: PET/CT: CT: Other:
Self exams:

Integrative Oncology: *Follow up as needed*   **Contact:** _____

☐ Acupuncture
Breath/relaxation techniques: ☐ Guided imagery   ☐ Progressive relaxation   ☐ Autogenics
Energy therapy: ☐ Reiki   ☐ Therapeutic Touch   ☐ Acupressure

Speech and Swallowing: *Practice what you have been taught by our staff*
                                                                    Contact: _____

- *Follow up with your speech and swallowing therapist after completing treatment*
- *If you had surgery, get a baseline swallowing test after your surgeon clears you for eating orally*
Speech Evaluation: ☐ Yes ☐ No
Results:
Swallowing Evaluation: ☐ Yes ☐ No
Results:
Acceptable diet choices:
☐ Thin Liquids   ☐ Thick liquids   ☐ Purees
☐ Soft Solids   ☐ Unrestricted diet

Dental Care: *See your dentist for routine checkups*   **Contact:** _____
   • Teeth/gums care: thoroughly brush your teeth; floss carefully and avoid gum irritation
   • Fluoride regimen: apply fluoride if advised
   • Other oral care:

Breathing: *Practice what you have been taught by our staff*
☐

Other:

ADJUSTING TO SURVIVORSHIP

Contact your social worker if you are experiencing distress
in any of the following areas   **Contact:** _____

☐ Body-image   ☐ Eating/sleeping patterns   ☐ Disinterest in activities that you enjoy
☐ Pervasive concerns and worry   ☐ Relationships with your family   ☐ Relationship with partner
                                 and friends
☐ Changes in mood   ☐ Sadness   ☐ Fears
☐ Nervousness

WELLNESS

Avoid: **Maintain:**
☐ Nicotine and Tobacco Products   ☐ Healthy nutrition
☐ Alcohol use   ☐ Physical activity
☐ Drug use   ☐ Screening for other cancers
☐ Overexposure to the sun

Screening for other cancers:
☐ Colonoscopy   ☐ Mammogram   ☐ PSA/Digital Rectal exam   ☐ PAP/HPV tests   ☐ Skin exam

ADDITIONAL INFORMATION

Organizations/Programs:	Contact Info:	Website:
Alcoholics Anonymous (AA)	Many local groups exist	http://www.alcoholics-anonymous.org
Narcotics Anonymous (NA)	Many local groups exist	http://www.na.org

Cancer Support Groups:	Contact Info:	Website:
American Cancer Society	1-800-ACS-2345	http://www.cancer.org
CancerCare	1-800-813-HOPE	http://www.cancercare.org
People Living With Cancer		http://www.cancer.net
National Cancer Institute (NCI)	1-800-4-CANCER	http://www.cancer.gov
NCI Office of Cancer Survivorship	1-301-402-2964	http://dccps.nci.nih.gov/ocs
Gilda's Club	1-888-GILDA-4-U	http://www.gildasclubnyc.org
LIVESTRONG	1-866-235-7205	http://www.livestrong.org

PERSONAL HEALTH RECORD
PROSTATE CANCER

Last Name: First Name:
DOB: Age: Gender: Date:
Day Phone: Evening Phone:
Address: City: State: Zip:
Email:
My Insurance: Policy #:

Spouse/Relative/Caretaker: Phone:
Health Care Agent: Phone:

MEDICAL INFORMATION

Gleason Score: PSA=   Date of diagnosis:
Staging   T: N: M:

My Health Care Team   **Phone:**   **Email:**
Medical Oncologist:
Radiation Oncologist:
Urological Surgeon:
Fellow:
General Urologist:
Nurse/Nurse Practitioner:
Integrative Oncology Nurse:
Pain/Symptom Management:
Social Worker:
Nutritionist:
Physical Therapist:
Patient Navigator:

Treatments received:
Surgical Procedures:

Chemotherapy: ☐ corticosteorids   ☐ paclitaxel   (mg)   ☐ mitoxantrone (mg)
                 (mg)
☐ paclitaxel   (mg)   ☐   (mg)   ☐ other
Freq: Total Dose:
Hormonal Treatments: ☐ Eulexin ☐ Casodex ☐ Zoladex   ☐ other
Radiation Therapy:
Area treated:
☐ External Beam Radiation Therapy   Last Date: Dose:
(EBRT)
☐ Brachytherapy   Last Date: Procedure: Dose:

FOLLOW-UP APPOINTMENTS:

Follow-ups: *Remember to follow up with your providers on a regular schedule*

☐ Surgical: ☐ Radiation Oncology: ☐ Medical Oncology:
☐ Cancer Supportive Services: ☐ Pain/Symptom Management: ☐ Nutrition:
☐ General Urologist   ☐ Physical Therapy: ☐ Social Work:

IMPORTANT FOLLOW-UP CARE:

Hot Flashes: number per day   interferes with comfort or functioning
Cognitive Impairment ("chemobrain")
Physical Therapy: *Practice the exercises you have been given by our*   **Contact:** _____
staff to manage the following
☐ Trouble urinating   ☐ Pain when urinating   ☐ Pain in pelvis   ☐ Fatigue

Nutritional Management: *See your nutritionist within 1 month post*
treatment to develop a plan for optimal nutrition and to manage symptoms   **Contact:** _____

Height: Current Weight: Ideal Body Weight: Weight History:
Weight gain or loss:

Follow up with the Nutritionist to address ongoing concerns related to nutrition, weight status and eating including any of the
following symptoms:
☐ Relying on comfort foods   ☐ Changes in taste
☐ Dry/sensitive mouth   ☐ Mouth sores
☐ Changes in taste

Treatment-Related Medications: *Remember to take your medicines as scheduled*

Exams: *Do the appropriate exams as scheduled*
Blood tests: Thyroid function:

Scans:
X-ray: PET/CT: CT: Other:
Self exams:

Integrative Oncology: *Follow up as needed*   Contact: _____

☐ Acupuncture
Breath/relaxation techniques: ☐ Guided imagery   ☐ Progressive relaxation   ☐ Autogenics
Energy therapy: ☐ Reiki   ☐ Therapeutic Touch   ☐ Acupressure

---

Speech and Swallowing: *Practice what you have been taught by our staff*
                                                          Contact: _____

- Follow up with your speech and swallowing therapist after completing treatment
- If you had surgery, get a baseline swallowing test after your surgeon clears you for eating orally
Speech Evaluation: ☐ Yes ☐ No
Results:
Swallowing Evaluation: ☐ Yes ☐ No
Results:
Acceptable diet choices:
☐ Thin Liquids   ☐ Thick liquids   ☐ Purees
☐ Soft Solids   ☐ Unrestricted diet

Dental Care: *See your dentist for routine checkups*   Contact: _____
- Teeth/gums care: thoroughly brush your teeth; floss carefully and avoid gum irritation
- Fluoride regimen: apply fluoride if advised
- Other oral care:

Breathing: *Practice what you have been taught by our staff*
☐

Other:

ADJUSTING TO SURVIVORSHIP

Contact your social worker if you are experiencing distress
in any of the following areas   Contact: _____

☐ Body-image   ☐ Eating/sleeping patterns   ☐ Disinterest in activities that you enjoy
☐ Pervasive concerns and worry ☐ Relationships with your family   ☐ Relationship with partner
                               and friends
☐ Changes in mood   ☐ Sadness   ☐ Fears
☐ Nervousness

WELLNESS

Avoid: **Maintain:**
☐ Nicotine and Tobacco Products   ☐ Healthy nutrition
☐ Alcohol use   ☐ Physical activity
☐ Drug use   ☐ Screening for other cancers
☐ Overexposure to the sun

Screening for other cancers:
☐ Colonoscopy   ☐ Mammogram   ☐ PSA/Digital Rectal exam   ☐ PAP/HPV tests   ☐ Skin exam

ADDITIONAL INFORMATION

Organizations/Programs:	Contact Info:	Website:
Alcoholics Anonymous (AA)	Many local groups exist	http://www.alcoholics-anonymous.org
Narcotics Anonymous (NA)	Many local groups exist	http://www.na.org

Cancer Support Groups:	Contact Info:	Website:
American Cancer Society	1-800-ACS-2345	http://www.cancer.org
CancerCare	1-800-813-HOPE	http://www.cancercare.org
People Living With Cancer		http://www.cancer.net
National Cancer Institute (NCI)	1-800-4-CANCER	http://www.cancer.gov
NCI Office of Cancer Survivorship	1-301-402-2964	http://dccps.nci.nih.gov/ocs
Gilda's Club	1-888-GILDA-4-U	http://www.gildasclubnyc.org
LIVESTRONG	1-866-235-7205	http://www.livestrong.org

PERSONAL HEALTH RECORD
SARCOMA

Last Name: First Name:
DOB: Age: Gender: Date:
Day Phone: Evening Phone:
Address: City: State: Zip:
Email:
My Insurance: Policy #:

Spouse/Relative/Caretaker: Phone:
Health Care Agent: Phone:

MEDICAL INFORMATION

Type of cancer: Date of diagnosis:
Staging   T: N: M:

My Health Care Team   Phone: Email:
Medical Oncologist:
Radiation Oncologist:
Thoracic Surgeon:
Fellow:
Pulmonologist:
Nurse/Nurse Practitioner:
Integrative Oncology Nurse:
Pain/Symptom Management:
Social Worker:
Nutritionist:
Physical Therapist:
Patient Navigator:

Treatments received:
Surgical Procedures:

Chemotherapy: ☐ doxorubicin   (mg)   ☐ dacarbazine   (mg)   ☐ mesna   (mg)
☐ gemcitabine   (mg)   ☐ vinorelbine   (mg)   ☐ irinotecan   (mg) ☐ docetaxel   (mg)
                                                                     ☐ other
Freq: Total Dose:
Radiation Therapy:
Area treated:
☐ External Beam Radiation Therapy   Last Date: Dose:
(EBRT)
☐ Brachytherapy   Last Date: Procedure: Dose:

FOLLOW-UP APPOINTMENTS:

Follow-ups: *Remember to follow up with your providers on a regular schedule*

☐ Surgical: ☐ Radiation Oncology: ☐ Medical Oncology:
☐ Cancer Supportive Services: ☐ Pain/Symptom Management: ☐ Nutrition:
☐ Pulmonologist   ☐ Physical Therapy: ☐ Social Work:

IMPORTANT FOLLOW-UP CARE:

Shortness of Breath   Blood when: number per day:
Taper and avoid nicotine products   Avoid alcoholic beverages
Physical Therapy: *Practice the exercises you have been given by our*   Contact: _____
staff to manage the following
☐ Fatigue/general   ☐ Pain   ☐ Shortness of Breath   ☐
deconditioning

Nutritional Management: *See your nutritionist within 1 month post*
treatment to develop a plan for optimal nutrition and to manage symptoms   Contact: _____

Height: Current Weight: Ideal Body Weight: Weight History:
Weight gain or loss:

Follow up with the Nutritionist to address ongoing concerns related to nutrition, weight status and eating including any of the
following symptoms:
☐ Relying on comfort foods   ☐ Breathing exercise; pulmonary rehabilitation
☐ Dry/sensitive mouth   ☐ Mouth sores
☐ Changes in taste

Treatment-Related Medications: *Remember to take your medicines as scheduled*

Exams: *Do the appropriate exams as scheduled*
Blood tests: Thyroid function:

Scans:
X-ray: PET/CT: CT: Other:
Self exams:

Integrative Oncology: *Follow up as needed*   Contact: _____

☐ Acupuncture
Breath/relaxation techniques: ☐ Guided imagery   ☐ Progressive relaxation   ☐ Autogenics
Energy therapy: ☐ Reiki   ☐ Therapeutic Touch   ☐ Acupressure

---

Speech and Swallowing: *Practice what you have been taught by our staff*   Contact: _____

- Follow up with your speech and swallowing therapist after completing treatment
- If you had surgery, get a baseline swallowing test after your surgeon clears you for eating orally
Speech Evaluation: ☐ Yes ☐ No
Results:
Swallowing Evaluation: ☐ Yes ☐ No
Results:
Acceptable diet choices:
☐ Thin Liquids   ☐ Thick liquids   ☐ Purees
☐ Soft Solids   ☐ Unrestricted diet

Dental Care: *See your dentist for routine checkups*   Contact: _____
   • Teeth/gums care: thoroughly brush your teeth; floss carefully and avoid gum irritation
   • Fluoride regimen: apply fluoride if advised
   • Other oral care:

Breathing: *Practice what you have been taught by our staff*
☐

Other:

ADJUSTING TO SURVIVORSHIP

Contact your social worker if you are experiencing distress
in any of the following areas   Contact: _____

☐ Body-Image   ☐ Eating/sleeping patterns   ☐ Disinterest in activities that you enjoy
                                ☐ Relationships with your family
☐ Pervasive concerns and worry and friends   ☐ Relationship with partner

☐ Changes in mood   ☐ Sadness   ☐ Fears
☐ Nervousness

WELLNESS

Avoid: Maintain:
☐ Nicotine and Tobacco Products   ☐ Healthy nutrition
☐ Alcohol use   ☐ Physical activity
☐ Drug use   ☐ Screening for other cancers
☐ Overexposure to the sun

Screening for other cancers:
☐ Colonoscopy   ☐ Mammogram   ☐ PSA/Digital Rectal exam   ☐ PAP/HPV tests   ☐ Skin exam

---

ADDITIONAL INFORMATION

Organizations/Programs:	Contact Info:	Website:
Alcoholics Anonymous (AA)	Many local groups exist	http://www.alcoholics-anonymous.org
Narcotics Anonymous (NA)	Many local groups exist	http://www.na.org

Cancer Support Groups:	Contact Info:	Website:
American Cancer Society	1-800-ACS-2345	http://www.cancer.org
CancerCare	1-800-813-HOPE	http://www.cancercare.org
People Living With Cancer		http://www.cancer.net
National Cancer Institute (NCI)	1-800-4-CANCER	http://www.cancer.gov
NCI Office of Cancer Survivorship	1-301-402-2964	http://dccps.nci.nih.gov/ocs
Gilda's Club	1-888-GILDA-4-U	http://www.gildasclubnyc.org
LIVESTRONG	1-866-235-7205	http://www.livestrong.org

PERSONAL HEALTH RECORD
TESTICULAR CANCER

Last Name: First Name:
DOB: Age: Gender: Date:
Day Phone: Evening Phone:
Address: City: State: Zip:
Email:
My Insurance: Policy #:

Spouse/Relative/Caretaker: Phone:
Health Care Agent: Phone:

MEDICAL INFORMATION

Type of cancer: Date of diagnosis:
Staging   T: N: M:

My Health Care Team   **Phone:**   **Email:**
Medical Oncologist:
Radiation Oncologist:
Thoracic Surgeon:
Fellow:
Pulmonologist:
Nurse/Nurse Practitioner:
Integrative Oncology Nurse:
Pain/Symptom Management:
Social Worker:
Nutritionist:
Physical Therapist:
Patient Navigator:
Sperm or testicular banking addressed prior to treatment?

Treatments received:
Surgical Procedures:

Chemotherapy: ☐ etoposide   (mg)   ☐ cisplatin   (mg)   ☐ mesna   (mg)
☐ ifosfamide   (mg)   ☐ bleomycin   (mg) ☐   ☐ other
Freq: Total Dose:

Radiation Therapy:
Area treated:
☐ External Beam Radiation Therapy (EBRT)   Last Date: Dose:
☐ Brachytherapy   Last Date: Procedure: Dose:

FOLLOW-UP APPOINTMENTS:

Follow-ups: *Remember to follow up with your providers on a regular schedule*

☐ Surgical: ☐ Radiation Oncology: ☐ Medical Oncology:
☐ Cancer Supportive Services: ☐ Pain/Symptom Management: ☐ Nutrition:

☐ Pulmonologist   ☐ Physical Therapy: ☐ Social Work:

IMPORTANT FOLLOW-UP CARE:

Shortness of Breath   Blood whens: number per day
Taper and avoid nicotine products   Avoid alcoholic beverages
Physical Therapy: *Practice the exercises you have been given by our staff to manage the following*   **Contact:**
☐ Fatigue/general deconditioning   ☐ Pain   ☐ Shortness of Breath   ☐

Nutritional Management: *See your nutritionist within 1 month post treatment to develop a plan for optimal nutrition and to manage symptoms*   **Contact:**

Height: Current Weight: Ideal Body Weight: Weight History:
Weight gain or loss:

Follow up with the Nutritionist to address ongoing concerns related to nutrition, weight status and eating including any of the following symptoms:
☐ Relying on comfort foods   ☐ Breathing exercise; pulmonary rehabilitation
☐ Dry/sensitive mouth   ☐ Mouth sores
☐ Changes in taste

Treatment-Related Medications: *Remember to take your medicines as scheduled*

Exams: *Do the appropriate exams as scheduled*
Blood tests: Thyroid function:

Scans:
X-ray: PET/CT: CT: Other:
Self exams:

Integrative Oncology: *Follow up as needed*   **Contact:** _____

☐ Acupuncture
Breath/relaxation techniques: ☐ Guided imagery   ☐ Progressive relaxation   ☐ Autogenics
Energy therapy: ☐ Reiki   ☐ Therapeutic Touch   ☐ Acupressure

---

Speech and Swallowing: *Practice what you have been taught by our staff*   **Contact:** _____

- Follow up with your speech and swallowing therapist after completing treatment
- If you had surgery, get a baseline swallowing test after your surgeon clears you for eating orally
Speech Evaluation: ☐ Yes ☐ No
Results:
Swallowing Evaluation: ☐ Yes ☐ No
Results:
Acceptable diet choices:
☐ Thin Liquids   ☐ Thick liquids   ☐ Purees
☐ Soft Solids   ☐ Unrestricted diet

Dental Care: *See your dentist for routine checkups*   **Contact:** _____
- Teeth/gums care: thoroughly brush your teeth; floss carefully and avoid gum irritation
- Fluoride regimen: apply fluoride if advised
- Other oral care:

Breathing: *Practice what you have been taught by our staff*
☐

Other:

ADJUSTING TO SURVIVORSHIP

*Contact your social worker if you are experiencing distress
in any of the following areas*   **Contact:** _____

☐ Body-image   ☐ Eating/sleeping patterns   ☐ Disinterest in activities that you enjoy
                        ☐ Relationships with your family
☐ Pervasive concerns and worry and friends   ☐ Relationship with partner
☐ Changes in mood   ☐ Sadness   ☐ Fears
☐ Nervousness

WELLNESS

Avoid: **Maintain:**
☐ Nicotine and Tobacco Products   ☐ Healthy nutrition
☐ Alcohol use   ☐ Physical activity
☐ Drug use   ☐ Screening for other cancers
☐ Overexposure to the sun

Screening for other cancers:
☐ Colonoscopy   ☐ Mammogram   ☐ PSA/Digital Rectal exam   ☐ PAP/HPV tests   ☐ Skin exam

---

ADDITIONAL INFORMATION

Organizations/Programs:	Contact Info:	Website:
Testicular Cancer Awareness Foundation		http://testicularcancerawarenessfoundation.org
Alcoholics Anonymous (AA)	Many local groups exist	http://www.acoholics-anonymous.org
Narcotics Anonymous (NA)	Many local groups exist	http://www.na.org

Cancer Support Groups:	Contact Info:	Website:
American Cancer Society	1-800-ACS-2345	http://www.cancer.org
CancerCare	1-800-813-HOPE	http://www.cancercare.org
People Living With Cancer		http://www.cancer.net
National Cancer Institute (NCI)	1-800-4-CANCER	http://www.cancer.gov
NCI Office of Cancer Survivorship	1-301-402-2964	http://dccps.nci.nih.gov/ocs
Gilda's Club	1-888-GILDA-4-U	http://www.gildasclubnyc.org
LIVESTRONG	1-866-235-7205	http://www.livestrong.org

PERSONAL HEALTH RECORD
THYMOMA

Last Name: First Name:
DOB: Age: Gender: Date:
Day Phone: Evening Phone:
Address: City: State: Zip:
Email:
My Insurance: Policy #:

Spouse/Relative/Caretaker: Phone:
Health Care Agent: Phone:

MEDICAL INFORMATION

Type of cancer: Date of diagnosis:
Staging   Masaoka Stage:

My Health Care Team   **Phone:**   **Email:**
Medical Oncologist:
Radiation Oncologist:
Thoracic Surgeon:
Fellow:
Pulmonologist:
Nurse/Nurse Practitioner:
Integrative Oncology Nurse:
Pain/Symptom Management:
Social Worker:
Nutritionist:
Physical Therapist:
Patient Navigator:

Treatments received:
Surgical Procedures:

Chemotherapy: ☐ doxorubicin   (mg) ☐ cisplatin   (mg) ☐ cyclophosphamide   (mg)
☐ etoposide   (mg)   ☐ ifosfamide   (mg) ☐ paclitaxel   (mg)
☐ other   Freq: Total Dose:

Radiation Therapy:
Area treated:
☐ External Beam Radiation Therapy
(EBRT)   Last Date: Dose:
☐ Intraopeartive Radiation Therapy   Last Date: Procedure: Dose:

FOLLOW-UP APPOINTMENTS:
Follow-ups: *Remember to follow up with your providers on a regular schedule*

☐ Surgical: ☐ Radiation Oncology: ☐ Medical Oncology:
☐ Cancer Supportive Services:
                           ☐ Pain/Symptom Management: ☐ Nutrition:
☐ Pulmonologist   ☐ Physical Therapy: ☐ Social Work:

IMPORTANT FOLLOW-UP CARE:
Shortness of Breath   Alpha-feto protein (AFP):   beta HCG
Taper and avoid nicotine products   Avoid alcoholic beverages
Physical Therapy: *Practice the exercises you have been given by our
staff to manage the following*   **Contact:** _____
☐ Fatigue/general deconditioning   ☐ Pain   ☐ Shortness of Breath   ☐

Nutritional Management: *See your nutritionist within 1 month post
treatment to develop a plan for optimal nutrition and to manage symptoms*   **Contact:** _____

Height: Current Weight: Ideal Body Weight: Weight History:
Weight gain or loss:

*Follow up with the Nutritionist to address ongoing concerns related to nutrition, weight status and eating including any of the
following symptoms:*
☐ Relying on comfort foods   ☐ Breathing exercise; pulmonary rehabilitation
☐ Dry/sensitive mouth   ☐ Mouth sores
☐ Changes in taste

Treatment-Related Medications: *Remember to take your medicines as scheduled*

Exams: *Do the appropriate exams as scheduled*
Blood tests: Thyroid function:

Scans:
X-ray: PET/CT: CT: Other:
Self exams:

Integrative Oncology: *Follow up as needed*   **Contact:** _____

☐ Acupuncture
Breath/relaxation techniques: ☐ Guided imagery   ☐ Progressive relaxation   ☐ Autogenics
Energy therapy: ☐ Reiki   ☐ Therapeutic Touch   ☐ Acupressure

Speech and Swallowing: *Practice what you have been taught by our staff*
                                                        Contact: _____

- *Follow up with your speech and swallowing therapist after completing treatment*
- *If you had surgery, get a baseline swallowing test after your surgeon clears you for eating orally*
Speech Evaluation: ☐ Yes ☐ No
Results:
Swallowing Evaluation: ☐ Yes ☐ No
Results:
Acceptable diet choices:
☐ Thin Liquids   ☐ Thick liquids   ☐ Purees
☐ Soft Solids   ☐ Unrestricted diet

Dental Care: *See your dentist for routine checkups*   **Contact:** _____
  - Teeth/gums care: thoroughly brush your teeth; floss carefully and avoid gum irritation
  - Fluoride regimen: apply fluoride if advised
  - Other oral care:

Breathing: *Practice what you have been taught by the staff*
☐

Other:

ADJUSTING TO SURVIVORSHIP

*Contact your social worker if you are experiencing distress
in any of the following areas*   **Contact:** _____

☐ Body-image   ☐ Eating/sleeping patterns   ☐ Disinterest in activities that you enjoy
                                ☐ Relationships with your family
☐ Pervasive concerns and worry   and friends   ☐ Relationship with spouse/partner
☐ Changes in mood   ☐ Sadness   ☐ Fears
☐ Nervousness

WELLNESS

Avoid: **Maintain:**
☐ Nicotine and Tobacco Products   ☐ Healthy nutrition
☐ Alcohol use   ☐ Physical activity
☐ Drug use   ☐ Screening for other cancers
☐ Overexposure to the sun

Screening for other cancers:
☐ Colonoscopy   ☐ Mammogram   ☐ PSA/Digital Rectal exam   ☐ PAP/HPV tests   ☐ Skin exam

ADDITIONAL INFORMATION

Organizations/Programs:	Contact Info:	Website:
Alcoholics Anonymous (AA)	Many local groups exist	http://www.alcoholics-anonymous.org
Narcotics Anonymous (NA)	Many local groups exist	http://www.na.org

Cancer Support Groups:	Contact Info:	Website:
American Cancer Society	1-800-ACS-2345	http://www.cancer.org
CancerCare	1-800-813-HOPE	http://www.cancercare.org
People Living With Cancer		http://www.cancer.net
National Cancer Institute (NCI)	1-800-4-CANCER	http://www.cancer.gov
NCI Office of Cancer Survivorship	1-301-402-2964	http://dccps.nci.nih.gov/ocs
Gilda's Club	1-888-GILDA-4-U	http://www.gildasclubnyc.org
LIVESTRONG	1-866-235-7205	http://www.livestrong.org

ENTERAL NUTRITION (TUBE FEEDING)

WHAT IS ENTERAL NUTRITION?

Enteral nutrition is using a feeding tube to help you get enough nutrition when you cannot eat well or are unable to eat. The feeding tube is placed very carefully into your stomach. It is called a *PEG* (percutaneous endoscopic gastrostomy). Sometimes, the doctors will place the tube in the area just past your stomach, called the jejunum. This is called a *PEJ* (percutaneous endoscopic jejunostomy). The doctor or nurse will show you how they put the tube in.

HOW DO I GET FOOD THROUGH A TUBE?

Once the tube is in the right place, liquid food is put down the tube. The food is like a shake and contains vitamins, minerals, and other nutrients your body needs. The food usually comes in cans, and the nutritionist will discuss how many to use per day to maintain good nutrition.

THESE ARE DIFFERENT WAYS TO USE THE PEG

Bolus Administration

The easiest way to give a feeding is called a bolus, which is all at once and is like eating a meal. Each can of feeding may take up to 15–30 minutes to go down the tube using a *syringe* or *gravity bag*. This kind of feeding is given four to six times a day, depending on how many cans you need. Specific instructions are given on the following pages.

Continuous Drip

This is when the feeding goes into the PEG tube for the entire day and/or night at a slow rate. A small, easy-to-use pump makes sure the right amount of food goes through the tube.

WHAT DO I NEED TO DO?

It's very important to keep the tube in the right place, so try to avoid pulling it or moving it by accident. You will need to give yourself regular feedings and water to *maintain your weight* and *get enough nutrition for energy and healing*.

Your nurse will show you how to take care of your tube and what to watch out for. Your supplies will be delivered to your home a few days after the PEG is placed.

Please make sure you ask any questions you have!

YOU AND YOUR FEEDING TUBE:
A READY REFERENCE GUIDE

TUBE TYPE: _____

APPEARANCE AND SITE CARE (DAILY)

Cleanse where tube exits skin and under the bumper with warm soap and water. Pat dry.

The site will usually have a dressing for the first 48 hours. Thin gauze pads may be used under the bumper after this.

Tube may become cloudy in appearance or develop black discoloration, which does *not* indicate a need for change of tube.

Scar tissue can develop around the tube, which is red and may bleed slightly if moved.

Secure the tube into the waistline of your pants or with a Spandage® to minimize its movement.

TUBE FEEDINGS

Formula: _____
Method: ❑ Syringe (Bolus) ❑ Gravity Bag (Bolus) ❑ Bag with Pump
　　　　　(Continuous)
Amount & Frequency: _____

Medications

Some medications *cannot be crushed*—ask your health care team about your medication if you are unable to swallow pills. If you need to put your medication through the tube, be sure the pills are finely crushed and dissolved with warm water before you start. Always let a syringe full of water flow through the tube before and after the medication is given. *Do not push fluid through... let it flow in.*

THINGS TO WATCH FOR

Call the health care team right away if you have...

- A blocked tube or if tube slips out
- Worsening/increasing pain at PEG tube site for more than one week after placement
- Signs/symptoms of infection—excessive redness, swelling, unusual drainage, or foul smell
- Fever of 100.5 degrees or higher
- Leakage or excessive bleeding around tube (spots of blood on gauze pad is *not* a concern)
- Vomiting, diarrhea, dehydration, constipation, excess fullness, or tasting feeds in your mouth

PHONE NUMBERS

Please call if you have concerns or questions.

PHYSICIAN: _____
Phone #: _____

PHYSICIAN: _____
Phone #: _____

NURSE: _____
Phone #: _____

DIETITIAN: _____
Phone #: _____

SOCIAL WORKER: _____
Phone #: _____

VENDOR: _____
Phone #: _____

HOW TO GIVE YOURSELF A TUBE FEEDING: BEFORE STARTING THE FEEDING

Gather supplies: Formula can(s), feeding bag and/or syringe, and 1 cup (8 oz.) of water.

Wash hands with soap and water before setting up the feeding.

Rinse top of the can and shake well before opening. Cans should be *room temperature.*

Sit up in a chair or raise the head of bed (do not feed while lying down).

Attach syringe to your feeding tube and let 1/2 cup (4 oz.) lukewarm water flow in.

FEEDING PROCEDURE

If using a syringe:

Open the can.

Remove the plunger from the syringe, pinch the PEG closed with thumb and finger to avoid leaks and attach the syringe to the feeding tube securely.

Hold the syringe in one hand and pour the can contents into the syringe with the other, slowly filling the syringe but not to the very top. Let the liquid flow in on its own—*do not* use the plunger to push it through.

NOTE: To control the flow of feeding:

—Lowering the syringe will slow the rate of feeding.

—Raising the syringe will speed up the rate of feeding.

It takes about 15–30 minutes for one can to flow in by gravity, depending on the rate of feeding. If any discomfort occurs, discuss with your health care team.

After the feeding, use the syringe to flush your PEG tube again with 1/2 cup warm water, or more if instructed to do so.

Pinch the PEG closed, detach the syringe, and close the port on the PEG tube.

Avoid lying down for an hour after feeding to prevent heartburn or backflow.

Rinse and dry the syringe after each feeding.

If using a gravity bag:

The bag should be hung on the IV pole at least 18 inches above the level of your stomach.

Close the clamp on the feeding bag.

Open the can and pour contents into the bag.

Open the clamp on the feeding tube bag to let the liquid fill the tubing completely, then close the clamp (do this over the sink or garbage pail).

Pinch the PEG closed, open the port and attach the bag tubing securely to it.

Open the clamp to start the feeding.

NOTE: To control the flow of the feeding, roll the clamp up to go faster and down to go slower.

It takes about 20–30 minutes for one can of feeding to be absorbed, depending on the rate of feeding. If any discomfort occurs, discuss with your health care team.

After the feeding is complete, close the clamp on the feeding bag and pinch the PEG tube before removing the bag to prevent a leak.

Use the syringe to flush your PEG tube again with 1/2 cup (4oz.) warm water (or more as instructed).

Detach the syringe and close the port on the PEG tube.

Avoid lying down for an hour after feeding to prevent heartburn or backflow.

After each feeding, rinse the feeding bag and tubing with warm water until the water runs clear. Dry with a paper towel and store in a clean place until the next feeding.

FIVE WISHES

*T*here are many things in life that are out of our hands. This Five Wishes document gives you a way to control something very important—how you are treated if you get seriously ill. It is an easy-to-complete form that lets you say exactly what you want. Once it is filled out and properly signed it is valid under the laws of most states.

What Is Five Wishes?

Five Wishes is the first living will that talks about your personal, emotional and spiritual needs as well as your medical wishes. It lets you choose the person you want to make health care decisions for you if you are not able to make them for yourself. Five Wishes lets you say exactly how you wish to be treated if you get seriously ill. It was written with the help of The American Bar Association's Commission on Law and Aging, and the nation's leading experts in end-of-life care. It's also easy to use. All you have to do is check a box, circle a direction, or write a few sentences.

How Five Wishes Can Help You And Your Family

- It lets you talk with your family, friends and doctor about how you want to be treated if you become seriously ill.

- Your family members will not have to guess what you want. It protects them if you become seriously ill, because they won't have to make hard choices without knowing your wishes.

- You can know what your mom, dad, spouse, or friend wants. You can be there for them when they need you most. You will understand what they really want.

How Five Wishes Began

For 12 years, Jim Towey worked closely with Mother Teresa, and, for one year, he lived in a hospice she ran in Washington, DC. Inspired by this first-hand experience, Mr. Towey sought a way for patients and their families to plan ahead and to cope with serious illness. The result is Five Wishes and the response to it has been overwhelming. It has been featured on CNN and NBC's Today Show and in the pages of *Time* and *Money* magazines. Newspapers have called Five Wishes the first "living will with a heart and soul." Today, Five Wishes is available in 23 languages

Who Should Use Five Wishes

Five Wishes is for anyone 18 or older — married, single, parents, adult children, and friends. Over 13 million Americans of all ages have already used it. Because it

works so well, lawyers, doctors, hospitals and hospices, faith communities, employer and retiree groups are handing out this document.

Five Wishes States

If you live in the **District of Columbia** or one of the **42 states** listed below, you can use Five Wishes and have the peace of mind to know that it substantially meets your state's requirements under the law:

Alaska	Illinois	Montana	South Carolina
Arizona	Iowa	Nebraska	South Dakota
Arkansas	Kentucky	Nevada	Tennessee
California	Louisiana	New Jersey	Vermont
Colorado	Maine	New Mexico	Virginia
Connecticut	Maryland	New York	Washington
Delaware	Massachusetts	North Carolina	West Virginia
Florida	Michigan	North Dakota	Wisconsin
Georgia	Minnesota	Oklahoma	Wyoming
Hawaii	Mississippi	Pennsylvania	
Idaho	Missouri	Rhode Island	

If your state is not one of the 42 states listed here, Five Wishes does not meet the technical requirements in the statutes of your state. So some doctors in your state may be reluctant to honor Five Wishes. However, many people from states not on this list do complete Five Wishes along with their state's legal form. They find that Five Wishes helps them express all that they want and provides a helpful guide to family members, friends, care givers and doctors. Most doctors and health care professionals know they need to listen to your wishes no matter how you express them.

How Do I Change To Five Wishes?

You may already have a living will or a durable power of attorney for health care. If you want to use Five Wishes instead, all you need to do is fill out and sign a new Five Wishes as directed. As soon as you sign it, it takes away any advance directive you had before. To make sure the right form is used, please do the following:

- Destroy all copies of your old living will or durable power of attorney for health care. Or you can write "revoked" in large letters across the copy you have. Tell your lawyer if he or she helped prepare those old forms for you. *AND*

- Tell your Health Care Agent, family members, and doctor that you have filled out a new Five Wishes. Make sure they know about your new wishes.

WISH 1

The Person I Want To Make Health Care Decisions For Me
When I Can't Make Them For Myself.

If I am no longer able to make my own health care decisions, this form names the person I choose to make these choices for me. This person will be my Health Care Agent (or other term that may be used in my state, such as proxy, representative, or surrogate). This person will make my health care choices if both of these things happen:

- *My attending or treating doctor finds I am no longer able to make health care choices, AND*
- *Another health care professional agrees that this is true.*

If my state has a different way of finding that I am not able to make health care choices, then my state's way should be followed.

The Person I Choose As My Health Care Agent Is:

First Choice Name

Phone

Address

City/State/Zip

If this person is not able or willing to make these choices for me, *OR* is divorced or legally separated from me, *OR* this person has died, then these people are my next choices:

Second Choice Name

Third Choice Name

Address

Address

City/State/Zip

City/State/Zip

Phone

Phone

Picking The Right Person To Be Your Health Care Agent

Choose someone who knows you very well, cares about you, and who can make difficult decisions. A spouse or family member may not be the best choice because they are too emotionally involved. Sometimes they **are** the best choice. You know best. Choose someone who is able to stand up for you so that your wishes are followed. Also, choose someone who is likely to be nearby so that they can help when you need them. Whether you choose a spouse, family member, or friend as your Health Care Agent, make sure you talk about these wishes and be sure that this person agrees to respect and follow your wishes. Your Health Care Agent should be **at least 18 years or older** (in Colorado, 21 years or older) and should **not** be:

- Your health care provider, including the owner or operator of a health or residential or community care facility serving you.

- An employee or spouse of an employee of your health care provider.

- Serving as an agent or proxy for 10 or more people unless he or she is your spouse or close relative.

I understand that my Health Care Agent can make health care decisions for me. I want my Agent to be able to do the following: **(Please cross out anything you don't want your Agent to do that is listed below.)**

- Make choices for me about my medical care or services, like tests, medicine, or surgery. This care or service could be to find out what my health problem is, or how to treat it. It can also include care to keep me alive. If the treatment or care has already started, my Health Care Agent can keep it going or have it stopped.

- Interpret any instructions I have given in this form or given in other discussions, according to my Health Care Agent's understanding of my wishes and values.

- Consent to admission to an assisted living facility, hospital, hospice, or nursing home for me. My Health Care Agent can hire any kind of health care worker I may need to help me or take care of me. My Agent may also fire a health care worker, if needed.

- Make the decision to request, take away or not give medical treatments, including artificially-provided food and water, and any other treatments to keep me alive.

- See and approve release of my medical records and personal files. If I need to sign my name to get any of these files, my Health Care Agent can sign it for me.

- Move me to another state to get the care I need or to carry out my wishes.

- Authorize or refuse to authorize any medication or procedure needed to help with pain.

- Take any legal action needed to carry out my wishes.

- Donate useable organs or tissues of mine as allowed by law.

- Apply for Medicare, Medicaid, or other programs or insurance benefits for me. My Health Care Agent can see my personal files, like bank records, to find out what is needed to fill out these forms.

- Listed below are any changes, additions, or limitations on my Health Care Agent's powers.

_____
_____
_____
_____
_____
_____

If I Change My Mind About Having A Health Care Agent, I Will

- Destroy all copies of this part of the Five Wishes form. *OR*

- Tell someone, such as my doctor or family, that I want to cancel or change my Health Care Agent. *OR*

- Write the word "Revoked" in large letters across the name of each agent whose authority I want to cancel. Sign my name on that page.

WISH 2
My Wish For The Kind Of Medical Treatment
I Want Or Don't Want.

I believe that my life is precious and I deserve to be treated with dignity. When the time comes that I am very sick and am not able to speak for myself, I want the following wishes, and any other directions I have given to my Health Care Agent, to be respected and followed.

What You Should Keep In Mind As My Caregiver

• I do not want to be in pain. I want my doctor to give me enough medicine to relieve my pain, even if that means that I will be drowsy or sleep more than I would otherwise.

• I do not want **anything** done or omitted by my doctors **or nurses with the** intention of taking my life.

• I want to be offered food and fluids by mouth, and kept clean and warm.

What "Life-Support Treatment" Means To Me

Life-support treatment means any medical procedure, device or medication to keep me alive. Life-support treatment includes: medical devices put in me to help me breathe; food and water supplied by medical device (tube feeding); cardiopulmonary resuscitation (CPR); major surgery; blood transfusions; dialysis; antibiotics; and anything else meant to keep me alive. If I wish to limit the meaning of life-support treatment because of my religious or personal beliefs, I write this limitation in the space below. I do this to make very clear what I want and under what conditions.

_____

_____

_____

_____

_____

In Case Of An Emergency

If you have a medical emergency and ambulance personnel arrive, they may look to see if you have a **Do Not Resuscitate** form or bracelet. Many states require a person to have a **Do Not Resuscitate** form filled out and signed by a doctor. This form lets ambulance personnel know that you don't want them to use life-support treatment when you are dying. Please check with your doctor to see if you need to have a **Do Not Resuscitate** form filled out.

Copyright (c) Aging with Dignity, www.agingwithdignity.org,
P.O. Box 1661, Tallahassee, FL 32301. (888) 5-WISHES.

Here is the kind of medical treatment that I want or don't want in the four situations listed below. I want my Health Care Agent, my family, my doctors and other health care providers, my friends and all others to know these directions.

Close to death:

If my doctor and another health care professional both decide that I am likely to die within a short period of time, and life-support treatment would only delay the moment of my death (Choose *one* of the following):

❏   I want to have life-support treatment.

❏   I do not want life-support treatment. If it has been started, I want it stopped.

❏   I want to have life-support treatment if my doctor believes it could help. But I want my doctor to stop giving me life-support treatment if it is not helping my health condition or symptoms.

In A Coma And Not Expected To Wake Up Or Recover:

If my doctor and another health care professional both decide that I am in a coma from which I am not expected to wake up or recover, and I have brain damage, and life-support treatment would only delay the moment of my death (Choose *one* of the following):

❏   I want to have life-support treatment.

❏   I do not want life-support treatment. If it has been started, I want it stopped.

❏   I want to have life-support treatment if my doctor believes it could help. But I want my doctor to stop giving me life-support treatment if it is not helping my health condition or symptoms.

Permanent And Severe Brain Damage And Not Expected To Recover:

If my doctor and another health care professional both decide that I have permanent and severe brain damage, (for example, I can open my eyes, but I can not speak or understand) and I am not expected to get better, and life-support treatment would only delay the moment of my death (Choose *one* of the following):

❏   I want to have life-support treatment.

❏   I do not want life-support treatment. If it has been started, I want it stopped.

❏   I want to have life-support treatment if my doctor believes it could help. But I want my doctor to stop giving me life-support treatment if it is not helping my health condition or symptoms.

In Another Condition Under Which I Do Not Wish To Be Kept Alive:

If there is another condition under which I do not wish to have life-support treatment, I describe it below. In this condition, I believe that the costs and burdens of life-support treatment are too much and not worth the benefits to me. Therefore, in this condition, I do not want life-support treatment. (For example, you may write "end-stage condition." That means that your health has gotten worse. You are not able to take care of yourself in any way, mentally or physically. Life-support treatment will not help you recover. Please leave the space blank if you have no other condition to describe.)

_____

_____

_____

_____

_____

*T*he next three wishes deal with my personal, spiritual and emotional wishes. They are important to me. I want to be treated with dignity near the end of my life, so I would like people to do the things written in Wishes 3, 4, and 5 when they can be done. I understand that my family, my doctors and other health care providers, my friends, and others may not be able to do these things or are not required by law to do these things. I do not expect the following wishes to place new or added legal duties on my doctors or other health care providers. I also do not expect these wishes to excuse my doctor or other health care providers from giving me the proper care asked for by law.

WISH 3
My Wish For How Comfortable I Want To Be.
(Please cross out anything that you don't agree with.)

- I do not want to be in pain. I want my doctor to give me enough medicine to relieve my pain, even if that means I will be drowsy or sleep more than I would otherwise.

- If I show signs of depression, nausea, shortness of breath, or hallucinations, I want my care givers to do whatever they can to help me.

- I wish to have a cool moist cloth put on my head if I have a fever.

- I want my lips and mouth kept moist to stop dryness.

- I wish to have warm baths often. I wish to be kept fresh and clean at all times.

- I wish to be massaged with warm oils as often as I can be.

- I wish to have my favorite music played when possible until my time of death.

- I wish to have personal care like shaving, nail clipping, hair brushing, and teeth brushing, as long as they do not cause me pain or discomfort.

- I wish to have religious readings and well-loved poems read aloud when I am near death.

- I wish to know about options for hospice care to provide medical, emotional and spiritual care for me and my loved ones.

WISH 4
My Wish For How I Want People To Treat Me.
(Please cross out anything that you don't agree with.)

- I wish to have people with me when possible. I want someone to be with me when it seems that death may come at any time.

- I wish to have my hand held and to be talked to when possible, even if I don't seem to respond to the voice or touch of others.

- I wish to have others by my side praying for me when possible.

- I wish to have the members of my faith community told that I am sick and asked to pray for me and visit me.

- I wish to be cared for with kindness and cheerfulness, and not sadness.

- I wish to have pictures of my loved ones in my room, near my bed.

- If I am not able to control my bowel or bladder functions, I wish for my clothes and bed linens to be kept clean, and for them to be changed as soon as they can be if they have been soiled.

- I want to die in my home, if that can be done.

WISH 5
My Wish For What I Want My Loved Ones To Know.
(Please cross out anything that you don't agree with.)

- I wish to have my family and friends know that I love them.

- I wish to be forgiven for the times I have hurt my family, friends, and others.

- I wish to have my family, friends and others know that I forgive them for when they may have hurt me in my life.

- I wish for my family and friends to know that I do not fear death itself. I think it is not the end, but a new beginning for me.

- I wish for all of my family members to make peace with each other before my death, if they can.

- I wish for my family and friends to think about what I was like before I became seriously ill. I want them to remember me in this way after my death.

- I wish for my family and friends and caregivers to respect my wishes even if they don't agree with them.

- I wish for my family and friends to look at my dying as a time of personal growth for everyone, including me. This will help me live a meaningful life in my final days.

- I wish for my family and friends to get counseling if they have trouble with my death. I want memories of my life to give them joy and not sorrow.

- After my death, I would like my body to be (circle one): buried   or   cremated.

- My body or remains should be put in the following location_____.

- The following person knows my funeral wishes: _____.

If anyone asks how I want to be remembered, please say the following about me:

_____
_____
_____

If there is to be a memorial service for me, I wish for this service to include the following
(list music, songs, readings or other specific requests that you have):

_____
_____
_____

(Please use the space below for any other wishes. For example, you may want to donate any or all parts of your body when you die. You may also wish to designate a charity to receive memorial contributions. Please attach a separate sheet of paper if you need more space.)

_____
_____
_____

Signing The Five Wishes Form

Please make sure you sign your Five Wishes form in the presence of the two witnesses.

I, _____, ask that my family, my doctors, and other health care providers, my friends, and all others, follow my wishes as communicated by my Health Care Agent (if I have one and he or she is available), or as otherwise expressed in this form. This form becomes valid when I am unable to make decisions or speak for myself. If any part of this form cannot be legally followed, I ask that all other parts of this form be followed. I also revoke any health care advance directives I have made before.

Signature:_____

Address:_____

Phone:_____ Date:_____

Witness Statement · (2 witnesses needed):

I, the witness, declare that the person who signed or acknowledged this form (hereafter "person") is personally known to me, that he/she signed or acknowledged this [Health Care Agent and/or Living Will form(s)] in my presence, and that he/she appears to be of sound mind and under no duress, fraud, or undue influence.

I also declare that I am over 18 years of age and am NOT:

- The individual appointed as (agent/proxy/surrogate/patient advocate/representative) by this document or his/her successor,
- The person's health care provider, including owner or operator of a health, long-term care, or other residential or community care facility serving the person,
- An employee of the person's health care provider,
- Financially responsible for the person's health care,
- An employee of a life or health insurance provider for the person,
- Related to the person by blood, marriage, or adoption, and,
- To the best of my knowledge, a creditor of the person or entitled to any part of his/her estate under a will or codicil, by operation of law.

(Some states may have fewer rules about who may be a witness. Unless you know your state's rules, please follow the above.)

Signature of Witness #1	Signature of Witness #2
Printed Name of Witness	Printed Name of Witness
Address	Address
Phone	Phone

Notarization · Only required for residents of Missouri, North Carolina, South Carolina and West Virginia

- If you live in Missouri, only your signature should be notarized.
- If you live in North Carolina, South Carolina or West Virginia, you should have your signature, and the signatures of your witnesses, notarized.

STATE OF_____   COUNTY OF_____

On this _____ day of _____, 20_____, the said _____,
_____, and _____, known to me (or satisfactorily proven) to be the person named in the
.oing instrument and witnesses, respectively, personally appeared before me, a Notary Public, within and for the State and County aforesaid, and acknowledged that they freely and voluntarily executed the same for the purposes stated therein.

My Commission Expires: _____

10   Notary Public

What To Do After You Complete Five Wishes

- Make sure you sign and witness the form just the way it says in the directions. Then your Five Wishes will be legal and valid.

- Talk about your wishes with your health care agent, family members and others who care about you. Give them copies of your completed Five Wishes.

- Keep the original copy you signed in a special place in your home. Do NOT put it in a safe deposit box. Keep it nearby so that someone can find it when you need it.

- Fill out the wallet card below. Carry it with you. That way people will know where you keep your Five Wishes.

- Talk to your doctor during your next office visit. Give your doctor a copy of your Five Wishes. Make sure it is put in your medical record. Be sure your doctor understands your wishes and is willing to follow them. Ask him or her to tell other doctors who treat you to honor them.

- If you are admitted to a hospital or nursing home, take a copy of your Five Wishes with you. Ask that it be put in your medical record.

- I have given the following people copies of my completed Five Wishes:

  _____
  _____
  _____

Residents of WISCONSIN must attach the WISCONSIN notice statement to Five Wishes.
More information and the notice statement are available at www.agingwithdignity.org or 1-888-594-7437.

Residents of Institutions In CALIFORNIA, CONNECTICUT, DELAWARE, GEORGIA, NEW YORK, NORTH DAKOTA, SOUTH CAROLINA, and VERMONT Must Follow Special Witnessing Rules.

If you live in certain institutions (a nursing home, other licensed long term care facility, a home for the mentally retarded or developmentally disabled, or a mental health institution) in one of the states listed above, you may have to follow special "witnessing requirements" for your Five Wishes to be valid. For further information, please contact a social worker or patient advocate at your institution.

Five Wishes is meant to help you plan for the future. It is not meant to give you legal advice. It does not try to answer all questions about anything that could come up. Every person is different, and every situation is different. Laws change from time to time. If you have a specific question or problem, talk to a medical or legal professional for advice.

Five Wishes Wallet Card

Important Notice to Medical Personnel:
I have a Five Wishes Advance Directive.

Signature

Please consult this document and/or my Health Care Agent in an emergency. My Agent is:

Name
Address   City/State/Zip
Phone

My primary care physician is:

Name
Address   City/State/Zip
Phone

My document is located at:

Cut Out Card, Fold and Laminate for Safekeeping

Here's What People Are Saying About Five Wishes:

"It will be a year since my mother passed on. We knew what she wanted because she had the Five Wishes living will. When it came down to the end, my brother and I had no questions on what we needed to do. We had peace of mind."

Cheryl K.
Longwood, Florida

"I must say I love your Five Wishes. It's clear, easy to understand, and doesn't dwell on the concrete issues of medical care, but on the issues of real importance—human care. I used it for myself and my husband."

Susan W.
Flagstaff, Arizona

"I don't want my children to have to make the decisions I am having to make for my mother. I never knew that there were so many medical options to be considered. Thank you for such a sensitive and caring form. I can simply fill it out and have it on file for my children."

Diana W.
Hanover, Illinois

To Order:

Call (888) 5-WISHES to purchase more copies of Five Wishes, the Five Wishes DVD, or Next Steps guides. Ask about the "Family Package" that includes 10 Five Wishes, 2 Next Steps guides and 1 DVD at a savings of more than 50%. For more information visit Aging with Dignity's website, or call for details.

(888) 5-WISHES or (888) 594-7437
www.agingwithdignity.org

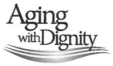

P.O. Box 1661
Tallahassee, Florida 32302-1661

Journal Page: Charting My Course

Journal Page: Charting My Course

Journal Page: My Bucket List

With no distractions or interruptions, think about things that you have always wanted to do but have not yet done and list them here:

Journal Page: My Bucket List

With no distractions or interruptions, think about things that you have always wanted to do but have not yet done and list them here:

Journal Page: My Bucket List

With no distractions or interruptions, think about things that you have always wanted to do but have not yet done and list them here:

Journal Page: My Bucket List

With no distractions or interruptions, think about things that you have always wanted to do but have not yet done and list them here:

MY PERSONAL AFFAIRS

- ❑ Last will and testament
- ❑ Health care proxy, living will, or other advance medical directive acceptable in your state
- ❑ Power of attorney
- ❑ List of bank accounts, pensions, life insurance policies (with review of the beneficiaries or "in trust for..." designations)
- ❑ Special accommodations for dependent children or elderly
- ❑ Thoughts about memorial services, burial or cremation, including list of invitees
- ❑ Wording of obituary
- ❑ Letters, audio or video recordings you would like to leave for loved ones on upcoming milestones in their lives: school graduations, marriages, births, or other such momentous personal occasions
- ❑ "How I want you to remember me" thoughts. Written or recorded. This is something almost always neglected because the people who love you the most are afraid to bring it up to avoid scaring you that you are closer to death than you would believe (another conspiracy of silence thing)
- ❑ "What I know that you may not": genealogy, family history, stories, Grandma's cookie recipes; whatever is significant in your family's life
- ❑ "Permission slips": Regarding very personal and deep family issues: permission to move from the family house when the time is right; permission for a spouse to date or remarry (grist for many a made-for-television movie), permission to go back to school to finish a degree. There are many variations on this theme.
- ❑ Thank you's

ABSTRACTS

EARLY PALLIATIVE CARE FOR PATIENTS WITH METASTATIC NON–SMALL-CELL LUNG CANCER

Jennifer S. Temel, M.D., Joseph A. Greer, Ph.D., Alona Muzikansky, M.A., Emily R. Gallagher, R.N., Sonal Admane, M.B., B.S., M.P.H., Vicki A. Jackson, M.D., M.P.H., Constance M. Dahlin, A.P.N., Craig D. Blinderman, M.D., Juliet Jacobsen, M.D., William F. Pirl, M.D., M.P.H., J. Andrew Billings, M.D., and Thomas J. Lynch, M.D.

N Engl J Med 2010;363:733–42.

Background

Patients with metastatic non–small-cell lung cancer have a substantial symptom burden and may receive aggressive care at the end of life. We examined the effect of introducing palliative care early after diagnosis on patient-reported outcomes and end-of-life care among ambulatory patients with newly diagnosed disease.

Methods

We randomly assigned patients with newly diagnosed metastatic non–small-cell lung cancer to receive either early palliative care integrated with standard oncologic care or standard oncologic care alone. Quality of life and mood were assessed at baseline and at 12 weeks with the use of the Functional Assessment of Cancer Therapy–Lung (FACT-L) scale and the Hospital Anxiety and Depression Scale, respectively.

The primary outcome was the change in the quality of life at 12 weeks. Data on end-of-life care were collected from electronic medical records.

Results

Of the 151 patients who underwent randomization, 27 died by 12 weeks and 107 (86% of the remaining patients) completed assessments. Patients assigned to early palliative care had a better quality of life than did patients assigned to standard care (mean score on the FACT-L scale [in which scores range from 0 to 136, with higher scores indicating better quality of life], 98.0 vs. 91.5; P = 0.03). In addition, fewer patients in the palliative care group than in the standard care group had depressive symptoms (16% vs. 38%, P = 0.01). Despite the fact that fewer patients in the early palliative care group than in the standard care group received aggressive end-of-life care (33% vs. 54%, P = 0.05), median survival was longer among patients receiving early palliative care (11.6 months vs. 8.9 months, P = 0.02).

Conclusions

Among patients with metastatic non–small-cell lung cancer, early palliative care led to significant improvements in both quality of life and mood. As compared with patients receiving standard care, patients receiving early palliative care had less aggressive care at the end of life but longer survival.

Continued

INTEGRATING SUPPORTIVE AND PALLIATIVE CARE IN THE TRAJECTORY OF CANCER: ESTABLISHING GOALS AND MODELS OF CARE

Eduardo Bruera and David Hui

J. Clinical Oncology 28 (25):4013–17 Sept. 1, 2010

Patients with advanced cancer frequently experience significant symptom burden and psychosocial distress. Palliative care has evolved as a discipline that addresses many of these concerns. Yet, palliative care referrals remain delayed as patients continue to focus on cancer treatments. Using a car analogy, we propose that the two seemingly opposing goals of care—receipt of cancer therapies and symptom management—can be addressed concurrently under an integrated care model. To ensure high quality and early access to supportive/palliative care services, oncologists need to be comfortable with the core competencies related to symptom management, psychosocial interventions, communication, and transition of care. For patients with severe distress, early referral to the interdisciplinary supportive/palliative care team is recommended. Through better integration and education, oncologists and supportive/palliative care specialists can work together to minimize the burden of progressive cancer.

TRUSTED INTERNET SITES

For general cancer information:

American Cancer Society: www.cancer.org

American Society of Clinical Oncology: www.asco.org

National Cancer Institute :   www.cancer.gov

National Comprehensive Cancer Network (especially patient guides to professional guidelines):   www.nccn.org

For specialty groups:

American Cancer Society: www.cancer.org

American Psychosocial Oncology Society: www.apos-society.org

American Society of Clinical Oncology: www.asco.org

American Society for Radiation Oncology: www.astro.org

The Bladder Cancer Advocacy Network: www.bcan.org

Breast Cancer Network for Strength: www.networkofstrength.org

Cancer*Care*:   www.cancercare.org

The Children's Cause for Cancer Advocacy: www.childrenscause.org

Coalition of Cancer Cooperative Groups: www.cancertrialshelp.org

C-3: Colorectal Cancer Coalition: www.FightColorectalCancer.org

Education Network to Advance Cancer Clinical Trials: www.enacct.org

International Myeloma Foundation: www.myeloma.org

Kidney Cancer Association: www.nkca.org

Lance Armstrong Foundation: www.laf.org

The Leukemia & Lymphoma Society: www.leukemia.org

Lymphoma Research Foundation: www.lymphoma.org

Multiple Myeloma Research Foundation: www.multiplemyeloma.org

National Breast Cancer Coalition: www.natlbcc.org

National Coalition for Cancer Survivorship: www.canceradvocacy.org

National Comprehensive Cancer Network: www.nccn.org

National Lung Cancer Partnership: www.NationalLungCancerPartnership.org

National Patient Advocate Foundation: www.npaf.org

North American Brain Tumor Coalition: www.nabraintumor.org

Ovarian Cancer National Alliance: www.ovariancancer.org

Pancreatic Cancer Action Network: www.pancan.org

Prevent Cancer Foundation: www.preventcancer.org

Sarcoma Foundation of America: www.curesarcoma.org

Susan G. Komen for the Cure Advocacy Alliance: www.komenadvocacy.org

U.S. TOO International Prostate Cancer Education and Support Network: www.ustoo.com

The Wellness Community: www.thewellnesscommunity.org

Index